Implementing Transference-Focused Psychotherapy Principles

Richard G. Hersh • Chiara De Panfilis
Editors

Implementing Transference-Focused Psychotherapy Principles

General Psychiatric Care for Personality Disorders

Springer

Editors
Richard G. Hersh
Department of Psychiatry
Columbia Vagelos College
of Physicians & Surgeons
New York, NY, USA

Chiara De Panfilis
Department of Medicine and Surgery
Unit of Neuroscience
University of Parma
Parma, Italy

ISBN 978-3-031-68061-8 ISBN 978-3-031-68062-5 (eBook)
https://doi.org/10.1007/978-3-031-68062-5

This Springer imprint is published by the registered company Springer Nature Switzerland AG
The registered company address is: Gewerbestrasse 11, 6330 Cham, Switzerland

In memory of Gerhard Dammann, beloved colleague and friend, whose dedication and expertise in the field of applied Transference-Focused Psychotherapy have inspired this book.

Foreword

Much time has passed since Otto Kernberg began to develop his structural understanding of personality disorders based on an evolving appreciation and development of object relations theory. Working at the famous Menninger Foundation in the United States in the 1950s and 1960s, Kernberg pondered the challenge of helping patients whose fragile ego strength did not allow for the application of the then-ubiquitous psychoanalytic model. Rather than abandon this model, he took on the task of appreciating and refining what is at its core and modifying the way the model is applied to the patient population we now refer to as "organized at the borderline level." For many years, Kernberg's work focused on treating patients in long-term individual psychotherapy with the goal of structural change in the personality. Practically speaking, structural change refers to the fact that we can expect to see change in a person's core subjective sense of self and others in addition to symptom change. Such change can lead to profound change in a person's quality of life.

Kernberg and his colleagues at the Weill Cornell Medical Center's Personality Disorders Institute described an evolving form of treatment, which came to be known as transference-focused psychotherapy (TFP) in a number of articles and books. The model of treatment appealed to therapists in many countries throughout the world. In 2012, adherents of this model came together to form the International Society for Transference-Focused Psychotherapy (ISTFP). The model was taught in an increasing number of psychiatry, psychology, and other therapy training programs. Some of these programs had only a limited capacity to provide long-term individual psychotherapy. Rather than decide that the model was not appropriate for their clinical circumstances, students of the model pointed out to their teachers that concepts and techniques from the model could be applied far beyond the context of individual psychotherapy. This feedback from students led to the development of the applied TFP that is described in its multiple manifestations in this book.

Applied TFP is based on the understanding that the TFP model is made up of many components that are employed as a coherent ensemble in the traditional model of TFP but can be used separately in specific clinical settings in applied TFP. These components are based on the object relations theory view of the mind that conceptualizes internalized representations of self and other as the core elements of mental/psychological structure. These elements determine the different experiences of self and other that a person feels at different points in time in response to external circumstances. When specific components of TFP are applied in different settings, the basic attitude toward the patient remains mostly unchanged: The therapeutic relationship receives particular attention, since it is assumed that early experiences in relationships are re-enacted in the transference. An understanding of the here-and-now in the therapeutic dyad can help to tolerate ruptures and to convey an empathic concern for the patient.

This concept of psychological/mental structure, which will be more fully elaborated in Chap. 2 of this book, led to the development of a clearly defined set of strategies, tactics, and techniques of treatment that can be applied in their fullest form in "classical TFP" (the long-term individual therapy form of TFP) or can be applied selectively in other clinical settings. This understanding that elements of TFP can be used without having to carry out the original complete therapy model freed colleagues up to creatively employ individual components according to the needs of the specific setting, whether it be a therapy of shorter duration, treatment in a hospital or day hospital, group psychotherapy, the prescribing of medication, consulting on a hospital medical service, and so on. Hersh and De Panfilis provide a comprehensive review of the development of applied TFP in Chap. 1 of this book.

While it is clear that most forms of applied TFP do not share the ambitious goals of "classical TFP" in terms of change in an individual's psychological structure, the advent and expansion of applied TFP has allowed clinicians outside the setting of intensive individual psychotherapy to use the concepts of internal representations of self and others and of the need for an appropriate structure in any form of clinical encounter between clinician and patient to increase their capacity for empathy with patients' internal experience, to improve communication, and to insist on a clear and adequate structure for all clinical encounters. The appropriate structure in TFP is protected by a treatment contract that takes external reality into account, i.e., the patient's behavior and life circumstances inside and outside the treatment. This distinguishes TFP from more traditional psychoanalytic work, which would focus exclusively on internal reality and abstain from structuring and protecting external reality. Aspects of this treatment contract can be employed most effectively in any setting where TFP principles are applied.

This volume was conceived by the late Gerhard Dammann, a leading figure in the early years of applied TFP. Gerhard and colleagues published groundbreaking papers that underscored the value they found in using TFP principles in their work with patients in higher acuity settings. Chiara De Panfilis and Richard Hersh have carried on in Dr. Dammann's tradition and have skillfully brought together the most important figures in the development of applied TFP. The contributors to this book include principal members of the TFP community in North America but most particularly from Western Europe where health care systems tend to give support of the full range and evidence-based treatments and to the range of levels of care needed by those patients suffering from serious personality disorders.

It is a testament to the depth of Otto Kernberg's model that its influence continues to expand. Kernberg's decades-long reflection on the nature of personality disorders and how to treat them always combined essential elements of psychoanalysis and of psychiatry. This volume is the best evidence to date of how the impact of his work can be reflected in treatment settings far beyond the individual therapy office.

It is fitting that the work that stemmed from his early observations in long-term hospital settings that, for all practical purposes, no longer exist in the United States, is being applied in creative ways in hospitals, day hospitals, and other clinical settings in many places throughout the world.

Department of Psychiatry
Weill Cornell Medical College and Columbia
Vagelos College of Physicians & Surgeons
New York, NY, USA

Frank Yeomans

Department of Psychoanalysis and Psychotherapy
Medical University of Vienna
Vienna, Austria

Stephan Doering

Contents

Part I Concepts and Models

1 **Introduction Toward Building a Transference-Focused Psychotherapy (TFP) Approach for Applied Fields of Mental Health** 3
Richard G. Hersh and Chiara De Panfilis

2 **Development and Evolution of Transference-Focused Psychotherapy (TFP): A Foundation for Expanding Treatment Applications** 27
John F. Clarkin, Eve Caligor, Julia Sowislo, Diana Diamond, and Frank Yeomans

3 **Transference-Focused Psychotherapy (TFP) Informed Psychoeducation** 49
Michael Rentrop, Maria Lidia Gerra, and Chiara De Panfilis

Part II Transference-Focused Psychotherapy (TFP) Principles in Specific Mental Health Treatment Settings

4 **Transference-Focused Psychotherapy (TFP) Informed Care within an Outpatient Community-Based Multi-professional Psychiatric Service** 85
Chiara De Panfilis, Paolo Ampollini, Giulia Ciccone, Francesca Palombi, and Sergio Dazzi

5 **Using Transference-Focused Psychotherapy (TFP) Principles in the National Health Service (NHS) in the United Kingdom (UK)** 111
Tennyson Lee and Jo-Anna Van den Bosch

6 **Using Transference-Focused Psychotherapy (TFP) Principles in Adult and Adolescent Day Hospital Settings** 135
Eulàlia Ripoll, Maya Krischer, and Joan Vegué Grilló

7 **Using Transference-Focused Psychotherapy (TFP) Principles in Short-Term and Extended Inpatient Psychotherapy Settings** 167
Birger Dulz, Bernhard Grimmer, Mathias Lohmer, Olga Wlodarczyk, and Gerhard Dammann

8 Transference-Focused Psychotherapy (TFP) Principles for Mental Health Professionals in Higher-Acuity Settings 197
Miguel Angel Gonzalez Torres and Luis Valenciano

9 Using Transference-Focused Psychotherapy (TFP) Principles in an Integrated Care Continuum 217
Maria Jesus Rufat and Joan Vegué Grilló

10 Transference-Focused Psychotherapy (TFP) Based Group Therapy 239
Bernhard Grimmer, Benjamin Kraus, Maya Krischer, Christiane Rösch, and Sandra Vohl

Part III Transference-Focused Psychotherapy (TFP) Principles with Specific Patient Populations

11 Using Transference-Focused Psychotherapy (TFP) Principles in the Treatment of Forensic Patients 265
Fritz Lackinger

12 Using Transference-Focused Psychotherapy (TFP) Principles in the Treatment of Medical and Personality Disorder Comorbidities 309
Richard G. Hersh, Mark Petrini, Elisa Bergonzini, and Maria Moscara

13 Using Transference-focused Psychotherapy (TFP) Principles in a Family Intervention for Adolescents with Personality Disorders 337
Alfons Icart and Teresa Ribalta

TFP Resources 361

Index 363

Contributors

Paolo Ampollini Department of Mental Health, Parma Local Health Agency, Parma, Italy

Elisa Bergonzini Department of Mental Health, Modena Health Agency, Modena, Italy

Jo-Anna Van den Bosch Mental Health of Older Adults Services, South London and Maudsley NHS Trust, London, UK

Eve Caligor Department of Psychiatry, Columbia Vagelos College of Physicians & Surgeons, New York, NY, USA

Giulia Ciccone Department of Mental Health, Modena Local Health Agency, Modena, Italy

John F. Clarkin Department of Psychiatry, Weill Cornell Medical College, New York, NY, USA

Gerhard Dammann Mental Health Services Thurgau, Münsterlingen, Switzerland

Sergio Dazzi Personality Disorders Lab, Parma, Italy

Diana Diamond Department of Psychiatry, Weill Cornell Medical College, New York, NY, USA

Birger Dulz German Society TFP (DGTFP)/TFP-Institute North (TIN), Hamburg, Germany

Maria Lidia Gerra Department of Mental Health and Pathological Dependencies, Parma Local Health Agency, Parma, Italy

Joan Vegué Grilló Centre Psicoteràpia Barcelona – Serveis Salut Mental (CPB-SSM). Grup TLP Barcelona, Barcelona, Spain

Bernhard Grimmer Department for Psychotherapy, Psychiatric Clinic Münsterlingen, Münsterlingen, Switzerland

Psychiatric Services Thurgau, Münsterlingen, Switzerland

University Hospital for Psychiatry and Psychotherapy, Paracelsus Medical University, Salzburg, Austria

Richard G. Hersh Department of Psychiatry, Columbia Vagelos College of Physicians & Surgeons, New York, NY, USA

Alfons Icart Grup TLP Barcelona, Barcelona, Spain

Fundació Orienta, Barcelona, Spain

Benjamin Kraus Psychiatric Services Thurgau, Münsterlingen, Switzerland

University Hospital for Psychiatry and Psychotherapy, Paracelsus Medical University, Salzburg, Austria

Maya Krischer Department of Child and Adolescent Psychiatry, Psychotherapy and Psychosomatics, University Clinic of Cologne, Cologne, Germany

Fritz Lackinger Vienna, Austria

Tennyson Lee DeanCross, Tower Hamlets Personality Disorder Service and Centre for Understanding Personality (CUSP), East London NHS Foundation Trust, London, UK

Mathias Lohmer TFP-Institute Munich, Munich, Germany

Maria Moscara Modena, Italy

Francesca Palombi Department of Mental Health, Parma Local Health Agency, Parma, Italy

Chiara De Panfilis Department of Medicine and Surgery, Unit of Neuroscience, University of Parma, Parma, Italy

Department of Mental Health, Parma Local Health Agency, Parma, Italy

Personality Disorders Lab, Parma, Italy

Mark Petrini Departments of Psychiatry and Medicine, Columbia Vagelos College of Physicians & Surgeons, New York, NY, USA

Michael Rentrop Kbo-Inn-Salzach-Klinikum, Wasserburg, Germany

Department of Psychiatry and Psychotherapy, Klinikum rechts der Isar, Technical University Munich, Munich, Germany

Teresa Ribalta TFP-A, Barcelona, Spain

Grup TLP Barcelona's, Barcelona, Spain

Fundació Orienta's, Barcelona, Spain

Eulàlia Ripoll Mental Health Center BPD Program, Centre Psicoteràpia Barcelona – Serveis Salut Mental (CPB-SSM), Barcelona, Spain

Christiane Rösch Psychiatric Services Thurgau, Münsterlingen, Switzerland

University Hospital for Psychiatry and Psychotherapy, Paracelsus Medical University, Salzburg, Austria

Maria Jesus Rufat Centre Psicoteràpia Barcelona – Serveis Salut Mental (CPB-SSM). Grup TLP Barcelona, Barcelona, Spain

Julia Sowislo Department of Psychiatry, Weill Cornell Medical College, New York, NY, USA

Miguel Angel Gonzalez Torres Psychiatry, Basurto University Hospital, Bilbao, Spain

Luis Valenciano CSM Molina de Segura, Murcia, Spain

Sandra Vohl Department of Child and Adolescent Psychiatry, Psychotherapy and Psychosomatics, University Clinic of Cologne, Cologne, Germany

Olga Wlodarczyk Department for Personality Disorders, Asklepios Clinic Nord Ochsenzoll, Hamburg, Germany

Frank Yeomans Department of Psychiatry, Weill Medical College, New York, NY, USA

Part I

Concepts and Models

Introduction Toward Building a Transference-Focused Psychotherapy (TFP) Approach for Applied Fields of Mental Health

1

Richard G. Hersh and Chiara De Panfilis

Transference-focused psychotherapy (TFP) for patients with borderline personality disorder (BPD) was developed over decades by a group of research clinicians guided primarily by psychoanalytic thinking, specifically object relations theory (ORT). These researchers initially identified important limitations in the practice of traditional psychoanalytic treatments with patients with BPD, treatments that were often identified as either ineffective or even counterproductive [1]. TFP's central elements, including its diagnostic assessment process, were informed by the work of Otto Kernberg, some of whose seminal writing on this topic predated the first inclusion of the borderline diagnosis in the DSM [2, 3]. With the marked increase in interest in BPD after the landmark event in 1980 of BPD's inclusion in the standard nosology, a growing emphasis emerged on the goal of conducting systematic research on treatments for patients with this disorder [4]. TFP as a manualized, extended, twice-weekly individual psychotherapy for patients with BPD has been described in a series of iterations; refinements in the treatment method have been informed by clinical observations and research outcomes [5, 6].

Specifically, the status of TFP as an empirically supported, evidence-based therapy [7] has been firmly established. In a preliminary study of behavioral change, the

Parts of some paragraphs are slightly modified excerpts from: Hersh, R. Applied transference-focused psychotherapy: an overview and update. Psychodyn Psychiatry. 2021: 49(2):273–295. https://doi.org/10.1521/pdps.2021.49.2.273.

R. G. Hersh (✉)
Department of Psychiatry, Columbia Vagelos College of Physicians & Surgeons, New York, NY, USA
e-mail: rh170@cumc.columbia.edu

C. De Panfilis
Department of Medicine and Surgery, Unit of Neuroscience, University of Parma, Parma, Italy
e-mail: chiara.depanfilis@unipr.it

R. G. Hersh, C. De Panfilis (eds.), *Implementing Transference-Focused Psychotherapy Principles*, https://doi.org/10.1007/978-3-031-68062-5_1

delivery of manualized TFP was found to decrease suicidal and parasuicidal behavior as well as hospitalization rates in a cohort of BPD patients, as compared to the year before the intervention [8]. Two independent randomized controlled trials [5, 9] further demonstrated that TFP is as effective as dialectical behavioral therapy (DBT) and supportive psychodynamic therapy (SPT) in reducing BPD symptoms [5] and more effective than therapy delivered by experienced community psychotherapists (ECP) in favoring treatment attendance and BPD remission, as well as in decreasing suicide attempts and hospitalizations [9]. Importantly, while metanalytic studies showed that all evidence-based psychotherapies are equally effective in decreasing BPD-specific symptoms (i.e., self-harm and suicide) [10], standard, twice-a-week individual TFP uniquely leads also to improvements in reflective function, attachment security and level of personality organization [11–13], as compared to other treatment modalities (i.e., DBT, SPT and ECP), indicating a specific and theoretically sound effect of standard TFP on intrapsychic changes in BPD patients.

The "Specializing The Generalist" Approach to PD Treatment

In the last decades, however, previous "horseracing" research approaches that compared the efficacy of different psychotherapies were replaced by a diverse line of research, which compared "specialist" psychotherapies to systematic, structured "generalist" approaches to BPD. Unexpectedly, well-structured generalist treatments (i.e., general psychiatric management – GPM-, structured psychiatric management- SPM- or SPT) performed as well as specialist psychotherapies on most borderline relevant symptomatic outcomes (see reference [14] for a review). These findings encouraged focusing on identifying the specific aspects or strategies of various empirically supported psychotherapies that represent their effective essential ingredients, which then could be usefully combined into a comprehensive integrated treatment or into enhanced, well-organized generalist interventions [14, 15]. This approach yields the potential to provide patients with personality disorder (PD) pathology practical, effective treatment options other than standard specialist psychotherapies. These integrated/generalist treatment options, in turn, may have the advantage of being less complex, narrowly focused and expensive, and more generalizable and scalable across diverse health systems and patient populations. For instance, research on service provision for BPD patients across 22 countries worldwide demonstrated that in no country was the number of certified clinicians in evidence-based treatments sufficient to meet the demands posed by BPD treatment seekers [16]. Weinberg et al. [17] examined the manuals of empirically supported psychotherapies for BPD (i.e., DBT, mentalization based treatment -MBT-, TFP, schema focused therapy -SFT-, GPM and systems training for emotional predictability and problem solving -STEPPS-) by comparing their common and specific treatment strategies. They found that common and effective strategies are a clear treatment framework, attention to affect, focus on treatment relationship, an active therapist, and exploratory and change-oriented interventions.

Therefore, *structured* generalist approaches that share common features with specialist approaches are likely to foster a good outcome for PD patients. Indeed, a clear and coherent structure of the treatment emerges as a major effective element of successful therapies for PD. For instance, metanalytic studies show that differences between "specialist" psychotherapy interventions and control conditions disappear in well-designed and implemented trials and where the control group was balanced for manualization of treatment or the involvement of the study team in treatment [10]. If this is the case, "reforms to clinical services, using existing resources, might be equally or more important than the delivery of any specific brand of psychotherapy" [18].

This shift of paradigm has important practical implications, since "specialist" psychotherapies may often be scarcely accessible across various mental health systems. Although specialized treatments are indicated and required for promoting meaningful change in some patients with PD pathology and are superior to unstructured generalized treatments, they are not always available in clinical practice.

For example, in countries where mental healthcare is publicly funded and provided by national health systems (NHS) to all citizens, public psychiatric services may find it difficult to deploy the necessary resources and time to provide PD patients with standard, formal individual psychotherapies. In these contexts, patients with PD thus run the risk of being treated at the margins, i.e., in caseloads of community mental health staff who may prioritize the needs of other patients, may lack specific skills to work with PD populations [19], and may exhibit more negative attitudes toward PD patients as compared to other psychiatric patients [20]. In those countries where the private health system is dominant, accessing appropriate psychotherapeutic treatment may be problematic for patients on both ends of the psychosocial spectrum, those socially disadvantaged and those well-resourced. Because the most severe PD patients are likely to also show the greatest psychosocial dysfunction, this phenomenon may paradoxically represent a barrier to effective treatment. These patients with limited resources may be misdiagnosed or may receive nonspecific treatments at the primary/emergency care level for extended periods. Conversely, certain more affluent patients may receive protracted unstructured, unproductive psychotherapy that does not fully take into account their levels of PD pathology, and/or expensive, complicated "state of the art" pharmacotherapy that too has limited positive yield and frequent concerning side effects.

Finally, in some well-resourced countries, multiple evidence-based therapies for BPD may be fully supported by the local health system; however, this seemingly privileged context may be associated with increased dropout rates. In this scenario, patients can easily end one treatment modality and select another equally available one, often in an uncoordinated shift, thus limiting treatment effectiveness.

Therefore, structuring general psychiatric services using effective elements drawn from specialist psychotherapies for PD may fill these gaps in treatment provision for PD patients.

Along these lines, central precepts of several evidence-based treatments for BPD have been applied in contexts other than the standard, individual psychotherapy setting for BPD. DBT theory and practice have been applied expansively, building on

Linehan's original conceptualization of the individual outpatient treatment model [21, 22]. DBT principles have been employed in psychiatric inpatient units and residential forensic programs, and with distinct patient populations including patients with BPD and co-occurring substance use disorders, patients with BPD and co-occurring depression disorders, and patients with eating disorders. Novel projects using DBT principles with families and DBT principles with patients in assertive community treatment (ACT) teams have also been proposed [23–26]. Similarly, the essential elements of MBT have been translated beyond use with individuals and the initially described partial hospital setting. MBT principles are now used in parenting programs, in the treatment of professionals in crisis, and with school populations [27]. In an effort to expand the scope of GPM for BPD, that intervention has been adapted for the inpatient psychiatric unit, the psychiatric emergency department, the consultation-liaison service, and the college mental health service [28]. Along these same lines, the patient population targeted by SFT has evolved. SFT principles have been used with patients with other personality disorders than BPD, as well as patients with eating disorders, anxiety disorders, and post-traumatic stress disorders [29].

The Rationale of This Volume

The overarching goal of this book is to bring together the many and varied applications of TFP principles used in contemporary practice *in clinical situations other than an extended, individual psychotherapy offered in a customary, outpatient treatment setting.* Thus, this volume will describe how general psychiatric treatment for PD can be implemented with key principles and insights from TFP across a variety of healthcare systems, countries, settings, and clinical experiences.

Why might TFP principles lend themselves to application in multiple ways for clinicians who may not prioritize, or even value, traditional psychoanalytic thinking? It is key to keep in mind that TFP as an individual psychotherapy departs consequentially from psychoanalysis and many psychoanalytic psychotherapies. TFP has a distinctive triad of "knowledge, attitude, and skills" that evolved directly from working with patients with severe personality disorder pathology [30]. Working with these severely ill patients yielded a deliberate and defined approach, grounded in rigorous diagnostic consideration. TFP is notable for its clear order and organization; it requires attention to well-defined steps, both in the assessment phase and during the course of treatment. Importantly, this emphasis on structuring the treatment represents a key and effective element that can be "generalized" to settings other than the standard outpatient psychotherapy format.

Preceding publications already described the application of TFP as an individual psychotherapy for the treatment of patients of varying ages and diagnoses. These adaptations have included: (1) the work of Caligor et al. describing the use of TFP principles for patients with higher-level personality pathology, (2) the work of Caligor et al. describing the use of TFP principles for patients across a full range of diagnoses and severity of illness, (3) the work of Normandin et al. on the adaptation of TFP for adolescents [31, 32], and (4) the work of Diamond et al. on the adaptation of TFP for patients with primary or co-occurring narcissistic disorders [33–35]. All of these publications focus on modifications of TFP principles, within a format of extended, individual psychotherapy, in populations other than BPD, building on a growing consensus about common factors in PD pathology across diagnoses and age ranges, as a collective movement in the research community has supported a hybrid categorical/dimensional model of personality disorder nosology as reflected in the DSM-5, Section III Appendix as the Alternative Model for Personality Disorders (AMPD) [36, 37].

However, at the same time that these interventions have been developed, researched, or refined, a new and different set of applications of key TFP principles *outside* the setting of an individual outpatient TFP has emerged. These kinds of applications are now referred to as "applied" TFP.

The Origins of This Volume

One of the most influential contributors to the development of applied TFP initiatives was the late Swiss psychiatrist and psychoanalyst Gerhard Dammann. As described later on in this chapter, Dammann was an early and influential proponent of expanding the scope of TFP principles beyond the standard, twice-a-week psychotherapy, in a number of ways, such as by integrating TFP elements with other psychotherapy approaches and by adapting them to the inpatient treatment of PD patients. In 2014, Gerhard Dammann's work prompted the International Society for TFP (ISTFP) to create a dedicated committee for "Inpatient TFP and TFP in psychiatric services", which he chaired until his premature passing away in 2020. Under his lead, the committee soon gathered contributions from several members and associations affiliated with the ISTFP worldwide, who had spontaneously developed various applied TFP initiatives. We will summarize some of these initiatives below in this chapter.

Importantly, the richness and diversity of such initiatives flourished in response to the specific features of the different healthcare settings on which they were grounded, each posing specific requests on how to apply TFP elements in the treatment of PD patients outside the format of standard individual therapy. As such, the committee included applied TFP contributions from several countries (i.e., Spain, Switzerland, the USA, Germany, Austria, Italy, the United Kingdom), different systems of care (i.e., publicly founded, mainly private, or mixed), diverse settings (i.e., acute and long-term inpatient treatment, day hospital, or community-based, outpatient treatment) as well as initiatives targeted to PD populations of different age ranges (i.e., adolescent, adult, and elderly) and with various comorbid conditions (i.e., trauma-related disorders and co-occurring medical conditions). Over time, the committee hosted lively discussions and exchanges among its members on how the standard TFP approach could be adapted to meet the diverse needs of these various settings. These discussions inspired Gerhard Dammann to propose gathering several of those diverse contributions on applied TFP in a book—this book.

Thus, this volume represents not only the realization of Dr. Dammann's seminal idea, but also an enduring tribute to his memory.

The Evolution of Applied TFP

As previously noted, the evolution of applied TFP has been a "grass roots" process, informed by the needs identified in disparate groups of practitioners and healthcare systems. Three trajectories, sometimes overlapping, in the field of applied TFP, have emerged: (1) the integration of TFP elements into a pluralistic approach to the treatment of patients with personality disorder pathology, (2) the use of TFP principles for teaching purposes both to trainees and to established clinicians, and (3) the reworking of TFP tenets for patients with co-occurring conditions and employed in treatment situations other than the standard outpatient individual psychotherapy (Table 1.1).

These developments do not reflect a "top down" directive but rather have developed organically, meeting particular needs, sometimes specific to a discipline, institution, or locale. The inclusion of TFP principles in a broad array of teaching initiatives has made these concepts available to many who can then use them flexibly in clinical practice; the integration of TFP elements with other schools of thought in contemporary psychotherapy has helped to "translate" TFP principles for use by those who are not familiar with a psychoanalytically informed language or approach; and the wider application of TFP principles for institutions and systems addresses understandable concerns about the limitations to access associated with a longer-term, expensive modality, not widely available.

1. The integration of TFP principles with other therapeutic interventions:

The integration of TFP with other psychotherapeutic schools reflects both the greater movement to theoretical pluralism of recent decades and the wide range of treatment settings where patients with PD pathology are now seen. As will be outlined, individual clinicians, groups of practitioners, and healthcare systems have borrowed elements of TFP theory to meld with their respective orientations (Table 1.2).

Gerhard Dammann highlighted the value of integrating TFP principles with other established theoretical approaches. He outlined the overlap of TFP and psychoanalytic interactional therapy [39]. He linked elements of TFP, developed in the

Table 1.1 Overview of applied TFP: Emerging areas of focus

1. Theoretical integration: Use of TFP principles either in tandem or in sequence with other evidence-based treatments for patients with personality disorder pathology
2. Teaching trainees and practising clinicians: Initiatives focused on teaching TFP principles to trainees and practicing clinicians
3. Specific patient populations/public health initiatives: Applications of TFP adapted for specific patient populations and/or utilized within general health care services.

Table 1.2 Theoretical integration

Brömmel & Dammann (2004) [38]: Integration of TFP and kathatymic imaginative psychotherapy (KIP)
Dammann (2004) [39]: Integration of TFP and psychoanalytic interactional therapy
Bernardo (2007) [40]: Integration of TFP and Gunderson's model of ambulatory care
Needham (2011) [41]: Integrative multidisciplinary treatment (IMT) combining TFP, MBT and DBT common factors
Higa & Gedo (2012) [42]: Sequencing of TFP and MBT in a case report
Rivera & Drake (2012) [43]: Integration of TFP and cognitive-behavioral treatment in a clinic setting
Ortega & Crespo (2013) [44]: Integration of TFP, MBT, and Gunderson's clinical guide
Martel & Lecours (2013) [45]: Integration of TFP and MBT
Kooiman, Kuipers & Huffstadt (2013) [46]: TFP combined with MBT for the psychiatric inpatient
Gunderson & Links (2014) [47]: TFP principles in the handbook for good psychiatry management for borderline personality disorder (GPM)
Schluter–Muller & Schmeck (2015) [48]: Integrating TFP in adolescent identity treatment (AIT)
Choi–Kain, Albert & Gunderson (2016) [49]: Overview of integration and sequencing of DBT, MBT, TFP, and GPM
Hörz–Sagstetter, Wernz & Rentrop (2017) [41]: TFP and couples counseling
Rösch & Grimmer (2017) [50]: TFP and DBT in a psychiatric inpatient unit
Schlutter–Muller (2017) [51]: TFP integrated with DBT for adolescent patients with personality disorder pathology

United States, with psychoanalytic interactional therapy, developed in Germany and studied in an inpatient population for patients with what were then called "Cluster B" disorders. With co-author Brömmel, he proposed the integration of TFP principles with katathymic imaginative psychotherapy, a treatment developed in the 1950s by the German psychiatrist Harnscarl Leuner that involves the use of guided imagery [38]. These two papers underscore the way in which TFP principles have been appreciated by clinicians in specific treatment milieus.

A more typical and mainstream example of the integration of TFP principles is reflected by the work of three Spanish clinicians. Bernardo outlined his clinic's use of TFP principles along with elements of the work of John Gunderson in their work with patients with BPD [40]. Ortega and Crespo built on this in their conceptualization of their clinic's approach, adding MBT theory to the blend of TFP and Gunderson's 2008 clinical guide [44, 52].

Higa and Gedo offered a model for treating patients with BPD that emphasizes the integration of theoretical orientations sequentially [42]. They presented a case study that stresses the use of MBT interventions in the opening phase of treatment, with a shift overtime to a more prominent focus on a TFP-informed attitude. Martel and Lecours also proposed what they call "an integrated conceptual framework" synthesizing MBT and TFP elements [45]. They suggested that an initial focus on mentalizing would address splitting and overtime lead to structural change in the patients with BPD. Another model for the integration and TFP and MBT was put forth by Kooiman et al., notably one in the inpatient setting [46]. In their work, Kooiman's group organized their inpatient program using TFP as the frame of reference, with adjunctive MBT elements. While acknowledging some fundamental differences in the two models as related to both theory and practice, they nevertheless maintained that an amalgam of the two provided optimization of their program.

The integration of TFP and MBT understandably grows out of their shared psychoanalytic foundations. An even broader movement toward integration has proposed the use of TFP, with or without MBT elements, in concert with primarily CBT-centered treatments. This approach to working with challenging patients was endorsed by Rivera and Drake in their explanation of their group work in a Canadian community day treatment program. Their program selectively chose aspects of TFP, MBT, and DBT, used in an intensive outpatient program [43]. Schluter–Muller advocated for the integration of TFP with DBT for adolescents with personality disorder diagnoses, building on an earlier description of adolescent identity treatment (AIT) and the place for TFP theory in that model [48, 51]. Rösch and Grimmer described their work in an inpatient psychiatry unit, which included both TFP and DBT elements in their program [50].

Choi-Kain and Gunderson outlined the benefits of adaptability by accentuating the possibilities of integrating and/or sequencing different methods [49]. Gunderson had acknowledged his appreciation of certain TFP elements in the development of GPM for the generalist clinician. In the GPM handbook, Gunderson and Links credited TFP as the source of their inspiration for monitoring countertransference, guarding boundaries, holding patients accountable for their avoidance and acting out, and realizing the value of interpretation [47].

In yet another arena, Hörz-Sagstetter, Wernz, and Rentrop supplemented existing theory about treatment for couples by describing a way of using TFP theory in that work [41]. They defined both the work with individuals and couples, and the specific aspects of TFP theory that can be used when addressing conflict in a couple.

2. Teaching TFP principles to trainees and practicing clinicians

TFP has been described as "the hardest to learn" of the evidence-based treatments for the disorder [47]. Learning TFP as individual psychotherapy requires exposure first to the didactics required to explain the theory and essential elements of the treatment, and then ongoing supervision, ideally with audiovisual recordings of sessions, over a sustained period. Such a treatment is labor-intensive and expensive; that said, interest in learning TFP has grown exponentially in recent years beyond the initial group of highly motivated individuals. The intrinsic value of TFP principles has spurred a range of teaching options for trainees and for providers established in the fields of psychiatry, psychology, social work, and medicine (Table 1.3).

Carsky and Yeomans described the ways that they used TFP principles in consultation, often in situations when therapists felt fearful, ineffective, or paralyzed [67]. Their consultative role did not aim to teach those clinicians TFP per se, but rather, they aimed to impart TFP principles to help in assessment, management, and use of countertransference. This paper outlined how core TFP elements including openness to making a PD diagnosis, a requirement of open communications with others

Table 1.3 Specific Patient Populations/Public Health Initiatives

Plafflin & Ross (2004) [53]: TFP for adolescent delinquents
Lackinger & Dammann (2005) [54]: TFP for BPD within the forensic population
Fontao, Pfafflin & Lamott (2006) [55]: TFP for the inpatient forensic population
Kernberg (2009) [56]: TFP groups in inpatient and day hospital settings
Schneider-Lehman (2009) [57]: TFP in trauma therapy
Lamott & Pfafflin (2009) [58]: TFP as part of integrated treatment in prisons and secure forensic hospitals
Draijer & Van Zorn (2013) [59]: TFP in trauma therapy
Kenkel & Seritan (2015) [60]: TFP in the geriatric population in institutional settings
Krischer & Normandin (2015) [61]: TFP for adolescent patients in a day clinic
Sollberger et al. (2015) [62]: TFP for BPD in a specialized inpatient service
Kruger & Meinters (2018) [63]: TFP in trauma therapy
Gaztambide (2018, 2019) [64]: TFP in minority communities
Lee & Hersh (2019) [65]: TFP in the National Health Service of the United Kingdom
Moscara & Bergonzini (2020) [66]: TFP in the consultation-liaison service of the general hospital

involved in a patient's progress, and the introduction of the idea of a treatment agreement, could be achievable and fruitful. Again, this teaching opportunity developed organically, given the clinicians' distress, the specific nature of the patient's pathology, and the reasonable and coherent model offered that is informed by TFP training.

Similarly, the demands made on psychiatry residents in their training spawned a proposal for the introduction of TFP training in that setting [30]. This program at the New York University School of Medicine went beyond the introduction of TFP as a psychotherapy training, to a broader proposal for the use of applied TFP principles in training sites, including inpatient psychiatry, forensic psychiatry, and consultation-liaison services. This use of applied TFP filled a documented gap in psychiatry trainees' education about the assessment and management of patients with PD pathology [68]. This paper outlined the distinction between the goals of training in TFP as individual psychotherapy and the goals of training in TFP for briefer clinician-patient interactions in settings not usually associated with the employment of psychoanalytically oriented methods. In a comparable vein, Bliss and McCardle delineated the practical needs of social workers seeing patients with PD pathology [69]. This article detailed the diverse requirements faced by social workers and the real-world limitations in practice patterns that might preclude fidelity to one particular manualized treatment. To this end, they put forth an eclectic model that included TFP, MBT, and DBT components. Such as model was studied by Needham and named integrative multidisciplinary treatment (IMT) for a public sector, teaching hospital site [70].

In a pilot program at Weill Cornell Medical College, psychiatry residents were introduced to TFP in an elective focusing on their work with patients with BPD. A review of this elective underscored the more general usefulness of TFP training for these novice psychotherapists. This review emphasized the wider range of skills conferred by familiarity with TFP and the use of TFP concepts in psychotherapy with a broad range of patients [71]. In a commentary, a leader in psychiatry residency education reinforced the possible value of the inclusion of TFP in the residency curriculum and offered suggestions for managing barriers to achieving such a goal [72]. Martin et al. stressed the potential benefits of TFP training for psychotherapists as part of their overarching endorsement of an introduction of TFP to psychiatrists in Australia [73]. They considered how TFP could fit both in psychiatry training and in Australian public and private services for patients with high-level needs now relatively underserviced.

Fundamentals of Transference-Focused Psychotherapy: Applications in Psychiatric and Medical Settings, published in 2016, was written for a broad audience [74]. The topics covered were the use of TFP principles in inpatient psychiatry, family involvement, crisis management, prescribing, the interface of medical and psychiatric disorders, and psychiatry education, which were identified as familiar, commonplace, and challenging for many practitioners. The target audience included many who would not necessarily ever access the TFP manual, but who could nevertheless use TFP principles in these contexts.

Many clinicians trained in general medicine and medical subspecialties see a significant number of patients with personality disorder pathology but have scant training in how to manage these patients. This need for guidance and information tailored for clinicians without mental health training led to the development of a curriculum for residents in internal medicine offered at the Columbia University Medical Center [75]. This weekly didactic program put an emphasis on making a personality disorder diagnosis based on limited information, establishment and maintenance of a treatment agreement, and monitoring of countertransference. These tools allowed medical providers to feel more empowered with the familiar "difficult patient," moving them from an expectable conflictual treatment relationship to one marked by collaboration and an explication of the respective obligations of both parties.

Three publications directly addressed the present-day reality of practice for many psychiatrists in the United States. While these publications may be useful to trainees, they should also have a genuine resonance for those already well-launched in their careers. Available data suggests that most psychiatrists will treat a significant number of patients with PD pathology in every clinical setting, from the outpatient office to higher acuity day programs, emergency rooms, or inpatient units. In addition, the role of the psychiatrist has notably evolved in recent years, with the majority of psychiatrists assuming a predominant, if not exclusive, role as prescriber. The application of TFP principles in prescribing for the patient with severe personality disorder pathology offered explicit, judicious guidance, keeping in mind common concerning patterns associated with this population including polypharmacy, lapses in treatment adherence, and problematic medication side effects [76]. Building on this theme, a review emphasized the value of core TFP tenets as a cornerstone of an effective risk management strategy [77]. Taken together, these articles aimed to reduce the well-described and concerning aversion many psychiatrists might have to both making a personality diagnosis and agreeing to assume responsibility for the care of patients with serious personality disorder pathology. A summary article for the general psychiatrist looked at all the component parts of TFP as an individual psychotherapy, itemizing those points that might be useful, even if the psychiatrist does not routinely provide individual psychotherapy [78].

3. The application of TFP principles to specific patient populations and treatment contexts

Applications of TFP to specific patient populations, as well as targeted coordinated public health initiatives, have occurred, for the most part, in Western Europe. These efforts emerged following the introduction of TFP principles for individual treatment and a number of groups then grafted TFP principles onto their work already in place. Applied TFP projects aimed at distinct populations or incorporated into public health initiatives have included work with (1) inpatient and outpatient forensic populations, (2) patients with trauma histories, (3) geriatric patients in institutional settings, (4) patients with substance use disorders, (5) medical inpatients seen by the consultation-liaison service, and (6) patients in historically underserved and marginalized minority communities. In the preceding discussion of treatment integration, a number of inpatient and day hospital settings were referenced. In those countries that continue to offer extended inpatient hospitalizations for patients with primary PD diagnoses, treatment milieus with a TFP focus and/or TFP-informed groups have been introduced for both adolescents and adults. A few locales have even used TFP principles across an entire integrated care curriculum.

The use of TFP principles with the forensic population began with attention to relapse prevention efforts. Pflafflin and Ross suggested that TFP's attention to a treatment agreement could be of use as part of a program to limit recidivism [53]. Lackinger and Dammann detailed ways that the treatment contracting process in TFP could be refined for use with forensic patients [54]. A pilot study by Fontao et al. of 18 months of TFP in an inpatient forensic setting yielded changes in personality dimensional scores and global psychopathology indices [55]. In their review of the use of those treatments empirically validated for patients with BPD for the forensic population, Lamott and Pfafflin compared experiences with TFP, MBT, and DBT. Most recently, Gibbels et al. reviewed the "state of the art" treatment options for actual and potential sexual offenders and included TFP among other interventions, while Lackinger has continued to contribute on the topic of integration of TFP principles for use with antisocial and pedophiliac offenders [79].

The utility of TFP principles in the treatment of patients with trauma histories was put forward by Schneider-Lehman in a discussion of the overlap between complex PTSD and BPD symptoms [57]. This notion was further elaborated in an analysis of the benefits of TFP for former child soldiers, a treatment intervention privileging exploration of aggression and its manifestations [59]. Kruger and Meinters offered a "multimodal therapeutic approach" to patients with trauma that adds adjunctive TFP components to a preexisting treatment model [63].

While the availability of longer-term inpatient treatment options has declined in recent years, in some well-resourced countries such opportunities remain for higher acuity adolescent and adult patients. Sollberger et al. conducted a randomized trial of psychiatric patients with BPD comparing what they call disorder specific treatment (DST), a variation of TFP, and DBT skills training modules with treatment as usual in their hospital in Basel, Switzerland. They found a significant improvement in the DST group after 12 weeks including a reduction in typical affective borderline symptoms and a reduction in identity diffusion [62]. A group led by Krischer in Cologne, Germany, has researched TFP for adolescents attending a day treatment program [61, 80, 32]. This program, which combines a primary TFP orientation with a complementary DBT skills group, has an objective of containment and stabilization, in advance of sustained office-based TFP to follow. Kernberg detailed the introduction of TFP group treatment in both the psychiatric day treatment and inpatient sites [56]. He introduced these groups as modified versions of "Bion's analysis of small group processes developed by Ezriel and Sutherland at the Tavistock Clinic."

The following ventures using TFP underscore ways that clinicians working with niche patient populations explore TFP principles in unexpected ways:

- Kenkel and Seritan reviewed psychotherapy options for geriatric patients in institutional settings and identified TFP as a reasonable choice, among others [60]. Their survey, with the inclusion of TFP, touched on an often-overlooked age group and offered direction to clinicians and staff, in the institutional environment who are much of the time insufficiently trained to work with BPD patients.
- Gaztambide analyzed the complex challenges for patients with BPD in communities of color [64]. He explored the interplay between "individual, communal and systemic complexities" contributing to barriers to recovery. He strongly advocated for a focus on TFP's meaningful activity requirement as a cornerstone of recovery for a group of patients facing challenges on multiple levels.
- Lee and Hersh offered an introduction to TFP keeping in mind the clearly defined requirements of the United Kingdom's National Health Service [65]. This system does not allow for psychotherapy treatment more frequently than weekly. They sketched a flexible adaptation of TFP principles, accommodating TFP adjusted to a once-weekly meeting, as well as applied TFP techniques to be employed in general psychiatry appointments.
- Moscara and Bergonzini proposed the integration of TFP principles in the work of the consultation-liaison psychiatry service of the general hospital [66]. This model used a vignette focusing on the clinical management of a patient with narcissistic psychopathology that interfered with medical management. The delicate negotiations required by the psychiatrist among the patient, his family, and the medical services are enhanced by a command of basic TFP theory.

Some Criticisms of Applied TFP

We have outlined earlier the rationale and utility for "applied" TFP and offered a review of existing initiatives in this field. As previously mentioned, the "applied TFP" approach is currently well established in the ISTFP. It is the focus of a dedicated committee within the ISTFP, and the leading developers of TFP as a formal outpatient psychotherapy are now recommending to further strengthen the applied TFP approach by disseminating critical concepts and techniques of TFP to a wider audience and various clinical settings, fulfilling in this way a crucial public health role (see, for instance, John Clarkin's preface to the volume *Fundamentals of Transference-Focused Psychotherapy: Applications in Psychiatric and Medical Settings*, by Hersh et al. 2016 [74]). This volume explicitly aims to take this next step.

However, some voices within the community of "standard" TFP therapists may not share this opinion. Actually, some criticisms of the "applied" TFP approach have been proposed, which we have tried to summarize below for the sake of transparency. In some ways, concerns expressed about support for the use of TFP principles in clinical situations other than in a standard, extended individual psychotherapy modality echo debates in the past about the extension of psychoanalytic principles. Similar concerns were raised about the risk of emerging psychoanalytic psychotherapies and the possibility that critical psychoanalytic theory and technique would be diluted in the process.

One criticism reflects the concern that "applied" TFP would basically distort the real nature of TFP as a psychoanalytically oriented therapy. This line of reasoning starts with the premises that (a) TFP was developed to treat PD within a psychoanalytic framework and (b) that central components of TFP, such as its strategies, tactics, and techniques alongside its focus on object relations, countertransference, transference analysis, and technical neutrality and with the need for a therapy contract, represent delineated elements of psychoanalytic theory and practice, adapted to treat people with PD because this group of patients, by and large, have not responded well to "classical" psychoanalytic therapy. What follows from these premises is that distinguishing between "direct", standard TFP and "applied" TFP may imply that TFP can be reduced to a series of easy-to-teach and easy-to-learn steps that can be disseminated to various different professionals and clinical settings. As described by British psychotherapist and TFP supervisor Frank Denning, rather than constituting an advantage and an advancement in the field of PD treatment, for the advocates of this criticism, this would represent a major threat to the status of TFP: it would imply that TFP as a model is inherently capable of being reduced in this way and, therefore, that TFP is not a real psychoanalytic model, since it can be quickly learned and then used in a way that has more in common with cognitive behavioral and other non-exploratory approaches. According to this view, understanding the internal object relations of PD patients by means of an extensive process of clarification, confrontation, and interpretation, would require extended training to enable the therapist to appreciate and fully understand the patients and their difficulties, informed by regular supervision in which the therapist's countertransference can be worked through. This would be simply impossible if, within an "applied" TFP framework, therapists are simply informed about certain techniques that they then deliver to the patient: ultimately, this would lead to loss of the complexity, depth, internal coherence, rigor, and ultimately value of TFP itself.

In response to this criticism, as editors of this volume we have already described earlier the rationale, the public health utility and the empirical evidence of efficacy of the "specializing the generalist" approach to PD treatment and, specifically, the rationale for informing this approach using TFP principles. This book will further describe how TFP strategies and techniques—including psychoanalytic concepts such as monitoring the countertransference—can and should be used in "applied" TFP. Here, we just want to mention that, although TFP surely represents a contemporary development of the psychoanalytic tradition, it includes substantial modifications with respect to psychoanalytic practice, as indicated by the following:

- Its manualized approach to therapy in order to ensure that TFP can be successfully taught and then practiced with adherence and competence by the therapists and that its efficacy can be reliably demonstrated.
- The lack of the requirement, in the TFP manuals, for advanced psychoanalytic training.
- The twice-a-week setting.
- Its clear definition of practical personal and treatment goals.
- Its constant focus not only in the here-and-now interaction between the patient and the therapist, but also on external reality.

As a psychoanalytically informed therapy, TFP retains an ambitious goal of treatment, that is, an enduring change in personality and personality functioning: in ORT terms, identity integration. Importantly, however, this intrapsychic goal will be reflected in the practical achievement of meaningful life goals outside the treatment. As such, TFP is an extended, highly structured psychodynamic treatment, which though expects clear and practical improvements in patients' everyday functioning. It is our opinion, as editors of this volume, that these unique features of TFP precisely favor and encourage an "applied" TFP approach to the general psychiatric care of PD populations. To do so, the component parts of TFP on their own should be made accessible and disseminated to various clinicians of differing training backgrounds and levels of experience.

While we do not assume nor imply that the "applied" TFP initiatives described in the present volume represent a therapeutic *alternative* to standard TFP, we firmly believe that all patients attending various and different clinical settings would benefit from a TFP-oriented therapeutic stance, regardless of the availability or accessibility to standard TFP. Indeed, this stance promotes hope and wish for change among PD patients and invites them to actively reflect on one's own difficulties rather than acting them out. This is opposite to other therapeutic attitudes that perpetuate a passive and negative view of PD psychopathology rooted in an obsolete disability model of personality pathology that is no longer supported—if it ever was —by findings of naturalistic longitudinal studies on the course and outcome of PD. In practical terms, it would be unethical not to use available and empirically supported therapeutical tools, such as those captured by TFP elements, when treating patients with PD who are not currently attending standard TFP. For instance, clinicians working within an "applied" TFP framework would anticipate, similarly to what happens in standard TFP, that a change is indeed expected, and would collaboratively work with the patient to identify meaningful treatment goals and to monitor their advancements toward those goals over the course of treatment, in a step-by-step fashion, even if the treatment occurs outside the standard, twice-a-week outpatient TFP setting.

Overview of This Volume

This current volume aims to include comprehensively the sites of exploration of the utility of TFP principles. The range of settings reflects different needs (individual, institution or healthcare system, public health jurisdiction) and different sources of support. The settings range from the most restrictive, including forensic units and inpatient psychiatry services, to outpatient mental health settings and primary care and medical subspecialty physicians' offices.

The contributing authors have been asked to detail their interventions using TFP principles by supplying, when possible and appropriate, the following information:

- Who are the clinicians involved?
- Who are the patients involved?
- What is the contemporary standard of care for clinicians treating this group of patients?
- What are the goals for imparting to these clinicians the principles of TFP for working with these patients?
- What is the source of institutional or government support for this initiative?
- What specific TFP principles might be of use to the clinicians working with these patients?
- What are the possible targets for measurement to gauge the effectiveness of instruction about applications of TFP principles?
- What are the didactic materials required to impart TFP principles to this target group of clinicians?
- What is the format for instruction of TFP principles to this audience of clinicians?
- What are useful, key publications on this specific subject?

TFP principles are not offered by these contributors as a panacea, but rather as practical ideas informed by an evidence-based treatment, reconsidered or reconfigured for a broader audience of clinicians. This approach fits with many of the most impassioned movements of our time: de-stigmatization of mental illness, advocacy for patients with PD diagnoses, attention to empirically validated interventions, and an openness to different schools of thought or theoretical orientations when doing so is in the best interest of patients and providers. This collective effort brings together clinicians with different backgrounds and from many countries; this heterogeneity confers an element of excitement and creativity to this proliferating approach to helping patients. While this book does not intend to represent a "manual" of applied TFP, it pursues the practical goal of providing mental health practitioners working in a variety of settings and institutions with specific "directions" on how to successfully import a TFP-oriented approach to the psychiatric care of PD patients into their specific treatment context.

The volume is organized along these lines.

Section I focuses on introducing current concepts and models of TFP. In Chap. 2, Caligor, Clarkin, Diamond, Sowislo, and Yeomans provide the reader with the basic theoretical principles and techniques of TFP for PD. This chapter outlines that the key principles of TFP, as an extended individual psychotherapy, include the therapist's openness to making a PD diagnosis; the therapist's ability to share with the patient his or her diagnostic impression using either standard diagnostic terms or other terminology to convey this impression; an early and specific discussion of the patient's personal goals and treatment goals; and the development and maintenance of a treatment agreement, which outlines the respective responsibilities of both parties involved. In addition, a focus on the three channels of communication—how the patient behaves, what the patient says, and how the therapist feels—is another critical component.

In Chap. 3, Rentrop, Gerra, and De Panfilis describe a TFP-informed model of psychoeducation for both patients and family members. Previous randomized controlled trials demonstrated that GPM-oriented psychoeducation is effective in decreasing symptom severity among BPD patients [81]. Furthermore, a structured psychoeducation intervention based on the "staying connected" relationship model increases the caregivers' perception of the quality of their interaction with their affected relative with BPD [82]. Given the centrality, in TFP, of sharing with the patient and their family the clinician's diagnostic impression, doing so in a structured fashion as described in this chapter's model of psychoeducation may represent an important step forward in the field of applied TFP.

Section II deals with how to apply TFP principles in specific mental health settings.

In Chap. 4, De Panfilis, Ciccone, Ampollini, Palombi, and Dazzi illustrate how to inform psychiatric care for severe PD with TFP principles in a community-based, publicly founded multi-professional mental health service. In this experience, instructing the various members of the mental health teams with the key elements of ORT and TFP allowed the staff to understand PD psychopathology as a consequence of the conflicting internal world of the patient, develop coherent responses toward the patients, and structure a multiphase TFP-oriented treatment approach even in the absence of standard psychotherapy.

In Chap. 5, Lee and van den Bosch illustrate the application of TFP principles within the UK National Health System. Starting in the beginning of 2000, UK policy implementation guidance encouraged the creation of dedicated services for PD [19]. The authors describe how TFP principles have been introduced into this context in several ways, i.e., as a modification of the standard twice-a-week setting in a once-a-week one, as an integration with other existing treatment modalities, and as a coherent approach to supervision of the multi-professional mental health teams.

Chapter 6 outlines how TFP principles may be applied to the treatment of PD populations in day hospital (DH) settings. Ripoll, Vegué, and Krischer describe how the multidisciplinary programs delivered by DH settings may benefit from applying

TFP principles to the therapeutic relationship between the patient and the various staff members. Notably, this chapter illustrates two distinct but consistent DH experiences in two different countries (Spain and Germany) and in two populations of different age ranges (adult and adolescent patients).

Chapters 7 and 8 are concerned with the application of TFP principles in inpatient settings.

In Chap. 7, Dulz, Grimmer, Lohmer, Wlodarczyk, and Dammann outline how TFP principles may be used to clarify and accurately interpret the transference and countertransference dynamics between the patient and various staff members of inpatient units for PD. This experience took place in German-speaking countries where long-term, psychodynamically oriented inpatient treatment for PD is still available (i.e., in Switzerland, Germany, and Austria). The authors also describe how TFP principles can assist in clinical decision-making during brief hospitalizations in acute psychiatric wards. Chapter 8 describes the introduction of TFP principles into the inpatient treatment for PD in the Spanish system of care. Valenciano and Gonzalez Torres illustrate how mental health professionals working in higher acuity settings such as general psychiatric wards and emergency rooms can successfully learn and apply TFP principles, with the aim to structure a tailored treatment for PD and prevent iatrogenic complications of inpatient stays.

Chapter 9 describes the application of TFP principles in an integrated care continuum such as the one provided in the Barcelona catchment area (Spain) by various mental health professionals belonging to a large specialized treatment team for PD. Rufat and Vegué describe how key TFP elements can be used to structure an individually tailored, ongoing treatment program for patients with borderline organization across different levels of care, such as the outpatient level, the DH level, the rehabilitation level, and the inpatient level. In this experience, adopting TFP principles ensures that the individual's treatment is organized around a shared treatment contract and specific treatment goals regardless of the level of care in which the patient is treated at a given moment. It also allows clinicians to consistently identify and address the object relation dyads between patients and the various professionals, with the final aim of fostering personality integration.

In Chap. 10, Grimmer, Kraus, Krischer, Rösch, and Vohl deal with the issue of applying TFP principles in a group therapy format. While TFP was originally conceived as an individual psychotherapy, the authors describe the relevance of ORT and TFP models in understanding the dynamics among group members and between group members and the leader during analytic group psychotherapy and propose original ways to translate TFP strategies techniques into the group therapy setting. This goal is accomplished by illustrating the elements of TFP-oriented group therapy for both adult and adolescent patients.

Section III concerns the application of TFP principles with specific patient populations.

In Chap. 11 Lackinger describes an original modification of TFP strategies for the forensic population. In the forensic setting, the application of TFP principles allows clinicians to refine the structural diagnosis of this severe patient population and to deploy a specific, novel TFP-oriented treatment approach, i.e., Transference-focused forensic psychotherapy (TFFP).

Chapter 12 illustrates how TFP principles can be effectively used in the treatment of PD patients with comorbid medical conditions. Indeed, PD patients are seen frequently in medical settings, where they are often described as "difficult" patients. Medically ill patients with personality pathology pose unique challenges to treating clinicians, such as poor compliance with medical prescriptions, high rates of health-care utilization, and a wide range of adverse health outcomes. Hersh, Petrini, Moscara, and Bergonzini describe two TFP-informed initiatives. The first one refers to an Italian experience highlighting the utility of using TFP principles during the psychiatric consultation of PD patients who are hospitalized for medical reasons. The second initiative consists of a US-based pilot training program that teaches internal medicine residents how to apply TFP principles in their usual practice to improve the clinical management of medically ill patients presenting with a co-occurring personality disorder pathology.

In Chap. 13, Icart and Ribalta propose a novel therapeutic family intervention for adolescents with borderline personality organization who display limited insight into their problem behaviors and, thus, find it difficult to adhere to individual psychotherapy. This intervention utilizes TFP principles to improve parental functions (PF) in families (i.e., TFP-PF) to facilitate the adolescents' process of differentiation and individuation; in turn, this will enhance the awareness of their difficulties and promote adherence to individual treatment.

Finally, Appendix 1, by Yeomans and Doering, summarizes helpful TFP resources and literature, with the aim to provide the reader with updated information about important developments in TFP theory and practice, which can further assist the clinicians in introducing TFP principles within their own psychiatric practice with PD patients.

Conclusion

This book describes a timely development for the treatment of patients with personality disorder pathology. As previously mentioned, outcome research points to the feasibility of "generalizing" effective ingredients of specialist psychotherapies to broader settings than the individual psychotherapy format. Thus, extending TFP principles beyond the individual psychotherapy modality fulfills a crucial public health role. In addition, current nosology research on PD diagnosis emphasizes the need to evaluate general features of PD along a continuum of severity of (dys)function in the self and interpersonal domains [83, 84], rather than focusing on diagnostic categories defined by often arbitrary criterion sets. Notably, such an approach is consistent with the diagnostic process of TFP, which stresses the need to evaluate the individual's level of personality organization in order to detect the presence of personality pathology. TFP then targets a broader patient group than the one captured by the sole DSM-5 BPD diagnosis, i.e., all patients functioning at a borderline level of personality organization. In this regard, several elements of TFP theory and practice have an intrinsic value that can be appealing to those clinicians who deal with heterogeneous populations of patients with severe PD and do not intend to practice extended individual psychotherapy treatments. This book outlines that these essential elements of TFP that can be applied in varying clinical situations include:

- using a structural approach to personality disorder diagnosis, which takes into account the patient's severity of illness and level of functioning;
- stressing the importance of sharing the clinician's diagnosis with the patient and family using straightforward language;
- employing a structured approach to treatment anchored from the beginning by a treatment contract describing the responsibilities of both treater and patients;
- maintaining an attitude as a therapist marked by curiosity and as well as an expectation for movement toward the patient's goals;
- ensuring safety over time for both patient and therapist allowing the therapist to both tolerate expectable confusion and to think clearly;
- endeavoring to make sense of the patient's symptoms and difficulties and respond with reflection and sensitivity.

Applied TFP has blossomed spontaneously, often the result of the personal enthusiasms of those students of TFP who become familiar with the essential elements listed above and then link what they have learned to the real-world predicaments they encounter. While applied TFP is in its fledging days, it holds out the promise of genuine versatility and benefit.

References

1. Kernberg O, Coyne L, Voth H. Psychotherapy and psychoanalysis: final report of the Menninger Foundation's psychotherapy research project. Bull Menninger Clinic. 1972;36(1–2):87–275.
2. Kernberg O. Structural interviewing. Psychiat Clin. 1981;4(1):169–95.
3. Kernberg O. Severe personality disorders. New Haven: Yale University Press; 1984.
4. American Psychiatric Association. Diagnostic and statistical manual of mental disorders. 3rd ed.; 1980.
5. Clarkin J, Levy K, Lenzenweger M, Kernberg O. Evaluating three treatments for borderline personality disorder: a multiwave study. Am J Psychiatry. 2007;164(6):922–8.
6. Yeomans F, Clarkin J, Kernberg O. Transference-focused psychotherapy for borderline personality disorders. Arlington: APA Publishing; 2015.
7. Chambless D, Dianne L, Hollon S. Defining empirically supported therapies. J Consult Clin Psychol. 1998;66:7–18.
8. Clarkin J, Foelsch P, Levy K, Hull J, Delaney J, Kernberg O. The development of a psychodynamic treatment for patients with borderline personality disorder: a preliminary study of behavioral change. J Pers Dis. 2001;15:487–95.
9. Doering S, Hörz S, Rentrop M, Fischer-Kern M, Schuster P, Benecke C. Transference-focused psychotherapy v. treatment by community psychotherapists for borderline personality disorder: randomised controlled trial. Br J Psychiat. 2010;196(5):389–95.

10. Cristea IA, Gentili C, Cotet CD, Palomba D, Barbui C, Cuijpers P. Efficacy of psychotherapies for borderline personality disorder: a systematic review and meta-analysis. JAMA Psychiat. 2017;74:319–28.
11. Levy KN, Meehan KB, Kelly KM, Reynoso JS, Weber M, Clarkin JF, Kernberg OF. Change in attachment patterns and reflective function in a randomized controlled trial of Transference Focused Psychotherapy for Borderline Personality Disorder. J Consul Clin Psychol. 2006;74:1027–40.
12. Buchheim A, Horz-Sagstetter S, Doering S, Rentrop M, Schuster P, Buchheim P, Pokorny D, Fisher-Kern M. Change of unresolved attachment in borderline personality disorder: RCT study of transference-focused psychotherapy. Psychoter Psychosom. 2017;86:314–6.
13. Fisher-Kern M, Doering S, Taubner S, Horz S, Zimmerman J, Rentrop M, Schuster P, Buchheim P, Buchheim A. Transference-focused psychotherapy for borderline personality disorder: change in reflective function. Br J Psychiat. 2015;207:173–4.
14. Livesley WJ, Dimaggio G, Clarkin JF. Integrated treatment for personality disorder: a modular approach: Guilford Publications; 2015.
15. Choi-Kan LW, Finch EF, Masland SR, Jenkins JA, Unruh BT. What works in the treatment of Borderline Personality Disorder. Curr Behav Neurosci Rep. 2017;4:21–30.
16. Iliakis EA, Sonley AKI, Ilagan GS, Choi-Kain LW. Treatment of borderline personality disorder: is supply adequate to meet public health needs? Psychiatr Serv. 2019;70:772–81.
17. Weinberg I, Ronningstam E, Goldblatt MJ, Schechter M, Maltsberger JT. Common factors in empirically supported treatments of borderline personality disorder. Curr Psychiat Rep. 2011;13:60–8.
18. Chanen AM, Jackson HJ, McCutcheon LK, Jovev M, Dudgeon P, Yuen HP. Early intervention for adolescents with borderline personality disorder: quasi-experimental comparison with treatment as usual. Aust New Z J Psychiat. 2009;43:397–408.
19. National Institute for Mental Health in England. Personality Disorders: no longer a diagnosis of exclusion. Policy implementation guidance for the implementation of services for people with personality disorder. 2003. https://personalitydisorder.org.uk
20. Chartonas D, Kyratsous M, Dracass S, Lee T, Bhui K. Personality disorder: still the patients psychiatrists dislike? BJPsych bulletin. 2017;41:12–7.
21. Linehan MM. Cognitive-behavioral treatment of borderline personality disorder. New York: Guilford; 1993.
22. Dimeff, LA, Koerner, K. Dialectical behavior therapy in clinical practice: applications across disorders and settings: Guilford Press; 2007.
23. Miller AL. Introduction to a special issue dialectical behavior therapy: evolution and adaptation in the 21st century. Am J Psychother. 2015;69(2):91–5.
24. Woodberry KA, Miller AL, Glinski J, Indik J, Mitchell AG. Family therapy and dialectical behavior therapy with adolescents: Part II: a theorical review. Am J Psychother. 2015;56(4):585–602.
25. Reynolds SK, Wolbert R, Abney-Cunningham G, Patterson K. Dialectical behavior therapy for assertive community treatment teams. In: Dimeff LA, Koerner K, editors. Dialectical behavior therapy in clinical practice applications across disorders and settings. Guilford Press; 2007. p. 298–325.
26. Riesen E, Aubry T. An evaluation of the delivery of dialectical behaviour therapy by the pinecrest queensway community mental health centre's assertive community treatment team. Centre for Research on Community Services.University of Ottawa; 2006.
27. Bateman AW, Fonagy PE. Handbook of mentalizing in mental health practice: American Psychiatric Publishing, Inc.; 2012.
28. Choi-Kain LW, Gunderson JG. Applications of good psychiatric management for borderline personality disorder: a practical guide: American Psychiatric Pub; 2019.
29. Taylor CD, Bee P, Haddock G. Does schema therapy change schemas and symptoms? A systematic review across mental health disorders. Psychol Psychother Theory Res Pract. 2017;90(3):456–79.

30. Zerbo E, Cohen S, Bielska W, Caligor E. Transference-focused psychotherapy in the general psychiatry residency: a useful and applicable model for residents in acute clinical settings. Psychodynam Psychiat. 2013;41(1):163–81.
31. Normandin L, Ensink K, Weiner A, Kernberg OF. Transference-focused psychotherapy for adolescents with severe personality disorders: American Psychiatric Pub; 2021.
32. Jahn C, Wieacker E, Bender S, Krisher M. Reduction of non-suicidal self-injury (NSSI) in adolescents with borderline personality disorder treated with TFP-A. Praz Kinderpsychol Kinderpsychiat. 2021;70:731–50.
33. Caligor E, Kernberg OF, Clarkin JF. Handbook of dynamic psychotherapy for higher level personality pathology: American Psychiatric Pub; 2007.
34. Caligor E, Kernberg O, Clarkin J, Yeomans F. Psychodynamic therapy for personality pathology. Washington, DC: APA Publishing; 2018.
35. Diamond D, Yeomans FE, Stern BL, Kernberg OF. Treating pathological narcissism with transference-focused psychotherapy: Guilford Publications; 2021.
36. Caligor E, Stern BL. Diagnosis, classification, and assessment of narcissistic personality disorder within the framework of object relations theory. J Personal Disor. 2020;34:104–21.
37. American Psychiatric Association. Diagnostic and statistical manual for personality disorders 5th edition (DSM-5). Washington, DC: American Psychiatric Publishing; 2013.
38. Brömmel B, Dammann G. Katathym Imaginative Psychotherapie (KIP) und Übertragungsfokussierte Psychotherapie (TFP) in der Behandlung von Borderline-Störungen. PTT-Persönlichkeitsstörungen: Theorie und Therapie. 2004;8(3):161–74.
39. Dammann G, editor. Interaktionelle Methode und übertragungsfokussierte Psychotherapie. Forum der Psychoanalyse; 2004. Springer.
40. Bernardo EG. Psychological treatment for borderline personality disorders. Clinica y Salud. 2007;18(3):347–61.
41. Hörz-Sagstetter S, Wernz C, Rentrop M. Übertragungsfokussierte Psychotherapie und Paarkonflikte. PTT-Persönlichkeitsstörungen: Theorie und Therapie. 2017;21(3):203–9.
42. Higa JK, Gedo PM. Transference interpretation in the treatment of borderline personality disorder patients. Bull Menninger Clin. 2012;76(3):195–210.
43. Rivera M, Darke JL. Integrating empirically supported therapies for treating personality disorders: A synthesis of psychodynamic and cognitive-behavioral group treatments. Int J Group Psychother. 2012;62(4):500–29.
44. Ortega CC, Crespo P. Aproximaciones actuales a la patología límite. Psicoterapia focalizada en la transferencia de O. Kernberg y otros modelos de psicoterapia psicoanalítica. Revista de Psicoanálisis de la Asociación Psicoanalítica de Madrid. 2013;68:125–54.
45. Martel D, Lecours S. Analyse critique du rôle accordé à l'interprétation du clivage dans la psychothérapie focalisée sur le transfert: contraste avec le traitement centré sur la mentalisation. Psychothérapies. 2013;33(3):177–94.
46. Kooiman C, Kuipers G, Huffstadt C. Transference-focused psychotherapie en mentaliseren in de klinische psychotherapie; een kwestie van vorm én vent. Tijdschrift voor Psychiatrie. 2013;55(12):939–48.
47. Gunderson JG and Links P. Handbook of good psychiatric management for borderline personality disorder. American Psychiatric Publishing; 2014.
48. Schlüter-Müller S, Schmeck K. Adolescent Identity Treatment (AIT). PTT-Persönlichkeitsstörungen: Theorie und Therapie. 2015;19(1):55–66.
49. Choi-Kain LW, Albert EB, Gunderson JG. Evidence-based treatments for borderline personality disorder: implementation, integration, and stepped care. Harvard Rev Psychiat. 2016;24(5):342–56.
50. Rösch C, Grimmer B. Störungsspezifische stationäre Behandlung von Persönlichkeitsstörungen. PTT-Persönlichkeitsstörungen: Theorie und Therapie. 2017;21(2):83–95.
51. Schlüter-Müller S. AIT (Adolescent Identity Treatment)–ein integratives Therapiekonzept zur Behandlung von Persönlichkeitsstörungen. Praxis der Kinderpsychologie und Kinderpsychiatrie. 2017;66(6):392–403.

52. Gunderson JG. Borderline personality disorder: a clinical guide: American Psychiatric Pub; 2009.
53. Pfäfflin F, Ross T. Zum umgang mit delinquenz in der borderline-therapie. PTT-Persönlichkeitsstörungen: Theorie und Therapie. 2004;8(1):49–54.
54. Lackinger F, Dammann G. Besonderheiten der Behandlungsbedingungen bei der übertragungsfokussierten Psychotherapie (TFP) persönlichkeitsgestörter Delinquenten. Recht & Psychiatrie. 2005;23(3):103–15.
55. Fontao MI, Pfäfflin F, Lamott F. Anwendung der Übertragungsfokussierten Psychotherapie (TFP) auf die Behandlung von Maßregelvollzugspatienten. Eine Pilotstudie. Recht & Psychiatrie. 2006;24(4):193–200.
56. Kernberg OF. Psychoanalytische Gruppenpsychotherapie. PTT-Persönlichkeitsstörungen: Theorie und Therapie. 2009;13(2):79–93.
57. Schneider-Lehmann A. Übertragungsfokussierte Psychotherapie und Traumatherapie. PTT-Persönlichkeitsstörungen: Theorie und Therapie. 2009;13(4):269–74.
58. Lamott F, Pfäfflin F. Psychotherapie für straftäter: Ein überblick = Psychotherapy for delinquents A review. Psychotherapeut. 2009;54(4):245–50.
59. Draijer N, Van Zon P. Transference-focused psychotherapy with former child soldiers: meeting the murderous self. J Trauma Dissociation. 2013;14(2):170–83.
60. Kenkel LE, Seritan AL. Psychotherapy. In: Hategan A, Bourgeois JA, Xiong GL, editors. Borderline personality disorder in older adults: Emphasis on care in institutional settings. Hauppauge: Nova Science Publishers; 2015. p. 89–98.
61. Krischer MK, Normandin L. Tagesklinische Behandlung von adoleszenten Borderline-Patienten mit Techniken der Übertragungsfokussierten Psychotherapie für Jugendliche: Konzept und erste Erfahrungen = Dayclinic treatment of adolescent borderline patients with techniques of the transference-focused psychotherapy for adolescents (TFP-A): concept and first experiences. PTT: Persönlichkeitsstörungen Theorie und Therapie. 2015;19(1):2–13.
62. Sollberger D, Gremaud-Heitz D, Riemenschneider A, Agarwalla P, Benecke C, Schwald O, et al. Change in identity diffusion and psychopathology in a specialized inpatient treatment for borderline personality disorder. Clin Psychol Psychother. 2015;22(6):559–69.
63. Krüger S, Meiners J. Übertragungsfokussierte Psychotherapie (TFP) und Therapie von Traumatisierungen. PDP-Psychodynamische Psychotherapie. 2018;17(3):147–56.
64. Gaztambide DJ. Lines of advance in treating people of color with borderline personality disorder: alloying the "gold" of vocational rehabilitation with the "copper" of psychodynamic psychotherapy. Psychoanal Social Work. 2019;26(1):50–68.
65. Lee T, Hersh RG. Managing the clinical encounter with patients with borderline personality disorder in a general psychiatry setting: key contributions from transference-focused psychotherapy. BJPsych Advances. 2019;25(4):229–36.
66. Moscara M, Bergonzini E. Integrating the principles of transference-focused psychotherapy with psychiatric consultation for patients admitted to a general hospital: a clinical application of a psychotherapeutic tool. Int J Appl Psychoanal Studies. 2021;18(1):18–29.
67. Carsky M, Yeomans F. Overwhelming patients and overwhelmed therapists. Psychodyn Psychiatry. 2012;40(1):75–90.
68. Sansone RA, Kay J, Anderson JL. Resident didactic education in borderline personality disorder: is it sufficient? Academic Psychiatry; 2013.
69. Bliss S, McCardle M. An exploration of common elements in dialectical behavior therapy, mentalization based treatment and transference focused psychotherapy in the treatment of borderline personality disorder. Clin Social Work J. 2014;42(1):61–9.
70. Needham B. Integrative multidisciplinary treatment: an intervention for complex mental health patients in a public sector, teaching hospital setting: University of Houston; 2011.
71. Bernstein J, Zimmerman M, Auchincloss EL. Transference-focused psychotherapy training during residency: an aide to learning psychodynamic psychotherapy. Psychodyn Psychiatry. 2015;43(2):201–21.
72. Chambers JE. Discussion of Transference-Focused Psychotherapy training during residency: an aide to learning psychodynamic psychotherapy. Psychodyn Psychiatry. 2015;43(2):223–8.

73. Martin L, Lloyd B, Cammell P, Yeomans F. Transference-focused psychotherapy in Australian psychiatric training and practice. Australasian Psychiatry. 2017;25(3):233–5.
74. Hersh RG, Caligor E, Yeomans FE. Fundamentals of transference-focused psychotherapy: applications in psychiatric and medical settings: Springer; 2017.
75. Petrini M. Management of personality disorders in primary care. Pri-med New York; 2015.
76. Hersh RG. Using transference-focused psychotherapy principles in the pharmacotherapy of patients with severe personality disorders. Psychodyn Psychiatry. 2015;43(2):181–99.
77. Hersh R. Augmenting psychiatric risk management: Practical applications of transference-focused psychotherapy (TFP) principles. Psychodyn Psychiatry. 2019;47(4):441–68.
78. Hersh RG. A psychodynamic approach for the general psychiatrist: using transference-focused psychotherapy principles in acute care settings. Psychiat Clin. 2018;41(2):225–35.
79. Gibbels C, Kneer J, Hartmann U, Krueger TH. State of the art treatment options for actual and potential sexual offenders and new prevention strategies. J Psychiat Pract. 2019;25(4):242–57.
80. Krischer M, Ponton-Rodriguez T, Gooran GR, Bender S. Transference focused psychotherapy for borderline-adolescents in a day clinic treatment program/Ubertragungsfokussierte Psychotherapie von BorderlineJugendlichen im tagesklinischen Setting. Praxis der Kinderpsychologie und Kinderpsychiatrie. 2017;66(6):445–64.
81. Ridolfi ME, Rossi R, Occhialini G, Gunderson JG. A clinical trial of a psychoeducation group intervention for patients with borderline personality disorder. J Clin Psychiatry. 2019;81(1):16069.
82. Grenyer BF, Bailey RC, Lewis KL, Matthias M, Garretty T, Bickerton A. A randomized controlled trial of group psychoeducation for carers of persons with borderline personality disorder. J Personal Disorders. 2019;33(2):214–28.
83. American Psychiatric Association. Diagnostic and statistical manual of mental disorders. 5th ed. Arlington; 2013.
84. Sharp C, Wall K. DSM-5 level of personality functioning: refocusing personality disorder on what it means to be human. Ann Rev Clin Psychol. 2021;17:313–37.

Development and Evolution of Transference-Focused Psychotherapy (TFP): A Foundation for Expanding Treatment Applications

2

John F. Clarkin, Eve Caligor, Julia Sowislo, Diana Diamond, and Frank Yeomans

Introduction

Personality pathology is ubiquitous, and every mental health professional must be alert to its presence and influence on the treatment formulation and process. One in ten individuals in Western societies have personality pathology. Approximately half of psychiatric outpatients manifest a diagnosed personality disorder, which is a key predictor of impairment and treatment outcome [1]. Inspired by the theoretical and clinical leadership of Otto F. Kernberg, colleagues at the Personality Disorders Institute (PDI), Weill Medical College of Cornell University, have developed a manualized but flexible, clinically informed, and empirically investigated treatment for patients with the range of personality pathology. This psychodynamic treatment, called transference-focused psychotherapy TFP is composed of three key elements: (1) a psychoanalytic model of personality pathology, (2) a clinical assessment procedure that focuses the intervention, and (3) an empirically driven model of psychotherapy. The evolution of this approach to personality pathology has spanned some 40 years and has involved an enrichment of the model of personality pathology with theoretical refinements and empirical research on the

J. F. Clarkin · J. Sowislo (✉) · D. Diamond
Department of Psychiatry, Weill Cornell Medical College, New York, NY, USA
e-mail: jclarkin@med.cornell.edu

E. Caligor
Department of Psychiatry, Columbia Vagelos College of Physicians & Surgeons, New York, NY, USA

F. Yeomans
Department of Psychiatry, Weill Medical College, New York, NY, USA

R. G. Hersh, C. De Panfilis (eds.), *Implementing Transference-Focused Psychotherapy Principles*, https://doi.org/10.1007/978-3-031-68062-5_2

pathology and its treatment. Since its original articulation as an intensive psychodynamic treatment for patients with borderline personality disorder (BPD), TFP has evolved into a transdiagnostic treatment for patients with problems in self-functioning and functioning with others as defined by the DSM-5 Alternative Model of Personality Disorder (AMPD; [2]).

At this point in its development TFP has been delivered in an intensive (2 sessions a week over 1 year or longer) individual treatment format, which is costly in terms of therapist and patient time. This treatment development for the individual has provided an opportunity to now apply what has been learned in less expensive and more efficient ways to a broader range of patients. In order to provide TFP to patients with a range of personality pathology and symptom disorders in multiple settings and different treatment formats as described in this book, it is essential to conceptualize and describe the core elements of this treatment approach. It is the aim of this chapter to describe the defining features and principles of TFP by explaining our current understanding of personality disturbance through the lens of object relations theory (ORT) and its treatment for patients across the range of personality pathology. This development of an object relations approach has been consistent with, and enhanced by, the remarkable advances in the understanding of personality pathology as reflected in the trajectory from DSM-III to DSM-5, the expansion of cross-sectional and longitudinal studies of the pathology, and the development of treatments applying cognitive-behavioral and psychodynamic strategies.

In this chapter, we introduce the theoretical foundation of the ORT model of personality functioning and pathology and highlight its relevance to assessment and treatment planning for TFP. We describe the theory and the system of classification of personality pathology that emerges within ORT, providing clinical illustrations, and comparing the ORT model with the model introduced in the AMPD in DSM-5. This articulation of ORT and the core of TFP provides a background for the expanded application of the treatment model to various treatment settings and formats as applied to patients with personality pathology and symptom disorders.

Origins of TFP in the Psychoanalytic Tradition

The clinical approach of TFP is grounded in contemporary object relations perspective, particularly the work of Otto Kernberg [3–6] that integrates contributions from British object relations theory [7–9] and American ego psychology [10–12] along with research in social cognition, neuroscience, attachment theory, mentalization theory and social psychology. The full exposition of this model as well as the empirical research in support of it is beyond the scope of this chapter and can be found elsewhere [4, 5, 13–15], but an integrative summary of key points of the model will be provided in this chapter.

As one of the general classes of psychodynamic psychotherapies, TFP shares the assumptions of these approaches [16]:

- Treatment of the patient as a unique individual
- Recognition of the complexity of factors bringing the patient to treatment
- Psychological causation and focus on the internal world
- Unconscious motivation and intentionality
- Defensive operations
- Internal representations and internalized relationship patterns
- Structural perspective (see below)
- The centrality of self-functioning and functioning with others
- Developmental perspective
- Continuity between normal and disrupted personality development

In contrast to the general class of psychodynamic treatments, however, TFP is focused specifically on patients with difficulties in self-functioning and functioning with others that are central to the range of personality disorders, difficulties that are grounded in their internal biased representations of self and others. TFP applies the four basic psychoanalytic technical therapeutic interventions [6] in a strategic way: (1) interpretation, (2) transference analysis, (3) technical neutrality, and (4) countertransference utilization. TFP is one of the most ambitious (in terms of treatment goals) and intensive psychodynamic psychotherapies. The treatment goal is improved self and interpersonal functioning, mediated by modification in the patient's representations of self in relation to others and the transformation of identity diffusion into normal identity.

Object Relations Theory: Model of Personality Pathology

Personality can be defined as the dynamic organization of relatively stable patterns of behavior, cognition, emotion, motivation, and ways of relating to and experiencing others [16]. Within the framework of an ORT model of personality, the most basic elements or building blocks of personality consist of internal object relations. In this formulation, the term "object" is used in the historic, psychoanalytical sense to refer to a person with whom the subject has a relationship. The term "internal" is used to mark an inner representation of a relationship within the subject's mind as opposed to an actual relationship in the outer world. Developmentally, internal representations emerge from actual experiences that get colored and exaggerated by unconscious processes such as wishes, fears, and fantasies.

Each internal object relation is composed of a mental representation of the self in relation to another person linked with a particular affect (inadequate self, linked by fear, to a critical other; a mistreated self, linked by rage, to an exploitive other; an accomplished self, linked by pride, to an admiring other). It is important to understand that within the ORT model, no representation of the self exists in isolation (e.g., small, childlike self) but is always connected to the affective experience of the relationship with a significant other (e.g., small childlike self in relationship with unavailable, neglecting caretaker and feelings of frustration versus in relationship with a loving and nurturing caretaker and feelings of gratification). Furthermore, when activated in a particular situation, internal object relations organize an individual's expectations and subjective experience. For example, a patient in which the above-mentioned internal object relation (childlike self in relationship with unavailable caretaker) gets activated might become frustrated over the therapist's absence due to vacation and perceive him or her as a neglecting figure.

According to the ORT model, the basic internal object relations come together in building higher order, core psychological structures (see Table 2.1 for an overview). Personality and personality disorders are understood in terms of the level of integration of those structures, with lower levels of integration characterizing the more severe personality pathologies. Identity (i.e., the experience of self and others) is considered the most important structure as the level of identity integration distinguishes between normal personality and personality pathology. A fully consolidated identity formation characterizes the normal personality as internal object relations coalesce to form an overarching, coherent, stable, realistic, affectively well-modulated and complex sense of self and significant others. This contributes to relationships that involve empathy, concern, and mutual dependence. In contrast, individuals with personality disorders suffer from the pathology of identity

Table 2.1 Structural Approach to the Nosology of Personality Pathology

	Normal personality organization	Neurotic personality organization	High-level borderline personality organization	Mid-level borderline personality organization	Low-level borderline personality organization
Identity	Integrated	Integrated	Mild-medium identity diffusion	Notable identity diffusion	Severe identity diffusion
Object relations	Long-lasting, interdependent relations	Long-lasting, interdependent relations	Some interdependent relations with conflict	Relations based on need fulfillment	Exploitative relationships
Defensives	Mature	Repression-based	Repression and splitting-based	Splitting-based	Splitting-based
Moral values	Moral conscience applied to behavior with flexibility	Rigid moral conscience	Uneven/ inconsistent moral behavior	Moderate pathology	Extreme pathology; absence of guilt
Aggression	Modulated; assertive without aggression	Modulated; inhibited	Some verbal aggression	Breaks in modulation; potential aggression against self and others	Potential aggression against others
Reality testing	Intact and stable; social reality testing intact	Intact and stable; social reality testing intact	Intact; some social reality testing deficits	Vulnerable to stress; transient psychotic states; social deficits	Vulnerable to stress; transient psychotic states; social deficits

formulation, reflecting failure of component object relations to form an overarching, integrated self-structure. In this situation, the sense of self and others is shallow, unstable, distorted, and accompanied by highly charged and poorly modulated affects. This contributes to an incapacity to invest in relationships and impairment of empathy and mentalization. Along with the central structure of identity, the model focuses on the following five inter-related structures:

- Object relations: internal working models of relationships; reflected in friendships, intimate relations, and sexuality
- Defenses: automatic responses to external stressors and internal conflicts; higher-level defenses introduce less distortion and are more adaptive; lower-level defenses distort subjective experience
- Aggression: manifested as both internal aggression and aggressive behavior toward self-and/or others
- Moral values: organized value systems; expressed in capacity for guilt and ethical ideals and behavior
- Reality testing: appreciation of conventional notions of reality

Pathology in these structures, particularly in the hallmark structure of identity, is thought to develop under the pervasive influence of splitting-based defenses. Splitting-based defenses (such as projective identification or primitive idealization) dissociate representations of self and others associated with positive affective experience from representations associated with negative affective experience. Developmentally, these mechanisms predominate in the mind of a young child, meaning that in early development experiences of the self in relation to others, they are organized according to a split between experiences that are rewarding, gratifying, and pleasurable and experiences that are frustrating and painful. However, in a nurturing environment, the child can eventually overcome this split and integrate both positive and negative attributes of self and others into more realistic, balanced, and mixed representations. Under adverse conditions (e.g., lack of empathy, neglect, or abuse) the defensive split can persist, and "good"/gratifying representations of self and others are kept separate in the mind from "bad"/frustrating representations. This accounts for the unstable, distorted, black and white, "all good" and "all bad" experiences that characterize identity pathology and personality disorders (PD).

Nosology: Levels of Personality Organization

The classification of personality pathology within the ORT model is consistent with the above-described theoretical conceptualization of personality, in contrast to other classification systems that are purely atheoretical (such as the DSM-5 model). The psychological structures described by the model can be used to make structural classification of personality disorders. While these structures are well integrated and developed in normal, healthy personality, PD is characterized by failure of integration of those structures: As the severity of personality disorder increases, the level of integration in core psychological structures decreases. Thus, a dimensional diagnosis of PD can be made by describing the (sometimes uneven) dysfunction in identity and the other related four personality structures. For example, in the more severe PD (1) identity is poorly consolidated, with experiences of self and others that are superficial, incoherent, contradictory, and distorted (2) relations with others are based on need fulfillment, exploitation and void of real intimacy and empathy (3) lower-level defensive operations (such as splitting) are predominant and lead to distortions in perceptions, as well as rigidity and failure of adaptation (4) control of aggression is impaired and can result in hateful, even lethal, attacks toward self and other (5) comprehension of moral values is lacking so that antisocial, including violent, behavior or frank psychopathy may predominate. Additionally (6) reality testing can be transiently lost. Alternative to this dimensional classification, the model also allows for a categorical, structural diagnosis, which describes a patient's level of personality organization. Here, patients can be classified as having a normal personality organization, a neurotic level of personality organization (NPO), a high borderline level of personality organization[1] (high BPO), middle borderline level of personality organization (middle BPO), and low borderline level of personality organization (low BPO). We describe these four prototypic levels of personality dysfunction in more detail as below:

The two structural approaches, namely the dimensional and the categorial ones, inform about the severity of personality dysfunction, spanning the normal to the most severe PD, which is crucial for treatment planning and prognosis. In addition to the structural diagnoses, the ORT model allows for a second-order diagnosis-based cluster of observable personality features or traits (examples of traits are conscientiousness and impulsivity). This approach is similar to the one taken in the DSM system, which lists several traits as diagnostic criteria for a personality disorder. Table 2.2 illustrates the relationship between structural and trait-based diagnoses in the ORT model. The broad category of patients with BPO ranges from patients with borderline, schizotypal, antisocial, paranoid, schizoid, and hypochondriacal personality disorders in the low to mid-BPO, to patients with avoidant, dependent, histrionic, and sadomasochistic personality disorders in the high BPO, to patients with obsessive-compulsive, depressive-masochistic, and hysterical personality disorder in the NPO. Patients with narcissistic personality disorder can have highly variable presentations, ranging from those in the most severely impaired category, ranging from lower, mid-, or even higher BPO. Notably, some individuals at the healthiest end of the narcissistic personality disorder spectrum may present as "neurotic" on superficial evaluation, but with a comprehensive assessment, these individuals will demonstrate more significant structural pathology consistent with BPO.

[1] We want to make clear the distinction between the DSM-5 borderline personality disorder (BPD) and the borderline level of personality organization (BPO). BPD is a specific personality disorder, diagnosed on the basis of a constellation of descriptive features. BPO is a much broader category based on structural features—in particular, pathology of identity formation. The BPO diagnosis subsumes the DSM-5 BPD, as well as all of the severe personality disorders.

Table 2.2 Severity of personality pathology: implications for treatment parameters

	Neurotic organization	High borderline organization	Mid-borderline organization	Low borderline organization
Level of Personality Functioning (LPFS)	Level 1	Level 2	Level 3	Level 4
Typical personality disorder diagnosis/ constellation	Obsessive Compulsive Depressive Hysterical	Dependent Histrionic Avoidant Narcissistic	Narcissistic Borderline Paranoid Schizoid	Narcissistic Borderline, and paranoid with antisocial features Antisocial
Nature of self/ other functioning	Integrated, realistic and continuous experience of self in relation to others; relationships characterized by mutuality. However, rigid functioning in areas of conflict.	Somewhat superficial and/or polarized experience of self in relation to others; some capacity for dependency but with conflict	Superficial, extreme, polarized, unstable sense of self in relation to others with gross distortion; need-fulfilling relationships	Caricature-like, extreme, highly polarized and chaotic sense of self in relation to others with gross distortion; exploitative relationships
Prognosis	Excellent	Good	Fair	Very guarded
Objectives of treatment	Flexible functioning in areas of conflict	Greater depth and stability in experience of self and others	Resolution of destructive behavior; greater depth in experience of self and others	Behavior control; modulation of aggression

Neurotic Personality Organization

The neurotic level of personality organization involves: (1) consolidated identity, (2) the predominance of repression-based and mature defenses, and (3) relatively well integrated and complex affective experience. NPO is distinguished from normal, healthy personality based on varying degrees of rigidity in personality functioning. The individual with normal personality organization can flexibly and adaptively manage external stressors and internal conflicts. In contrast, the individual with NPO tends to rely on rigid and to some degree maladaptive responses, which reflect the impact of repression-based defenses on psychological functioning. Individuals organized at a neurotic level (similar to those at a normal level) benefit from a sense of self and significant others that is stable, well-differentiated, realistic, and coherent, along with a capacity for full, deep, and mutual relationships. Although moral functioning is fully internalized in NPO, it may be overly rigid, which appears in excessive self-criticism. Furthermore, there may be difficulty combining intimacy with sexuality. Aggression tends to be well integrated and modulated, and reality testing is stable and secure.

Borderline Personality Organization

The hallmark feature of BPO is a pathology of identity formation (1). As mentioned above, this goes hand in hand in conjunction with (2) the predominance of splitting-based defenses, and (3) poorly integrated affect states with a preponderance of poorly modulated aggression. BPO manifests as a shallow, unstable, polarized ("black and white"), distorted, and discontinuous experience of self and others. These fragmented and poorly integrated views of self and others are the result of the operation of splitting-based defenses (e.g., splitting, idealization/devaluation, projective identification, denial). Individuals organized at a borderline level have pervasive difficulties that compromises their functioning in many if not all domains.

Three Levels of BPO The borderline level of personality organization covers a relatively broad spectrum of personality pathology. Individuals at the higher (healthier) end of the BPO spectrum have some capacity for dependent, but compromised, relationships, generally have only minor impairments in moral functioning, and are for the most part not overtly aggressive. In contrast, individuals at the low end of the BPO spectrum, have extremely compromised object relations, extreme impairment in moral functioning with antisocial features, and are overly aggressive, while those in the middle BPO spectrum have moderately compromised pathology of object relations and variable moral functioning. Their pathology of aggression is less severe than that characteristic of the low BPO spectrum. Distinctions within the range of BPO are highly clinically significant, determining prognosis and guiding treatment planning.

BPO and Reality Testing In contrast to those with psychotic disorders, individuals organized at a borderline level have generally intact reality testing. However, in areas of conflict or in states of emotional activation, reality testing may be transiently compromised. Those with more severe pathology (i.e., low and to some extent mid-BPO personality organization) are particularly susceptible to these transient break downs of reality testing.

In addition, the pathology of identity formation, which characterizes BPO, is associated with deficits in *social reality testing*, namely in the capacity to accurately perceive social cues and to infer others' intentions and internal states. In contrast, social reality testing is highly developed and stable in individuals organized at a neurotic level, as well as in the normal personality.

Alternative Model of Personality Disorders in DSM-5

A comparison of the ORT model with other current models of social and interpersonal behavior, such as the cognitive-affective processing model and the interpersonal processing model, provides perspective [17, 18]. Specifically, in terms of assessment and approaches to diagnosis it is informative and timely to compare the ORT model of personality pathology with the Alternative Model of Personality Disorder (AMPD) in DSM-5 [2].

DSM-5 retains the categorical DSM-IV-TR definition and classification of PD in Section II of the DSM-5 while introducing an alternative approach to PD in Section III of the manual. The AMPD represents a paradigm shift within the DSM approach to personality disorder, introducing: (1) a clear definition and criteria for personality disorder, (2) a dimensional, in contrast to categorical, approach to personality disorders, (3) a definition of the essential nature of personality pathology in terms of personality *functioning* in contrast to traits and symptoms, and (4) a privileging of the dimension of severity.

The AMPD introduces as general criteria for personality disorder (1) significant impairments in self-functioning (identity and self-direction) and interpersonal functioning (empathy and intimacy) (Criterion A) in conjunction with (2) the presence of one or more pathological personality traits (Criterion B). Impairment in self and interpersonal functioning is classified dimensionally according to severity of impairment, from mild, or subsyndromal, through extreme, using the Level of Personality Functioning Scale (LPFS).

While the development of the ORT model [5, 19] predated introduction of the AMPD by several decades, there is considerable compatibility between the two models. Both models embrace a dimensional view, both identify self and interpersonal functioning as core features of healthy and pathological personality functioning, and both privilege severity of impairment in the clinical assessment.

In addition to the significant overlap between the ORT and AMPD models, there are also important distinctions between the two models, which are highly relevant to clinical work. First, the AMPD omits defenses entirely, which reflects the intention on the part of the DSM-5 work group to develop a model that is empirically based, purely descriptive, and purposefully atheoretical. Second, the ORT model but not the AMPD identifies moral functioning and management of aggression as central domains of personality functioning. In the ORT model, aggression and moral functioning help locate the patient on the spectrum of severity. The greater the extent of aggression and less concern and remorse related to that aggression the higher the level of structural pathology (i.e., severity) and the poorer the prognosis. Second, the ORT model recognizes that varying degrees of moral functioning deficits are involved not only in the antisocial personality disorder but potentially in all severe personality disorders, in particular patients presenting with borderline, narcissistic, and paranoid personality disorders and malignant narcissism [20, 21]. Pathology of moral functioning is a hallmark of the most extreme, low BPO.

Third, while the AMDP takes on a descriptive approach, the ORT model is embedded in an overarching, dynamic theory of personality functioning [16, 19] and attends to the underlying structural and dynamic features that organize descriptive features.[2] This approach enables clinicians to anticipate problems (e.g.,

[2] For example, self-injurious behavior is seen not simply as a trait, but rather as an expression of poorly integrated and poorly modulated aggression linked to pathogenic internal object relations;

deception and withholding, destructive acting out) that are likely to emerge in the treatments of patients with severe to extreme personality pathology.

Description of Treatment Model and Clinical Approach

TFP is a theory-based, empirically supported, intensive treatment for the full range of personality pathology. Based on ORT, the treatment focus is on the pathology of self-functioning and related problems in interpersonal functioning, the hallmarks of all PD, and reflecting the underlying pathology of identity formation ("identity diffusion").

TFP has been described in manual form for adults with less severe PD [22], with BPD [23], and with narcissistic personality disorder [24]. Most recently, TFP has been described for adolescents with severe personality disorders [25]. In a major advance and central to the aim to describe the core of the treatment approach in this chapter, TFP has been presented in a transdiagnostic form as applied to the full range of severity of personality pathology [16].

Model of Change

The hypothesized mechanism of change in TFP for patients at a borderline level of organization is increased affect regulation achieved through mentalization, i.e., the growing ability of the patient to put momentary affect arousal, especially in social interactions, into a more benign and broader contextual understanding of self and others [26].

In the TFP model, negative affects are central to the pathogenies as they activate splitting-based defenses and related dissociated processes. Splitting-based defenses in turn consolidate the sharp separation of negative and positive experiences and representations of self and others. These dynamics interfere with identity integration and consolidation, thereby introducing instability into interpersonal relations. Taking this centrality of negative affect into account, the TFP treatment model posits a major role for affect activation, followed by affect containment, in the clinical process [27, 28].

The emergence of affectively charged object relations in the treatment is supported by the TFP treatment frame and the technically neutral stance of the TFP therapist. Once activated, the affectively charged perceptions of self and others may materialize in the patient's interactions with the therapist and/or in his descriptions of current interpersonal relationships. Those are the main foci of clinical attention in the therapy. For example, a therapist calls attention to a patient's

similarly, deceitfulness, rather than an isolated trait, is seen as an expression of pathology and failure of integration of systems organizing moral functioning, intimately linked to pathology of self and interpersonal functioning; black and white thinking is not viewed simply as a cognitive trait, but also as an expression of the impact of splitting-based defenses.

conviction that his therapist must see him as weak and "pathetic;" at another time, the therapist may put into words this patient's opposite experience that the therapist no doubt feels diminished by the patient's "superior" social class. As these perceptions of self in relation to others are identified and explored, affects are contained, and extreme and distorted perceptions of self and others are contextualized. Ideally, as affects are tempered and extreme perceptions of self and others gradually modified, dissociated experiences of self and others coalesce over time, leading to identity consolidation. The interpretive process, described and illustrated below, organizes these developments, and guides clinical interventions to promote integrative processes.

Principle Intervention Strategies and Techniques

Patient Assessment Because both normal and pathological personality functioning is integral to treatment prognosis and outcome for all mental disorders, it is clinically sound to do a complete assessment of personality functioning and symptom picture for all patients. A complete clinical assessment includes descriptive features of personality functioning (presenting symptoms, pathological personality traits, and psychiatric history), and structural diagnosis leading to the identification of the patient's level of personality organization [16], as both aspects inform treatment planning. Research has demonstrated that severity, captured in the ORT model by level of personality organization (i.e., normal, neurotic, borderline organization), is most effective in predicting prognosis and outcome [29]. The presence of the dominant observable clinical constellations such as paranoia, narcissism, antisocial structure, and behaviors provides the clinician with an understanding of the dominant object relations that are likely to unfold in the treatment.

The structural diagnosis of levels of personality organization can be made by using the Structured Interview for Personality Organization-Revised (STIPO-R; [30]). The STIPO-R is a semi-structured interview version of Kernberg's Structural Interview [31]. It contains 55 items that assess the five domains of personality structure essential for treatment planning (i.e., identity, object relations, defenses, aggression, and moral values). The complete STIPO-R interview guide and scoring sheet can be found on www.borderlinedisorders.com

Case Formulation The case formulation is essential to combine information from the patient assessment to formulate a hypothesis about the causes of the patients' difficulties, which is conceptually essential to plan appropriate intervention [32]. With information from the assessment process concerning the severity of personality dysfunction, combined with patient goals (and patients' therapy motivation), the assessor can decide if TFP is indicated. In addition, the information on patients' level of personality organization enables the clinician to anticipate aspects of the treatment process that could potentially follow (see Table 2.3).

Table 2.3 Levels of personality organization and impact on treatment planning and process

	Neurotic organization	High borderline organization	Mid-borderline organization	Low borderline organization
Objectives of treatment	Increase flexible functioning in areas of conflict	Greater depth and stability in experience of self and others	Resolution of destructive behavior; greater depth in experience of self and others	Behavior control; modulation of aggression
Structuring of treatment	Less need for structured contract	Explicitly agreed upon treatment contract	Carefully constructed treatment contract is essential	Contracting must be extensive; focus on secondary gain and safety of patient and therapist
Treatment alliance	Clarity about seeking help from expert; open to working alliance	Ambivalence about seeking help and depending on expert interfere with initial alliance; early alliance unstable or superficial	Suspicion, with fear of critical attack or exploitation by therapist interferes with alliance; alliance built during course of treatment	Relatively fixed view of therapist as corrupt, arrogant, exploitative limits the capacity to form an alliance
Transference process	Develops gradually and is affectively well-modulated. Realistic quality and relative stability over time	Early idealized transferences can keep paranoid object relations out of treatment	Develops rapidly, is affectively charged and extreme Confusing and chaotic quality with role reversals and abrupt shifts Early transferences predominantly paranoid	Affectively charged; predominantly paranoid
Countertransference	Relatively well integrated in the form of thoughts or associations. Therapists affected in subtle and socially appropriate ways which may be almost imperceptible at first	Subtler than in mid/low BPO Therapist feels less controlled and has more inner space to reflect	Can be extremely uncomfortable, difficult to contain, experienced as imposed on; Therapist feels controlled and driven to action	Extremely uncomfortable; Therapist feels controlled and driven to action

As mentioned above, the structural diagnosis has direct and reliable implications for treatment planning and prognosis. Individuals organized at a neurotic level of personality organization have a very favorable prognosis and can benefit from relatively unstructured treatments. Usually, these patients can easily establish and maintain a therapeutic alliance, transference distortions develop gradually and are subtle. Their psychodynamic treatment will be organized around the goal of reducing rigidity in personality functioning [22].

In contrast, individuals organized at a borderline level (particularly at a low borderline level), require a highly structured treatment setting. These patients have great difficulty establishing and maintaining a therapeutic alliance; transference distortions develop rapidly. Usually, transference is very affectively charged and extreme, and as such might lead to disruption of the treatment. For patients with BPO, the treatment goal is structured around ameliorating identity diffusion and promoting normal identity consolidation [16, 23].

In general, more progress toward identity integration is expected with high and mid-level BPO as compared to low-level BPO. This progress will manifest in changes in the transference relationship and in improved friendships, intimacy, and work.

Treatment Structure With the information from a thorough assessment, the TFP therapist shares the diagnostic impression, linking identity and personality functioning to the patient's presenting complaint. Next, the patient and therapist jointly identify treatment goals, which are focused on improving concrete aspects of self and interpersonal functioning. Therapy goals help organize the treatment and relate the treatment to the patient's day-to-day functioning.

Before treatment formally begins, the TFP therapist and the patient agree upon a "treatment contract," which consists of a verbal agreement articulating the responsibilities of both therapist and patient. The treatment agreement establishes the treatment frame and the necessary conditions for treatment while providing the structure needed for effective treatment of individuals with personality pathology [33]. In general, the extent to which the treatment is structured in the treatment contract increases with severity. More precisely, severe personality pathology requires an elaborate and highly structured treatment agreement. The goal of this agreement is to contain behavioral dysregulation (acting out) that would otherwise threaten the patient and treatment.

Typically, under the contract, patients are responsible for coming to the sessions on time and discussing as freely as possible what is on their mind. Furthermore, the contract contains procedures for managing any self-destructive or suicidal behavior. It also stresses that the patient is responsible for engagement in school or work during the treatment period, whether it be part-time volunteer work or full-time paid engagement. This engagement in meaningful activity is more relevant for poorly functioning mid and low-level BPO patients than for better functioning neurotic and most high-level BPO patients. The therapist is responsible for listening intently to the feelings, thoughts, and concerns of the patient and to comment when deemed helpful. By structuring the treatment with explicit roles and behaviors for therapist and patient, the contract helps to identify effective interaction and deviations from it.

Therapeutic Neutrality The basic stance of a TFP therapist is therapeutic neutrality. The therapist is a focused, neutral observer who does not take sides in relation to the patient's internal conflicts, and from this position fosters the patient's observation and understanding of his/her own conflicts. As the therapist allies him/herself with the patient's capacity for self-observation, the patient's capacity to articulate, observe, and reflect on her own conflicts is encouraged. The patient's enhanced ability to reflect, in turn, decreases impulsive, reflexive action, and increases self-observation and affect regulation in times of stress. From this point of view, technical neutrality is not a passive or noncommittal attitude toward the patient. Instead, while maintaining a neutral, non-judgmental stance in relation to the patient's conflicts, the TFP therapist manifests interest and curiosity in relation to the patient as an individual and as per his/her experience. By maintaining technical neutrality, the therapist protects a strategic position that allows for the patient's more active clarification and reflection on her/his own conflicts.

Interpretive Process The process of interpretation most defines TFP, and four discernable levels of intervention in the interpretive process have been described [27, 34]. These levels take on individualized content and process with each patient.

First Phase in the Interpretive Process The therapist highlights the patient's experience of the self and other (including the therapist) to elaborate the dominant object relation (e.g., the patient experiences himself as a victim in the hands of an aggressive, victimizing other/therapist). First, the therapist focuses on inquiring into areas of vagueness, omission, or contradiction in the patient's depiction of self and others, without calling into question the patient's experience (i.e., staying within the patient's subjectivity while maintaining therapeutic neutrality). This special mode of inquiry facilitates further affective reactions of the patient toward the therapist. Next, the therapist puts these reactions, namely the patient's dominant affective experience of himself in relation to the therapist, into words.

Clinical Vignette Early in the treatment of a low BPO patient, the therapist is exploring his patient's experience of a recent exchange. The patient had canceled a session, then called the therapist last minute expecting to keep the now canceled appointment. The therapist had missed the patient's call and did not retrieve the message for several hours, at which point the appointment had been missed. At their next meeting, the patient berates the therapist, insisting that any normal person would know to check messages, and accusing the therapist of being irresponsible, dismissive, and callous. The therapist clarifies the patient's experience and observes that in response to his interventions, the patient is becoming increasingly aggressive, devaluing, contemptuous, and paranoid. To provide containment of the patient's highly charged affect and to communicate empathy by putting words to the patient's experience the therapist comments: "I can see that you experience me as dismissive and uncaring, while you feel mistreated, disregarded and uncared for." This process, when done well, results in the patient feeling understood by the therapist, while promoting affect containment and enhanced affect regulation in the moment.

Second Phase in the Interpretive Process The TFP therapist observes and identifies role reversals between self and object representations within the object relation dyad articulated in the first phase. Often, the patient does not experience those reversals consciously but enacts them in behavior. For example, while the patient perceives herself as a bullied victim in the hands of an aggressive, powerful other, the patient comes to aggressively attack and bully the therapist. In this process, the patient still sees herself in the familiar role of victim, while, without reflection and largely out of awareness, behaving as a victimizer and attacker. An alert therapist points out these role reversals, helping the patient to tolerate awareness of dissociated (typically aggressive) aspects of his behavior and experience, and then inviting her/him to reflect upon their possible meaning.

Clinical Vignette After repeated exchanges in which the therapist put into words the patient's experience in the transference in the form of the dominant object relation of a dismissive, contemptuous, and callous therapist in relation to a mistreated, devalued, and uncared for patient, the dyad joined by mutual hostility, the patient began to seem less agitated in her sessions and ultimately more reflective. At this point the therapist decided to hazard a more advanced intervention, calling the patient's attention to her own, dismissive behavior in relation to the therapist: "I understand that I seem contemptuous and dismissive. At the same time, I wonder if you can step back for a moment and consider that your behavior, raising your voice and berating me for being unprofessional and uncaring, might leave me feeling dismissed and mistreated as well."

By bringing the role reversal to the patient's attention, the therapist is inviting the patient to go beyond her immediate, concrete experience; the patient is supported in her capacity to step back and consider alternative perspectives while forming cognitive connections between dimensions of behavior and experience that have been previously dissociated. This intervention promotes mentalization, inviting the patient to reflect on dissociated aspects of her behavior and internal experience, and to consider its impact on the experience of the other. In sum, tactfully calling attention to role reversals functions as a bid for reflection, inviting the patient to observe the way her mind works and how it influences her behavior, and to explore this reality further within the therapeutic relationship.

Third Phase in the Interpretive Process The therapist makes a connection between two contradictory object relations (typically idealized and persecutory experiences of self and other) that have been defensively dissociated and invites the patient to observe and reflect on those.

Clinical Vignette While her sessions remained stormy, things were beginning to improve in the patient's life. During this period, the patient began a session by once again berating the therapist for being callous, accusing the therapist of treating her as if she were "less than human." The therapist empathized with the patient's experience of him as callous and uncaring and they explored those familiar feelings. After a pause, the patient looked down and sheepishly acknowledged that between sessions she had begun to secretly think of the therapist as "cool, a nice person, that you really care about me and care for me as no one ever has." While appreciating the value of the patient's sharing this highly positive experience in the transference, the therapist was aware that it was embedded in ongoing splitting, in contrast to representing the greater integration of paranoid and idealized representations that is the goal of treatment. The therapist intervened: "I appreciate your sharing these positive feelings, helping me to understand that when you are away from me, and perhaps in our session today as well, you experience me as caring and nurturing, able to take almost perfect care of you. At the same time, I remember that you often have a very different experience of me, as you did even at the beginning of our session today, when I seem callous and uncaring, treating you as if you were 'less than human.'"

This level of intervention calls attention to the discontinuous and polarized nature of the patient's experience in the transference, helping the patient to appreciate that her experience is internal and subjective, in contrast to material and concrete, and that subjective experience is constructed and symbolic. (For example, it is not possible that the therapist is, in fact, both the absolute best caretaker and the absolute worst as he has seemed at different moments.)

Fourth Phase in the Interpretive Process The therapist generates hypotheses about the meaning of the patient's transference experience and the anxieties and motivations driving the patient's defenses.

Clinical Vignette The therapist continued to call the patient's attention to the dissociation between idealized and paranoid aspects of her experience. With time, the patient's customary splitting approached becoming ego-dystonic, which is to say it struck the patient as both notable and curious that she had such different, contradictory experiences of the therapist at different times, and she was aware that this was a characteristic of her experience in her other important relationships as well. The therapist sensed a new attitude on the part of the patient, reflecting both an awareness that they were observing an aspect of her mental functioning and a curiosity about her experience. The therapist offered a trial interpretation, providing the patient with a way to understand why she might keep separate her positive view of the therapist, splitting it off from her more familiar, paranoid, experience: "It seems that at this moment, as you have a positive feelings for me, you need to see me not simply as caring, but as *perfectly* caring and *perfectly* nurturing and attentive, as if you feel you must split off any possibility of negative feelings or any memory of your experience of me as callous and dismissive. It is as if you fear the positive feelings you have at this moment might be swamped by even a hint of the negative ones that can be so powerful, so you need to split them off entirely."

In this process, the level of interpretations must match the patient's cognitive-affective level. More precisely, patients at different levels of personality organization have different cognitive-affective capacities. These capacities in turn color their object relations and their ability to regulate and integrate affects and thus set the limits for speed and degree of treatment progress. To capture the process of interpretation in research, we have articulated a manual to rate the steps of the interpretative process [35].

Process of Treatment TFP has been shown in one treatment development study [36] and two randomized clinical trials [37, 38] to demonstrate significant symptom change (e.g., aggression), reduction in hospitalizations, and change in personality functioning in comparison to alternative treatments. Most clinically relevant is the process or trajectory of change and mechanisms of change. TFP is associated with significant increases in reflective functioning (RF) [28, 39–41], and the treatment focus on patient understanding of self in relationship to others leads to lower emotional arousal during the session and higher RF post-treatment [42, 43]. With a clear understanding of the mechanisms of change, a focused therapist can provide a more efficient treatment, and the teaching and supervision of TFP can be more precise and effective.

There are discernible stages in the progression of TFP with severe personality disorder patients. Treatment is preceded by careful diagnostic assessment as described above. After completing the clinical assessment of symptoms and levels of personality organization, the therapist shares his or her diagnostic impression and discusses treatment options.

If a course of TFP is deemed appropriate, the patient and therapist negotiate a verbal treatment contract. This stage is followed by the early treatment phase, during which patients tend to challenge the treatment frame, criticize the treatment, or even threaten discontinuation of treatment. More specifically, in patients with BPD, serious and potentially lethal behaviors are most common during this treatment phase. In patients with NPD either a scathing devaluation of the therapist or, alternatively, a dismissive, neglectful attitude that fails to register the therapist as an individual, are most common.

As treatment progresses, out-of-session destructive behavior decreases, making it possible to shift clinical attention to understanding the underlying conflicted object relations that drive these behaviors. This attenuation of destructive behavior is achieved by the structure of the treatment frame, a consistent focus on destructive acting out, and limit setting. At the same time that disruptive acting out in the patient's daily life decreases, the dysfunctional views of self and others get expressed in a conflicted relationship with the therapist where they can be actively examined.

The usual further progression in TFP is reduction of problem behaviors and the patient's growing acknowledgment of aggressive affects as parts of self rather than projected onto others. Consequently, idealized and persecutory object relations become less extreme and affectively charged and begin to transiently coalesce. These changes in object relations manifest in an improved therapeutic relationship and growing productive involvement in work and relationships in the patient's life. In our clinical experience, enhanced capacity for intimate relationships is often the last domain to develop.

Teaching and Supervision of TFP

Training in TFP has typically involved two elements: (1) attendance in a didactic course enhanced by extensive reading and viewing of videotaped sessions that focuses on the basics such as a model of personality pathology, assessment, and treatment elements and (2) supervision in the treatment of several cases. The most important learning is generally in the supervision experience since the relatively straightforward concepts become more complex and less clear when the affects that emerge in the therapy sessions may make it difficult to keep in mind and adhere to the principles and techniques.

Learning TFP has been found to be beneficial across a broad range of therapist levels. TFP has been experienced by some as a good introduction to learning psychodynamic psychotherapy [44] while others have found it a useful addition to full psychoanalytic training that allows competency in treating patients with levels of personality disorder that are not effectively treated by less structured analytic approaches.

Therapists learning TFP as it was originally formulated for patients with BPO, often at the mid to lower levels, are strongly advised to participate in peer supervision groups as part of their practice. The other main models of therapy for BPD, dialectical behavior therapy (DBT; [45]) and mentalization-based therapy (MBT; [46]), make similar recommendations. This recommendation is based on the level of affect that can emerge in therapy sessions. From the TFP point of view, elements of a patient's internal world that are dissociated from the patient's awareness can be activated in the therapist's countertransference. Awareness and therapeutic use of countertransference reactions may be the most challenging part of TFP. The intense affects that can emerge in sessions create the ever-present risk of either therapist enactments of countertransference or of blind spots to countertransference. Peer consultation groups are especially helpful in dealing with these countertransference issues. A description of the TFP consultation or supervision process can be found elsewhere [47].

TFP Compared to Other Treatment Approaches

Clinicians across multiple treatments orientations emphasize mental representations of self and others as central to guiding interpersonal behavior. This central role in conceptualizing self-other representations is integral to treatment orientations as diverse as cognitive [48], meta-cognitive [49], interpersonal [50], attachment [51–53], and object relations perspectives [54]. These mental representations of self and others are referred to as cognitive-affective units, schemas, interpersonal copies, internal working models, and internalized object relations dyads, and in process terms such as reflective functioning.

However, different models of psychotherapy target mental representations of self and others in diverse ways: DBT [45] uses a cognitive-behavioral approach with emphasis on techniques like skills development and mindfulness. MBT [53] focuses on modulating affects in the therapy sessions. In contrast, TFP allows the safe emergence of affect-driven perceptions of self and others (including the therapist) by providing a treatment frame. In this model, the affect arousal in the sessions is considered crucial as it enables the modification of extreme cognitions and related affects in the "hot" and immediate experience of others. This approach is consistent with current understanding of primitive affects and their contribution to numerous forms of psychopathology. As stated by Panskeep and Biven [55], "The intense re-experiencing of emotional episodes opens up new treatment possibilities because it provides therapists an emotional 'closeness,' especially within a secure therapeutic alliance, that is optimal for therapeutic change."

Expanding the Utilization of Core Aspects of TFP

In an impressive application of TFP concepts and principles, the members of ISTFP have utilized the core aspects of TFP in different treatment settings, formats, and with an expanded range of patients diagnoses and problem conditions. This book provides a summary of this development.

The basic elements of TFP developed in intensive (sessions two times a week for a year or more), individual treatment format on an outpatient basis for patients with varying levels of personality organization are described here as articulated and investigated at the PDI. It remains to be seen how these elements can be used productively and effectively in other settings, treatment formats, and for an extended range of patients with combinations of levels of personality organization and symptom constellations.

Thorough patient assessment and case formulation as described here will be essential to the process. With the theoretical background of ORT, the assessor can link the level of personality organization to realistic treatment goals. Flexible and creative application of structuring the treatment episode and utilization of the interpretive process will be essential.

Summary and Conclusion

The intensive use of TFP treatment for patients with BPD and typical co-morbid conditions of paranoid, narcissistic disorders, and antisocial traits has been investigated over the last 40 years. This development has involved refinements in the ORT model, the clinical assessment of patients with a range of personality pathology, and TFP treatment in the individual treatment format. With this theoretical background and extensive assessment and treatment experience, TFP is now prepared to expand its defining features and principles of intervention to a wider range of treatment settings, formats, and patient diagnoses. With the defining features and principles of clinical intervention described in this chapter, TFP is a developed methodology available for expanding its utilization. Experience gained from the TFP methodology can be used in a total treatment approach or can be integrated with other approaches in the treatment of personality-disordered patients. TFP provides a multifaceted platform for flexible application across the severity of personality pathology, diverse medical and psychiatric treatment settings, and in different treatment formats.

References

1. Bach B, Kerber A, Aluja A, Bastiaens T, Keeley JW, Claes L, et al. International assessment of DSM-5 and ICD-11 personality disorder traits: toward a common nosology in DSM-5.1. Psychopathology. 2020;53(3–4):179–88.
2. American Psychiatric Association. Diagnostic and statistical manual of mental disorders. 5th ed. Washington, DC: American Psychiatric Publishing; 2013.
3. Kernberg OF. Transference and countertransference in the treatment of borderline patients. J Natl Assoc Private Psychiatr Hosp. 1975;2:14–24.
4. Kernberg O. Object-relations theory and clinical psychoanalysis. New York: Aronson; 1976.
5. Kernberg OF. Severe personality disorders: psychotherapeutic strategies. Yale: Yale University Press; 1984.
6. Kernberg OF. Treatment of severe personality disorders: resolution of aggression and recovery of eroticism. Washington, DC: American Psychiatric Association Publishing; 2018.
7. Joseph B. Psychic equilibrium and psychic change: selected papers of Betty Joseph. Psychology Press; 1989.
8. Fairbairn WRD. Psychoanalytic studies of the personality. London/New York: Routledge; 2013.
9. Klein M. Envy and gratitude and other works 1946–1963: Edited by: M. Masud R. Khan. London: The Hogarth Press and the Institute of Psycho-Analysis; 1975. p. 1–346.
10. Erikson EH. Childhood and society. New York: WW Norton & Company; 1993.
11. Erikson EH. The problem of ego identity. J Am Psychoanal Assoc. 1956;4(1):56–121.
12. Jacobson E. The self and the object world: vicissitudes of their infantile cathexes and their influence on ideational and affective development. Psychoanal Study Child. 1954;9(1):75–127.
13. Kernberg OF. Contemporary controversies in psychoanalytic theory, techniques, and their appli. New Haven: Yale University Press; 2008.
14. Caligor E, Kernberg OF. A psychoanalytic theory of personality disorders. In: Major Theories of personality disorders. 2nd ed. New York: The Guilford Press; 2005. p. 114–45.
15. Diamond D, Yeomans FE, Stern BL, Kernberg OF. Treating pathological narcissism with transference-focused psychotherapy. New York: Guilford Publications; 2021.

16. Caligor E, Kernberg OF, Clarkin JF, Yeomans FE. Psychodynamic therapy for personality pathology: treating self and interpersonal functioning. Washington, DC: American Psychiatric Association Publishing; 2018.
17. Meehan KB, Clarkin JF, Lenzenweger MF. Conceptual models of borderline personality disorder, part 1: overview of prevailing and emergent models. Psychiatr Clin. 2018;41(4):535–48.
18. Meehan KB, Clarkin JF, Lenzenweger MF. Conceptual models of borderline personality disorder, part 2: a process approach and its implications. Psychiatr Clin. 2018;41(4):549–59.
19. Kernberg OF, Caligor E. A psychodynamic theory of personality disorders. In: Lenzenweger MF, Clarkin JF, editors. Major theories of personality disorder. 2nd ed. New York: Guilford Press; 2005. p. 114–56.
20. Kernberg OF. Borderline conditions and pathological narcissism. Lanham: Rowman & Littlefield; 1985.
21. Akhtar S. Paranoid personality disorder: a synthesis of developmental, dynamic, and descriptive features. Am J Psychother. 1990;44(1):5–25.
22. Caligor E, Kernberg OF, Clarkin JF. Handbook of dynamic psychotherapy for higher level personality pathology. Washington, DC: American Psychiatric Publishing; 2007.
23. Yeomans FE, Clarkin JF, Kernberg OF. Transference-focused psychotherapy for borderline personality disorder: a clinical guide. Washington, DC: American Psychiatric Publishing; 2015.
24. Diamond D, Yeomans FE, Levy KN. Psychodynamic psychotherapy for narcissistic personality disorder. In: Campbell K, Miller JD, editors. The handbook or narcissism and narcissistic personality disorder: theoretical approaches, empirical findings, and treatment. New York: Wiley; 2011. p. 421–33.
25. Normandin L, Ensink K, Weiner A, Kernberg OF. Transference-focused psychotherapy for adolescents with severe personality disorders. Washington, DC: American Psychiatric Publishing; 2021.
26. Levy KN, Clarkin JF, Yeomans FE, Scott LN, Wasserman RH, Kernberg OF. The mechanisms of change in the treatment of borderline personality disorder with transference focused psychotherapy. J Clin Psychol. 2006;62(4):481–501.
27. Caligor E, Diamond D, Yeomans FE, Kernberg OF. The interpretive process in the psychoanalytic psychotherapy of borderline personality pathology. J Am Psychoanal Assoc. 2009;57(2):271–301.
28. Levy KN, Meehan KB, Kelly KM, Reynoso JS, Weber M, Clarkin JF, et al. Change in attachment patterns and reflective function in a randomized control trial of transference-focused psychotherapy for borderline personality disorder. J Consult Clin Psychol. 2006;74(6):1027.
29. Bach B, Simonsen S. How does level of personality functioning inform clinical management and treatment? Implications for ICD-11 classification of personality disorder severity. Curr Opin Psychiatry. 2021;34(1):54–63.
30. Clarkin JF, Caligor E, Stern BL, Kernberg OF. The structured interview for personality organization-revised (STIPO-R). Unpublished manuscript, Weill Medical College of Cornell University Available from www.borderlinedisorders.com. 2016.
31. Kernberg OF. Structural interviewing. Psychiatr Clin N Am. 1981;4(1):169–95.
32. Persons JB. Case formulation-driven psychotherapy. Clin Psychol Sci Pract. 2006;13:167–70.
33. Delaney JC, Yeomans F. Functions of the treatment contract in TFP. Psychodyn Psychiatry. 2021;49(2):322–38.
34. Clarkin JF, Caligor E, Sowislo JF. An object relations model perspective on the alternative model for personality disorders (DSM-5). Psychopathology. 2020;53(3):134–41.
35. Keefe JR, Sowislo JF, Clarkin JF. Transference-focused psychotherapy adherence rating scale. 2020.
36. Clarkin JF, Foelsch PA, Levy KN, Hull JW, Delaney JC, Kernberg OF. The development of a psychodynamic treatment for patients with borderline personality disorder: a preliminary study of behavioral change. J Personal Disord. 2001;15(6):487–95.
37. Clarkin JF, Levy KN, Lenzenweger MF, Kernberg OF. Evaluating three treatments for borderline personality disorder: a multiwave study. Am J Psychiatry. 2007;164(6):922–8.

38. Doering S, Horz S, Rentrop M, Fischer-Kern M, Schuster P, Benecke C, et al. Transference-focused psychotherapy v. treatment by community psychotherapists for borderline personality disorder: randomised controlled trial. Br J Psychiatry. 2010;196(5):389–95.
39. Fischer-Kern M, Doering S, Taubner S, Hörz S, Zimmermann J, Rentrop M, et al. Transference-focused psychotherapy for borderline personality disorder: change in reflective function. Br J Psychiatry. 2015;207(2):173–4.
40. Buchheim A, Hörz-Sagstetter S, Doering S, Rentrop M, Schuster P, Buchheim P, et al. Change of unresolved attachment in borderline personality disorder. Psychother Psychosom. 2017;86(5):314–6.
41. Hörz-Sagstetter S, Mertens W, Isphording S, Buchheim A, Taubner S. Changes in reflective functioning during psychoanalytic psychotherapies. J Am Psychoanal Assoc. 2015;63(3):481–509.
42. Kivity Y, Levy KN, Wasserman RH, Beeney JE, Meehan KB, Clarkin JF. Conformity to prototypical therapeutic principles and its relation with change in reflective functioning in three treatments for borderline personality disorder. J Consult Clin Psychol. 2019;87(11):975.
43. Kivity Y, Levy KN, Kelly KM, Clarkin JF. In-session reflective functioning in psychotherapies for borderline personality disorder: the emotion regulatory role of reflective functioning. J Consult Cin Psychol. 2021;89(9):751.
44. Bernstein J, Zimmerman M, Auchincloss EL. Transference-focused psychotherapy training during residency: an aide to learning psychodynamic psychotherapy. Psychodyn Psychiatry. 2015;43(2):201.
45. Linehan MM. Cognitive-behavioral treatment of borderline personality disorder. New York: Guilford Publications; 2018.
46. Bateman A. Mentalization-based treatment for borderline personality disorder: a practical guide. Oxford: Oxford University Press; 2006.
47. Yeomans F, Caligor E, Diamond D. The development of transference-focused psychotherapy and its model of supervision. Am J Psychother. 2023;76(1):46–50.
48. Pretzer J, Beck JS. Cognitive therapy of personality disorders: twenty years of progress. In: Contemporary cognitive therapy: theory, research and practice. New York: Guilford Press; 2004. p. 299–318.
49. Dimaggio G, Semerari A, Carcione A, Procacci M, Nicolo G. Toward a model of self pathology underlying personality disorders: narratives, metacognition, interpersonal cycles and decision-making processes. J Personal Disord. 2006;20(6):597–617.
50. Benjamin LS. Interpersonal theory of personality disorders: the structural analysis of social behavior and interpersonal reconstructive therapy. In: Lenzenweger MF, Clarkin JF, editors. Major theories of personality disorder. 2nd ed. New York: Guilford; 2005. p. 157–230.
51. Levy KN. The implications of attachment theory and research for understanding borderline personality disorder. Dev Psychopathol. 2005;17(4):959–86.
52. Meyer B, Pilkonis PA. An attachment model of personality disorders. In: Lenzenweger MF, Clarkin JF, editors. Major theories of personality disorder. New York: Gulilford; 2005. p. 231–81.
53. Bateman AW, Fonagy P. Mentalization-based treatment of BPD. J Personal Disord. 2004;18(1):36.
54. Clarkin JF, Lenzenweger MF, Yeomans F, Levy KN, Kernberg OF. An object relations model of borderline pathology. J Personal Disord. 2007;21(5):474–99.
55. Panksepp J, Biven L. The archaeology of mind: neuroevolutionary origins of human emotions, Norton series on interpersonal neurobiology. New York: WW Norton & Company; 2012.

Transference-Focused Psychotherapy (TFP) Informed Psychoeducation

3

Michael Rentrop, Maria Lidia Gerra, and Chiara De Panfilis

Introduction

In both standard, classical transference-focused psychotherapy (TFP) and "applied" TFP interventions for patients with personality disorder (PD) diagnoses, there is an emphasis on the establishment of a clear treatment structure. This treatment structure, or frame, follows organically from the initial stages of the intervention. The term "applied" TFP refers to the use of TFP principles outside the setting of an extended individual outpatient psychotherapy, such as, among others, inpatient settings, medical settings, crisis management, and prescription of pharmacotherapy [1]. The next chapters of this volume will describe several "applied" TFP initiatives across various countries, systems of care and settings (i.e., day hospital, community-based outpatient care, group therapy, forensic settings, medical and psychiatric hospitalization). All these initiatives share with classical individual TFP a deliberate approach toward structuring the clinical interventions when

M. Rentrop
Kbo-Inn-Salzach-Klinikum, Wasserburg, Germany

Department of Psychiatry and Psychotherapy, Klinikum rechts der Isar, Technical University Munich, Munich, Germany
e-mail: michael.rentrop@kbo.de

M. L. Gerra
Department of Mental Health and Pathological Dependencies, Parma Local Health Agency, Parma, Italy
e-mail: magerra@ausl.pr.it

C. De Panfilis (✉)
Department of Medicine and Surgery, Unit of Neuroscience, University of Parma, Parma, Italy
e-mail: chiara.depanfilis@unipr.it

R. G. Hersh, C. De Panfilis (eds.), *Implementing Transference-Focused Psychotherapy Principles*, https://doi.org/10.1007/978-3-031-68062-5_3

dealing with patients with borderline personality disorder (BPD) or, more broadly, borderline personality organization (BPO).[1] This approach begins even before the TFP or "applied" TFP treatment starts, with an extended assessment phase. Central elements of this pre-treatment phase are a structural diagnosis of personality disorder followed by an open discussion of the clinician's diagnostic impression with the patient (and, if appropriate, with the family members and other treaters), with psychoeducation (PE) about course, prognosis, and treatment options for the disorder [2]. These initial steps represent a pathway toward creating a clear treatment framework, rooted in an honest informed consent process: patients (and family members) are advised about the nature of the PD pathology, the related limits of some treatments (i.e., psychopharmacotherapy, unstructured psychotherapy), and the appropriateness of those interventions promoting patients' responsibility and motivation for change. The topic of sharing the PD diagnosis with associated PE about the disorder, in straightforward language, is therefore of paramount importance in TFP as well as in any TFP-informed treatment, in a variety of settings and clinical situations. In clinical practice, this task is generally carried out by the TFP therapist or the treating clinician, on an individual basis. However, to our knowledge, a structured way to provide PE informed by TFP principles has not yet been described.

This chapter will illustrate a TFP-oriented model of group PE for patients with BPD and other DSM-5 Cluster BPD diagnoses (excluding antisocial PD). This model aims to provide to this heterogeneous group of patients a "solid foundation" of basic information about the PD diagnosis. Furthermore, it aims to counter fatalistic attitudes of both patients and clinicians when dealing with these disorders, and to support patients' motivation to stay engaged in useful treatments, including individual and group psychotherapies. This PE intervention is intended to be proposed to patients after a PD diagnosis has been made by the treating clinician and communicated to the patient. PE aims to prepare patients for standard TFP, or for any "applied TFP" interventions (as those described in this volume) in those settings where classical standard TFP might not be feasible.

Because the overwhelming majority of research done in the PD field has been focused on patients with BPD, in this chapter we will refer primarily to PD patients with a BPD diagnosis, as we consider BPD to be the prototypical presentation of moderate to severe personality disorder pathology. In some cases, we will specifically use the term BPO to describe a broader group of patients with different subtypes of personality disorder pathology, and in some selected cases will specifically name other PD categories such as narcissistic personal disorder (NPD), when indicated.

---

[1] See Chap. 2 in this volume for the distinction between BPD and BPO. The BPO category includes the DSM-based BPD diagnosis as well as other severe PD characterized, at the structural level, by identity diffusion.

Psychoeducation for Borderline Personality Disorder

PE has a long tradition in the field of general clinical psychiatry. Several PE programs, usually rooted in cognitive-behavioral therapy, have been implemented and widely disseminated for various mental health disorders. PE is a structured intervention for patients and caregivers, which aims (1) to provide information about the illness and its treatment, (2) to motivate patients to cope with the illness, and (3) to improve treatment adherence and efficacy [3].

Extensive evidence has demonstrated that structured individual and familiar PE programs improve the treatment outcome and the course of schizophrenia [4], bipolar disorder [5–7], major depression [8, 9], and eating disorders [10, 11]. However, research focusing on the validation of individual and family PE for BPD is more limited.

Existing Research on PE in BPD

PE for Patients with BPD

Zanarini and colleagues [12] studied a cohort of 50 women with BPD, either assigned to a PE workshop on BPD diagnosis (n = 30) or a waiting list (n = 20). PE was associated with a significantly greater decline in general impulsivity and in storminess of close relationships, as assessed by the Zanarini Rating Scale for DSM-IV BPD (ZAN-BPD) [13]. However, PE did not result in significant improvement in psychosocial functioning, suggesting that PE programs may represent a form of pre-treatment.

A subsequent study by the same research group [14] recruited 80 women with BPD, who were randomized either to the PE treatment group (n = 40) or the control group (n = 40). The treatment consisted of a web-based PE intervention, laid out like a book, detailing information on different aspects of BPD psychopathology. At 3-month follow-up, this program led to a greater decline in impulsivity as well as a greater increase in psychosocial functioning compared to the control group; these outcomes persisted even at a 12-month follow-up.

Ridolfi and colleagues [15] performed a randomized controlled trial of a PE program based on Good Psychiatric Management (GPM), a generalist model for treating BPD. Ninety-six outpatients with BPD were randomized either to receive six weekly sessions of a group-format PE (n = 48) or assigned to a waiting list for PE and to treatment as usual (n = 48), thus serving as a control group. The group receiving PE significantly improved in all sectors of BPD psychopathology as measured by the ZAN-BPD, as compared to the control group, and this effect persisted after 2 months.

Finally, the systems training for emotional predictability and problem solving (STEPPS) group therapy, which includes a strong psychoeducation component, has been found to be more effective than treatment as usual in reducing affective, cognitive, interpersonal and impulsive symptoms in BPD [16].

PE for Carers of Patients with BPD

In a randomized clinical trial conducted by Grenyer and colleagues [17], 33 carers attended a 10-week long manualized PE program, based on a relationship model ("staying connected," project air strategy for personality disorders) [18, 19]. The outcomes were compared to those of a control group assigned to a waiting list (n = 35). Carers who participated in the PE program reported more improvements in their relationship with the relative with BPD, greater decrease in expressed emotion, and greater improvements in their perception of being able to play an active role in interacting with BPD service providers, than the waitlist group.

Hoffmann and colleagues [20, 21] evaluated the efficacy of the family connections intervention, a 12-week multiple-family education program. The first pilot study [20] included 44 participants, who completed pre-, and post-baseline self-report evaluations. Family members experienced decreases in their levels of burden and grief and increases in their level of empowerment over the duration of the program and these changes were maintained 3 months after the program had ended. To replicate these findings, the subsequent study enrolled a second cohort of 55 family members of BPD patients. Again, participants showed significant improvements on all well-being variables, including substantial decrease in depression levels [21].

Another study [22] used the "Making Sense of BPD" model, which is a manualized group psychoeducational program consisting of three sessions of developmentally tailored PE for the family and friends of youth with BPD features. After this program, the 23 included participants reported a significant decrease in subjective burden and an increase in personality disorder knowledge, although objective burden and distress remained unchanged [23].

Finally, in a pilot study that included both BPD patients (n = 30) and close relatives and caregivers of BPD patients (n = 33) Pitschel-Walz et al. [24] evaluated the effectiveness of a 10-sessions psychoeducational group program. After completing the program, both relatives and patients reported reduced levels of burden and an increased knowledge about the disorder as compared to baseline. Additionally, BPD patients experienced an increase in hope that psychotherapy may help to achieve long-term stability. The reduction of burden among the relatives was correlated with higher levels, at baseline, of patients' symptom severity and carers' burden. There was no change in quality of life. The participants and therapists generally rated the psychoeducational sessions as positive and helpful, especially regarding those PE sessions that focused on increasing communication skills and coping with crises.

Why Psychoeducation Is Important? The Goals of PE in BPD

Improving Knowledge About the Disease

Integrating PE in the treatment paradigm for patients with BPD is of critical importance because there are still many misconceptions about this disorder. The primary goal of PE therefore consists in providing reliable information on the condition.

Although BPD is a complex mental health disorder, with a lifetime prevalence approaching 3%, and a prevalence in psychiatric settings of, respectively, 11%

among outpatients and 22% among inpatients [25, 26], it may often be underdiagnosed in ordinary general psychiatry practice. Difficulties in diagnosing BPD may be due to different reasons [27]. First, the heterogeneity of the construct of BPD, reflected in the various possible combinations of DSM categorical criteria [28], is considered the main factor contributing to the apparent inconsistency of this diagnosis. Second, various BPD symptoms may overlap with those characterizing other disorders that are more familiar to general psychiatrists, like mood disorders [29], post-traumatic stress disorders, substance use disorders, and eating disorders, which could be more easily recognized, thereby failing to account for the clinical complexity of BPD. Finally, the stigma of intractability surrounding BPD could be another factor contributing to misdiagnosis. This concept creates a vicious cycle because having a diagnosis represents the first step for the treatment of BPD [30]. This might be particularly true for young patients with BPD (i.e., adolescents and young adults). While it is currently acknowledged that BPD can be best conceptualized as a developmental disorder with an onset in adolescence, many clinicians are still reluctant to make and disclose a BPD diagnosis, due to mistaken beliefs that personality pathology is transient or normative among young people or concern that the diagnosis is stigmatizing. Importantly, however, delaying a diagnosis because of fear of stigma in youths prevents access to care and leads to worse short- and long-term outcomes [31]. Thus, making a BPD diagnosis and communicating it timely to the affected individuals and their carers is of paramount importance.

Bolstering Hope for Change

The second goal of PE is to motivate patients to best manage their condition, thus reinforcing a realistic hope for change.

During the past decade, longitudinal research has challenged the assumption that BPD is a lifelong, chronically disabling disorder [32, 33]. Rather, BPD has a good long-term prognosis: symptomatic improvement over time occurs in most patients [34, 35]. However, impairments in psychosocial functioning seem to persist despite a significant decrease in the number of BPD criteria met [36]. This further strengthens the conclusion that, as evidence-based treatments are available, there is no rationale for delaying diagnosis and treatment provision. Providing patients with this updated information about the BPD course aims to enhance their motivation and engagement in treatment. Most importantly, this clarifies that change is indeed not only possible, but also expected: despite a currently challenging clinical presentation, it is anticipated that as treatment progresses things can go better for patients, and life can "make sense."

Empowering the Patient in Shared Treatment Decision-Making with Mental Health Professionals

PE aims to enable patients to discuss BPD with their treatment providers from an "expert to expert" perspective and to make shared decisions about treatment planning. This process is generally applicable to the treatment of all patients with psychiatric disorders, regardless of diagnosis, but it is particularly important for patients with BPD [37]. Most existing psychotherapies, or even well-structured generalist treatments for BPD, emphasize the need that patient and health care providers agree on a treatment plan; this ensures that patients are actively engaged in their own treatment and assume responsibility for it. This treatment plan represents the framework of treatment; it should include the definition of the personal treatment goals, the viable options for crisis management, and the modalities of others' involvement (i.e., health professionals, family members) in the therapeutic proccss (i.e., project air strategy for personality disorders [38]). In standard TFP, for instance, a treatment contract outlining the patient's and therapist's responsibilities and how to address potential threats to the treatment is negotiated before treatment starts. This strategy is intended to prevent premature treatment discontinuation by patients, which is frequent in naturalistic treatment settings. According to Barnicot and co-workers [39], treatment drop-out can approach 60% among BPD patient populations and may occur disproportionately during the early stages of treatment [40].

A TFP-Informed Psychoeducational Program

In this chapter, we will describe a TFP-oriented model of group PE, which can represent a potential structured pre-treatment intervention for patients with certain PD presentations. This model has been inspired by the extensive experience of working within a structured group psychoeducational program for BPD in Munich, Germany. That program has been manualized [41] and patients with BPD were helped by both expanding their knowledge about the disorder and engendering hope for their recovery [24]. While the Rentrop et al. program [41] included information drawn from various BPD theories, such as the biosocial theory of BPD [42], the PE intervention proposed here mainly focuses on the key elements of personality pathology according to TFP theory and practice. The model described in the current chapter is grounded in TFP principles, and is intended, among other aims and scopes, to facilitate patients' adherence and commitment to standard TFP or to "applied" TFP interventions. It is up to this point a proposal, which still needs evaluation as well in standard TFP as also in "applied" TFP services. It possibly may also be offered in places without comparable TFP services as a stand-alone first step in treatment. TFP therapists or TFP-oriented clinicians can refer BPO patients to this PE program following completion of the structural diagnostic process, including an evaluation of PD severity/level of functioning, and the communication of their diagnostic impression to the patient. Therefore, the PE program proposed here can start in the pre-treatment phase, when clinicians are identifying treatment goals and negotiating the treatment contract with their patients, and continue during the initial phase of treatment, if the clinician and patient have agreed on a contract and thus, therapy could start (Fig. 3.1). In this way, PE can motivate, prepare, and inform patients about the TFP treatment.

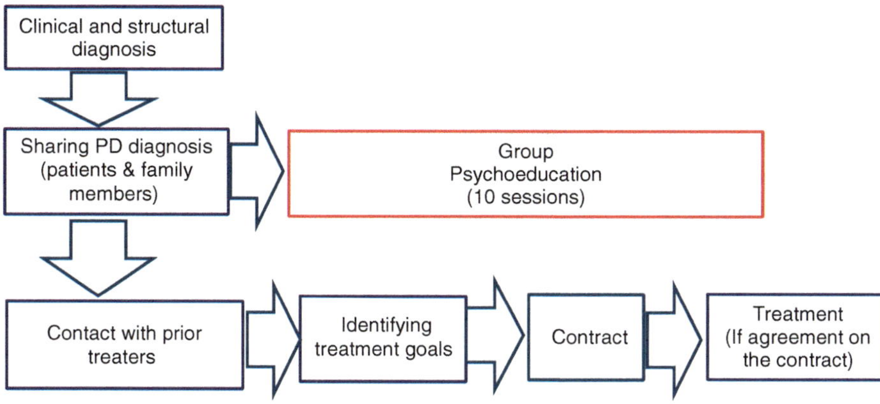

Fig. 3.1 Timing of PE within a standard TFP or "Applied" TFP treatments

Structure of the PE Program

The proposed PE program consists of 9 weekly group outpatient sessions, each lasting 60–75 min. In inpatient settings, the group program may be carried out twice-weekly. The sessions focus on establishing the group and treatment frame (Session 1), making and sharing a PD diagnosis (Session 2), exploring the complex topic of how personality disorders develop (Session 3), describing common comorbidities (Session 4), illustrating the role of pharmacotherapy (Session 5) and of psychotherapy interventions (Sessions 6 and 7), addressing crisis management (Session 8). Finally, Session 9 will be devoted to open questions/clarification and evaluation of the program.

The group typically includes 8–10 patients diagnosed with BPD and/or other Cluster B diagnoses functioning at a mid to low BPO level (excluding antisocial PD). Since to date, most of the available knowledge on diagnosis, treatment, course, and comorbidities of Cluster B PDs relies on existing research on BPD, as noted earlier, the information on available findings referenced in the sessions outlined above will then be used as a proxy for other moderate to severe PD presentations and complemented with additional specific information on other PD diagnoses, depending on the composition of the group.

The group is conducted by two experienced clinicians (e.g., psychiatrist, psychologist, nurse), with previous clinical experience with PD patients and with patients' group management. The group climate is kept informal; the aim is to collect information from group members and give additional skilled information, but with simplicity [43]. Most importantly, a PE group is not a psychotherapeutic group program but a collaborative group helping to share information and learn from each other.

Participants sit in a circle facing a board. They are invited to develop didactic material on the specific meeting topic, under the guidance of the group coordinators. Information is collected collaboratively from various group members:

participants share their individual experiences about the specific topic of the meeting. Such an exchange among group members has the objective of strengthening commitment to treatment. The coordinators summarize all the gathered information in a diagram on a flipchart (no overhead slides are used) and clarify the information if necessary. One of the participants, in turn, is asked to write a summary of the content of the session to provide material that can be reviewed at home and shared with family members.

The meetings have a common structure with: (1) greetings of participants and "warm-up" exercise (see description below), (2) identification of the goals of the session, (3) development and discussion of the didactic material of the day, and (4) summary and conclusion.

Warm-Up Exercise of the Meetings

In PE group programs, particularly with patients suffering from schizophrenia, an "emotional flashlight" is usually employed as a warm-up exercise ("How do I feel today?"). Such an approach is not helpful for BPD patients, whose subjective experience is most often characterized by intense negative affects and distorted, polarized, views of self and others that are split-off from positive effects and self-other representations.

Increasing empirical evidence indicates that patients with BPD exhibit a specific bias toward underestimating positive social cues in their environment. It has been shown that these patients often do not register others' accepting, trustworthy, or cooperating behavior toward them and, instead, react negatively to them at the subjective, physiological, and neural levels [44–51]. Thus, BPD patients may benefit from interventions aimed at accurately appraising and recognizing positive aspects of their internal and external reality. One way in which the PE program presented here pursues this aim is by asking patients, as a warm-up exercise, to consider "What was the best thing happening to me since our last meeting?" During the first meetings many group members tend to answer with a terse "nothing." In this case, they are then asked to take a closer look, metaphorically-speaking, as if using a magnifier or, if necessary, an electron microscope, to identify some positive occurrence in their lives during the preceding days.

First Meeting: Group and Treatment Frame

The coordinators start the meeting by introducing the general rules of the program. They emphasize the need for confidentiality and mutual respect and highlight the responsibilities of the participants. Participants are asked not to talk openly about suicidal ideation and self-harming behavior during the group meetings. Furthermore, they are instructed not to discuss details of abuse or trauma-related experiences in the group. Because these themes tend to trigger other group members, they should be discussed exclusively in the context of an individual treatment setting, in an atmosphere of privacy. These requirements are consistent with the attitude conveyed in the TFP literature that patients with significant PD pathology may have more control over their behavior than is often assumed. Patients in the group are asked to do their best to resist urges to self-harm, a maladaptive coping strategy often employed by patients with borderline pathology to manage overwhelming negative feelings that develop over time. If this unfortunate myth is not addressed, patients may assume that they cannot control themselves, and, therefore, will not be motivated to employ their optimal expressions of self-regulation [52].

The consequences of violation of the rules are discussed, as well as the strategies that would be used to manage potential situations of emotional overload. The group therapist clarifies that if any participant starts talking about self-harm or suicidal behavior or ideation, the therapist will immediately stop that group member. In the case of someone coming to the PE session in a crisis, help would be offered, for example, leaving the group for a moment with one of the therapists. In extreme circumstances, a participant could even be suspended from the PE group for repeated violations of the requirements of the program. In this way, establishing emergency regulations and negotiating an agreement on the rules of the group also represents the first test of a therapeutic contract.

Then, the coordinators and the patients introduce themselves, using interactive strategies of self-presentation. Often PD patients have difficulties presenting themselves in rounds of introduction. Identity diffusion makes the task of describing oneself particularly hard for them. Therefore, a sheet of paper with cues may be helpful (e.g., name / how long have I dealt with my PD / what are my treatment experiences / what do I expect from participating in this PE program).

Second Meeting: Personality Disorder Diagnosis

This session addresses the topics of the meaning of "personality disorder" and of "borderline personality organization." It also describes general symptoms of PD according to the alternative model for personality disorders (AMPD) of the Diagnostic and Statistical Manual of Mental Health Disorders (DSM-5) [28].

The first part of the meeting is designed to gather information from the participants about the PD diagnoses they have received, including the possibility that derogatory terms about individuals with PD diagnoses might have been used over the course of previous treatments. Participants are also invited to report other disorders they might also have been diagnosed with, prior to, or in addition to, the PD diagnosis. A lack of familiarity about the PD in general, and BPD in particular, may emerge, supporting the need for a clear definition of the disorder.

The process begins with the definition of the term "personality disorder." For many PD patients "personality disorder" sounds offensive, suggesting weakness of their character. To offer a global definition, we start by invoking Kurt Schneider's description proposed in a different era: personality disorder means that a person has certain familiar characteristics that are somehow expressed in an extreme way, so that the individual and those around them experience distress [53].

The general diagnosis of PD is then reviewed and described by the group coordinators following the AMPD, through a stepwise process [54].

Participants are informed that the DSM-5 AMPD definition of PD describes impairments in the fields of (a) identity (Who am I?), e.g., difficulties in identifying and describing oneself in a reliable way that is steady over time, as well as challenges in the consistent pursuit of personal goals and (b) difficulties in interpersonal relationships, e.g., partnerships, friendships and work relations.

This information is complemented by explaining the concept of "borderline personality organization" which has theoretical roots in psychoanalytic object relations theory (ORT) [55].

The group coordinators will first discuss with the participants how personality can be defined. Generally speaking, personality is the automatic instinctive way that we think, feel, and act, that comes naturally to us. We became who we are because over time, based on repeated interactions with others, we incorporate a series of images of ourselves in relation to others.

Personality is precisely about these internalized images of self and others that we incorporate over the course of development. This gives us a sense of self and a sense of others that may or may not be accurate. In PD pathology this sense is often not accurate: the internal images of self and others do not necessarily correspond to external reality. In this case, individuals live more in response to their internal image than to what is really going on around them [56].

The coordinators further explain to the participants, using straightforward language and a flipchart, that according to a TFP-oriented model of personality pathology, personality disorders can be evaluated by considering seven dimensions of personality functioning, which are depicted in Table 3.1.

The assessment of these seven dimensions of personality functioning can help the clinician determine the level of personality organization and therefore the severity of illness. The coordinators can give practical examples of the information that can be derived from this assessment. For instance, individuals functioning at a

Table 3.1 Diagnostic "toolbox" for explaining borderline personality organization

Dimension of personality functioning	Explanation
Identity	Stable ability to tell about one's own main positive and negative traits, to have consistent values, interests, and goals
Relationships (Quality of object relations)	Ability to keep up partnerships and friendships over time
Defense mechanisms	Unconscious ways of dealing with psychological distress; coping strategies that can be either adaptable and sustaining, or problematic, leading to instability
Aggression	Tendency toward aggressive behavior against oneself or others
Coping versus rigidity	Ability to cope with new circumstances versus inflexibility
Moral values	Stabile inner knowledge of right and wrong that is neither too harsh nor too lax
Reality testing	Ability to differentiate between a shared reality and delusional thoughts and hallucinations; capacity to read social cues

borderline level of personality organization could find it difficult to have a clear sense of what kind of work would sustain them and this could be a source of distress. Difficulties in intimate relationships can also emerge, such that they could see the partner they date mostly as someone who can satisfy them sexually, but not someone they would care about. The diagnostic toolbox helps the clinician identify an individual's strengths and weaknesses.

The coordinators will illustrate, using plain language, the concept of defense mechanisms, which are defined as unconscious psychic mechanisms employed to cope with conflicts. Some of those may be adaptive and mature, others may have a neurotic quality (i.e., repression-based defenses), while others are immature in the sense that they develop in early childhood and usually diminish in most people over time (i.e., splitting-based defenses). Higher functioning adults typically more often use mature and repression-based defenses rather than splitting-based defenses. Repression refers to tending to forget about some aspects of life, like the danger in daily activities, and risks in relationships (e.g., being cheated on). This unconscious exclusion of unpleasant or unwanted thoughts, feelings, or memories from awareness aims to protect the mind from excess anxiety. Although it may limit the expression of an individual's personality, it generally does not result in reality distortions. Conversely, splitting refers to the tendency to keep contradictory aspects of oneself and of others divided, resulting in a view of self and others that is all good or all evil but never with both positive and negative aspects at the same time. In some persons splitting may dominate even in adulthood, leading to distorted and polarized views of oneself and others, which is seen as a key feature indicating difficulties in personality organization.

BPO is further illustrated by explaining the meaning of the term "identity diffusion."

The coordinators will draw graphical illustrations (Fig. 3.2) of, respectively:

(a) Model of a healthy person with integrated identity
(b) Model of a person with identity diffusion

The group coordinators will explain that with identity diffusion, images of self and others are organized in an extreme or caricatured version, meaning a totally negative perception of self and others, linked by a strong negative affect, or a totally positive perception of self and others, linked by a purely positive affect.

The coordinators will then:

- Encourage the patients in the group to provide feedback about whether they recognize themselves and others in their life in any of those dyads, at times.
- Emphasize that having these extremely negative or positive internal views of self and others prevents PD patients from accurately appraising and judging actual external reality. In everyday life, these dyads might be activated and determine the subjective experience of the patients. Because what we feel about ourselves and others determines, in any given situation, how we behave and how we think, in patients with personality disorders, the fact that the internalized images of self

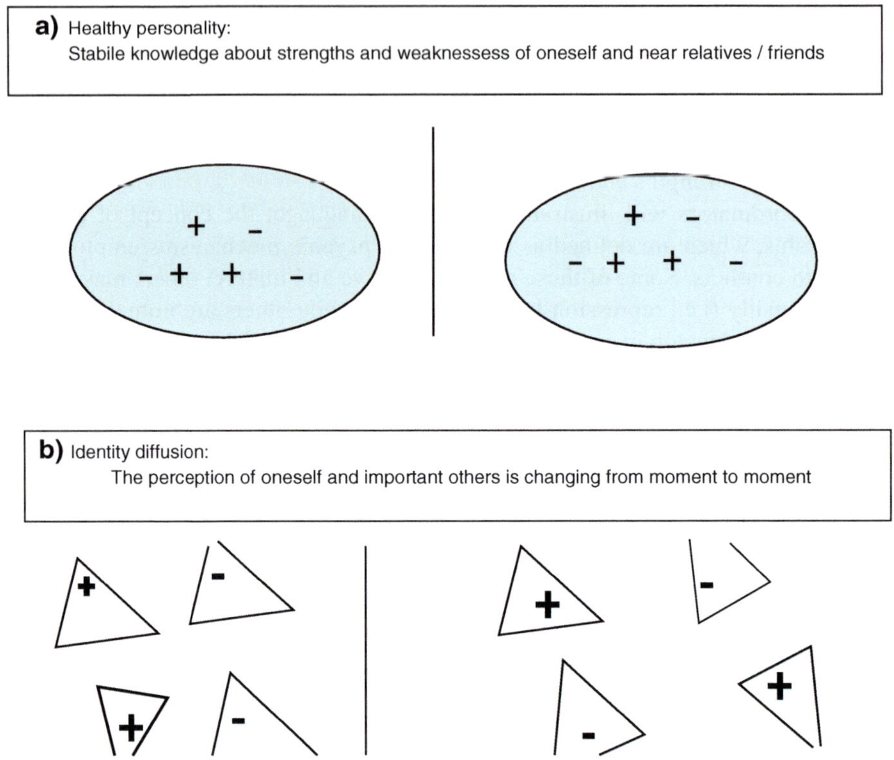

Fig. 3.2 Illustrations of Integrated and Split personality organizations

and others do not correspond accurately to reality, is problematic. The self and others are seen and perceived not according to their real characteristics, but according to the internal views of self and others that get activated in that moment. This can determine dramatic cognitive and emotional responses to the slightest trigger event [56].

- Point out that because of the presence of these two different, split-off types of self-other representations (i.e., all negative/devalued vs all positive/idealized) in some PD patients, the mind of people with PD might have "absolute qualities". Thus, individuals with BPD exhibit an all-or-nothing and uncompromising view of self and others. This causes them to rely on particularly high internal standards when judging and experiencing themselves and others—i.e., they have perfectionistic standards of what means to be human. Therefore, if one does not fit this very ideal view of what a person should be then they see themselves as a failure, worthless and not deserving to exist [57].
- Clarify that this same line of reasoning also applies to significant others, such that if the other does not meet the unrealistic expectation of BPD patients to provide them with unlimited love, the other would automatically be perceived as malevolent and attacking. In BPD, this phenomenon results from powerful

defense mechanisms: accepting and recognizing that others can be of *some* help to the patient would mean relinquishing the internal hope to find someone who would be *perfectly* helpful. Tragically, this prevents BPD patients from benefiting from mutual interpersonal exchanges. Here, the discussion of the idealized dyad can be particularly fruitful. The group coordinators can also use the Diogenes metaphor to explain the attitude of BPD patients toward others. Diogenes was a famous ancient Greek philosopher who is remembered, among other things, for his search for "a perfectly honest and trustworthy man," which he did by carrying a lantern in broad daylight in the marketplace, claiming he was looking for an honest person but could not find one. In the same vein, BPD patients endlessly seek gratifying relationships with others, which then fail because of others' inability to meet patients' unrealistic expectations of "perfect" acceptance and love (Fig. 3.3).

Some patients within the group may have also received a diagnosis of narcissistic personality disorder (NPD) or narcissistic traits. It can be helpful for the coordinators to provide some information about narcissistic disorders. First, they will clarify that the term narcissism has multiple meanings. Healthy narcissism refers to liking what one does, deriving gratification from one's accomplishments, and generally experiencing a sense of satisfaction from work and love. Some patients may have narcissistic traits, sometimes characterized by self-importance and attention-seeking

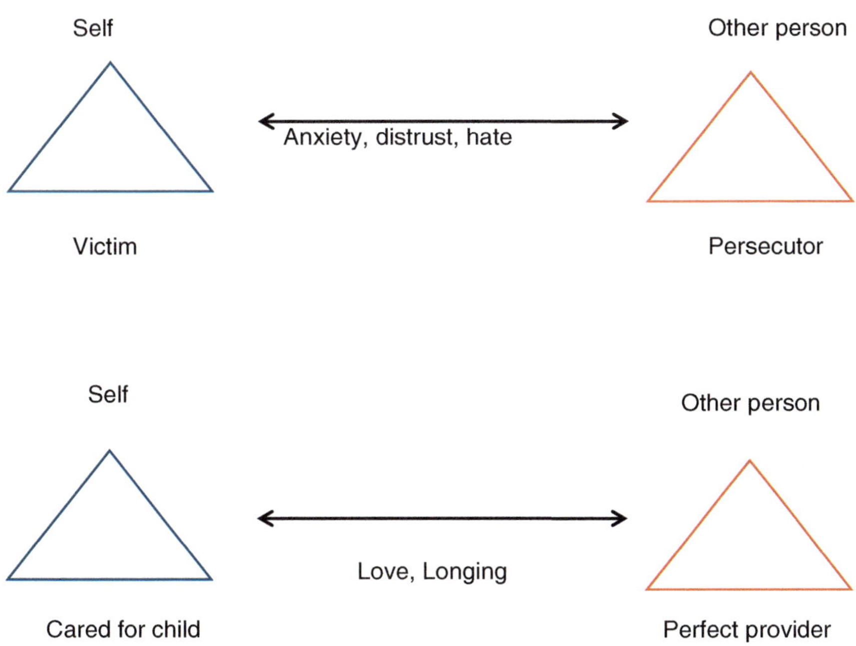

Fig. 3.3 Split-off dyads

behavior. Narcissistic traits can be circumscribed, as with the patient who finds it easy to use energy to be successful vocationally, but who may show a limited emotional investment in other people. The term NPD, as defined in the DSM-5, describes a specific profile of pathological narcissism. This subtype of narcissism is marked by superficial grandiosity, which may reflect the patient's inner world of emptiness and inferiority. The patient with NPD may typically exhibit vulnerability to personal slights but at the same time find it difficult to empathize with others and take into account others' needs. This can lead to challenges in establishing mutual relationships. The arrogant stance that characterizes individuals with NPD can represent an attempt to identify with an ideal, all good, sense of who they are, which is extremely hard to maintain over time and may imply a denial of dependency needs. The main pathological theme in narcissistic disorders can thus be understood as prominent fluctuations in self-esteem.

The second part of the meeting focuses on symptoms. The group coordinators will explain that individuals with BPO may describe symptoms that reflect different PD diagnoses, reflecting the well-documented phenomenon of high rates of PD comorbidity. Furthermore, there is a wide range of possible symptoms, or heterogeneity, of PD presentations. Again, as a group task, the coordinators will clarify with the participants those PD symptoms they may have experienced themselves or heard about in the past [58]. The main task of the coordinator is to document what is shared in a useful way. As a practical matter single symptoms should be gathered on the right side of the flipchart and umbrella terms should be placed on the left side (Table 3.2).

All these themes are then expanded on and discussed with the participants. For instance, one of the most characteristic features of BPD is affective instability or

Table 3.2 Symptoms (as collected by group members)

Behavior	Cutting myself Suicide attempts Unpredictable for my friends and family
Identity	Do not know who I am Hating myself Having difficulties describing my relatives and friends Low self-esteem
Emotion	Inner tension Emotional instability Being angry very often Going up and down Anxieties Stressed out Rage when others do not give me what I think to deserve
Thoughts	Black and white Paranoid Fear of humiliation Fear of rejection
Perception	Feeling like the world is not real Hearing voices when stressed

emotion dysregulation. Mood shifts often occur in response to interpersonal events, involving conflict and/or actual or potential interpersonal rejection, and are mostly characterized by angry outbursts, rather than by elation or long-lasting sadness, with slow recovery from distress [59]. These rapid mood changes are often recognized by patients as chronic unpleasant aversive inner tensions, without any specific emotional quality. In the TFP model of BPD, these affective outbursts are secondary to identity diffusion and the patient's use of splitting as a defense. Difficulties in establishing a realistic internal self-image and image of others lead to a distorted perception of self and others, causing intense affects of extreme quality.

Impulsive and self-destructive chronic behavioral patterns represent another core feature of BPD, including recurrent self-harm (particularly cutting), suicide attempts, overdoses, substance abuse, bulimia and shoplifting. The patients are informed about the clinicians' understanding of self-cutting not as suicidal behavior, but as a behavior that can help the patient cope with intense, negative affect states. Moreover, in BPD suicidality frequently has a communicative function, representing the only way that the patient can imagine being heard.

The group coordinators will make it clear to the participants that although this urge might be extremely intense, especially during particularly distressing affect states, it can nonetheless be resisted. Participants are encouraged to share their experiences about those behaviors they have found useful in resisting the urge to self-harm (e.g., self-distraction, talking to a friend, not talking to someone else, going for a walk, etc.). This strengthens the message that self-harm is not necessary and can be resisted. Participants will also be informed that during the course of treatment that might follow with a clinician practicing TFP or a TFP-informed intervention, if the patient finds it particularly difficult to resist self-harm, they can be referred to a DBT skills training group. Finally, the cognitive and perceptual symptoms of BPD include the psychotic or psychotic-like symptoms that occur when patients are particularly stressed [60]. Transitory, odd thinking, non-delusional paranoia, unusual perceptual experiences, and depersonalization, can be relatively common and, over 70 years ago, contributed to the definition of "borderline" when describing those patients who exhibited both neurotic and psychotic symptoms [61]. In TFP interventions, these states are often understood as episodes of particularly intense splitting and dissociation (i.e., paranoid thinking about someone as the expression of viewing the other as a totally negative and malevolent person, without being able to see more positive aspects). Patients with BPD may also have difficulties in social reality testing, meaning that they can find it difficult to accurately "read" the reasons underlying others' behavior toward them (e.g., "My friend looked at her clock when we were out for a coffee together, it means that she wanted to get rid of me."), and/or accurately appreciate the impact of their own behavior on others (e.g., "There were no reasons at all for my boyfriend to break up with me; he's a betrayer, a monster, I was so loving and affectionate to him, though I'll admit we had lots of arguments and I threatened him repeatedly").

Third Meeting: Development of BPD

The goal of this session is to provide information on the complex topic of how PDs develop, in an attempt to address unfortunate patterns of ascribing PD pathology to whatever diagnosis is in fashion or automatically, and without support, to trauma.

The patients are involved in an exercise aimed at identifying risk factors for BPD. The opening question of this section is an invitation to the participants to share their thoughts about this. Again, all contributions are collected and written down on a flip chart.

First, the proposed contributing factors are integrated using a bio-psycho-social framework [62]. (As noted earlier, most of the research on the development of PD pathology has focused on BPD. Relevant available information on the bio-psycho-social factors linked to the development of BPD and other PD diagnoses is reviewed.)

The coordinators' task is to assign the patients' input into several fields of biological, social, or psychological factors.

As an example, in the case of BPD, "bio" can refer to documented rates of heritability of the disorder; genetic loading does not always result in the expression of the disorder, but can contribute to an elevated vulnerability to develop it in adolescence. "Psycho" can refer to the growing literature on attachment styles and their link to the development of BPD. Finally, "social" can connote the well-described link between the development of BPD and lower socio-economic status.

Information is provided on the biological correlates of BPD, including genetic, structural, and neurochemical vulnerabilities. The group coordinators will be clear that this research field is rapidly evolving with various accumulating novel findings. In general, however, it is well established that the interaction between genetic factors and adverse childhood experiences influences brain development through altered hormones and neuropeptides. Adverse childhood experiences may modulate gene expression and lead to stable personality traits. However, no specific genetic variants associated with BPD have been identified yet. While BPD is more common in people with a family history of BPD, with a 46% heritability, the transmissible risk is linked with a different way of experiencing and dealing with intense affects, rather than with the disorder itself. The concepts of familial risk and heritability of BPD will also lead to a discussion of pregnancy for women with BPD. Focusing on biological factors that are implicated in BPD will be useful in reducing stigma [63], although the etiology of BPD is more complex and cannot be attributed only to genes [25].

In turn, the roles of environmental risk or protective factors are highlighted, which may diversely influence the expression of specific genetic and biological vulnerabilities. The subtle role of early bonding is described, suggesting that the risk factors for BPD are deeply rooted in early insecure attachment relationships, which represent developmental precursors of difficulties with representation and identity formation in BPD [64].

It is important to emphasize that the presence of the disorder should not cause parents or patients to feel guilty, given the likelihood that more central to the emergence of the pathology is the possible mismatch between child temperament and parental style.

Finally, the topic of developmental trauma will be addressed. Several studies have retrospectively investigated the history of developmental trauma in patients with BPD, suggesting that patients with BPD report significantly higher rates of traumatic childhood experiences (i.e., neglect or abuse), compared with controls. However, traumatic experiences do not always lead to the development of BPD and BPD can develop without traumatic experiences. Moreover, splitting mechanisms may lead patients with BPD to perceive even a supportive family attitude as malevolent or abusive [65]. The group coordinators will highlight that BPD is a developmental disorder in nature in the sense that primary caregivers might not have been able to meet the needs of the child or help them work through their problems. Sometimes this may have happened because of suboptimal, inconsistent, or traumatic parenting, but at other times this may have occurred not because of a noticeable deficiency in the parenting but because of the unusual challenge in meeting the needs of a child with extreme temperamental tendencies and reactivity.

The TFP model is then proposed as a theoretical model to understand the essence of the disorder and integrate various causal factors in a comprehensive view of PD pathogenesis (Fig. 3.4). For this aim, the coordinators encourage the group to look back at the definition of PD proposed in the previous meeting. Key terms like

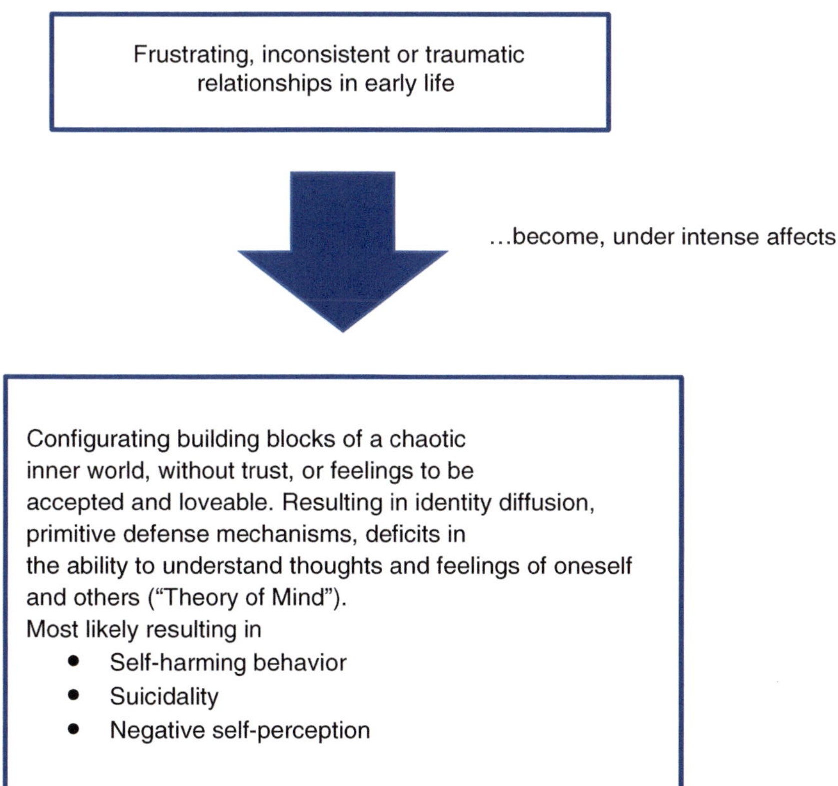

Fig. 3.4 TFP model of psycho-social mechanisms in the origin of BPD

identity, identity diffusion, quality of object relations, defense mechanisms, and reality testing are repeated.

The TFP model of PD development emphasizes the importance of relationships in the first years of life. The coordinators will communicate to the group, in straightforward language, that every person incorporates these early experiences into his/her psychic structure in the form of dyads (meaning two persons interacting). When the early relationships are unreliable, inconsistent, or even traumatic, all these difficult relationships are integrated into our psychic structure or inner life. In a healthy development of the psychic structure, children up to 5 years will learn to understand thoughts and feelings of another person and they will develop an integrated picture of their main attachment figures, being mostly friendly and satisfying but sometimes also frustrating and frightening. These critical developmental steps fail in some people. Instead of being able to integrate a "mostly good but sometimes difficult" picture of the counterpart, these individuals will consider only one quality of another at a time, in an "all good or all evil" way of perception.

At the same time, the group coordinators will clarify that this interplay between genetics (i.e., temperamental traits of negative affect, reactivity, or aggression) and psychological risk factors (i.e., trauma, neglect) does not necessarily lead to a stable, enduring disorder that can never be modified. People can improve despite their genetic tendencies or a history of early trauma. A BPD diagnosis does not mean the individual is "disabled"; rather, BPD patients may have limitations in regulating behavior, thoughts, and emotions, but nonetheless can learn how to do that [66]. Therefore, in TFP, the etiology of the patient's personality pathology is not as crucial as a more helpful understanding of how the patient's mind works. For instance, considering trauma as the sole central problem for a patient with a PD diagnosis would risk missing out on other important aspects of their personality that directly impact their behavior and functioning. It may be important to explore with the patient with a history of trauma, both the details of the patient's experience as a victim, but also, in an appropriately cautious and thoughtful way, the patient's own behavior that can be victimizing of others. One of the unfortunate aspects of trauma is that it prevents individuals from having a healthy acceptance of their own aggressive side, which is a normal side. For this reason, "detoxifying" aggression is central to TFP. In the same vein, genetic tendencies toward intense affects can be "reframed" and used productively, as in the support for a patient's ambitions [67, 68].

Fourth Meeting: Common Comorbidities

This meeting focuses on the comorbidities frequently seen in patients with PD diagnoses. It aims to provide information on various mental health disorders that routinely co-occur with PD functioning at a mid-low borderline level of personality organization. Examining comorbidities can help clarify for patients with a PD diagnosis how best to understand the range of symptoms they experience. Sometimes these symptoms are best understood as part of the PD itself, as in identifying interpersonally mediated affective instability as a symptom of a PD, and not as a separate mood disorder. Other times, it is useful for the PD patient to understand genuine comorbidities, such as a distinct substance use or anxiety disorder, which merit appropriate treatments distinct from an intervention for the PD.

The other diagnoses previously assigned to the participants, which were discussed in the second meeting of this psychoeducation intervention, are listed in order of frequency. This list of other diagnoses reflects the complexity of the DSM-5 criteria for PD diagnoses. The wide range of symptoms including alterations in mood states, disordered eating behavior, social anxiety, substance abuse, and psychotic-like phenomena, understandably leads clinicians, over time, to identify multiple, distinct, co-existing psychiatric disorders in these PD patients [69]. In many cases, the diagnosis of PD can be considered as a primary diagnosis and these comorbidities are regarded as secondary to the personality disturbance. However, in actuality, most people with, BPD, for instance, meet the criteria of coexisting conditions such as mood disorders (83%), anxiety disorders (85%), or substance use disorders (78%). In line with certain clinical guidelines for BPD [70, 71] most of the presentations (i.e., depression, post-traumatic stress disorder, or anxiety) that can be treated within a well-structured treatment program for BPD should not preclude the patient from accessing the BPD treatment in a useful way. In these cases, no available evidence indicates that BPD treatment should be altered when the person has a co-occurring psychiatric condition, nor that treatments for comorbid conditions should be altered when a person also has BPD. However, certain co-occurring disorders such as severe alcohol or substance use disorders, eating disorders (particularly anorexia nervosa or an avoidant/restrictive food intake disorder with severe weight loss and malnutrition), major depression with neurovegetative symptoms or sustained psychosis, may interfere with the patient's ability to use TFP and even be life-threatening, and thus may preclude BPD therapy. In these cases, those other conditions should be managed first, for instance by referring the patient to the corresponding appropriate service, since these disorders need to be well-controlled before BPD can be treated successfully [25]. In TFP, as well as in "applied" TFP interventions, the clinicians will make sure to include the requirement to address these co-occurring conditions in the treatment contract and will start and then continue therapy for BPD and other PD only if there is evidence that the patient is adequately addressing these comorbidities. This would also mean that the TFP therapist or the TFP-oriented clinicians will establish contact and share information with the other professionals who are treating the patient for, for example, their substance use or eating disorder specialist. This would also avoid splitting (e.g., the TFP clinician is seen as "all good" and the clinician treating the other condition is "all bad," or vice versa).

Fifth Meeting: Pharmacological Treatment

The goal of this session is to explain to the patients, using plain language, the current state-of-the-art pharmacotherapy for patients with a PD diagnosis. Most of the information will necessarily rely on existing research about medication use in BPD, as treatment studies or practice guidelines for other DSM PD categories are not available. In the case of extensive use of medication in the group, a second meeting on this topic will be needed.

The patients are asked to report which medications they were prescribed during their previous treatments, and for what reasons. Again, all contributions are collected and written down on a flip chart. The coordinator will write the single medications on the right side of the flip chart and umbrella terms of the corresponding pharmacological classes should be placed on the left side.

The coordinators will discuss with the group the available empirical evidence on this topic, with the aim of fostering informed decision-making and a collaborative patient-prescriber relationship. The meeting starts with explaining that existing clinical guidelines converge in recommending that medications should not be used as primary therapy for BPD, because they have only modest and inconsistent effects, and do not change the nature and course of the disorder [70–73]. Consistently, no psychotropic drug is currently approved for BPD or any other PD. Medications can be considered to target discrete co-occurring conditions (i.e., a major depression episode, or severe anxiety disorder). Medications such as atypical antipsychotics and sedating antihistamines could also be considered for crises using a single drug and a minimum effective dose for not longer than 1 week, as part of an overall treatment plan agreed on in advance. In any case, medications should be used one at a time, their efficacy should be regularly reviewed, and they should be stopped before starting another medicine [70, 71]. However, it should be mentioned that despite these clear-cut guidelines, several studies across various countries robustly demonstrated that over 90% of BPD patients receive at least one medication, with polypharmacotherapy rates as high as 70–80%. BPD patients, on average, receive 2.7 medications at the same time: 80% of patients receive at least two medications, and 50% three or more medications [74, 75]. Thus, the meeting will also address the factors that could explain this paradoxical heavy use of pharmacotherapy in the context of no or little evidence of the efficacy of medications. On the one hand, the number of psychopharmacological trials available for reviewing the efficacy of the various medications is limited (the most recent Cochrane meta-analysis could include only 46 randomized controlled trials [76]). Further, it is difficult to draw firm conclusions from the existing meta-analytic reviews because of the small number of studies of each pharmacological class of agent, the small sample sizes in most studies, and the heterogeneity of the outcomes considered. This results in mixed findings of insufficient evidence to be proposed as treatment options in the guidelines [76]. A prudent but flexible and pragmatic approach to pharmacotherapy in BPD is likely indicated. Medications should never be used as the sole treatment for BPD; they should only be prescribed when necessary (e.g., for symptom relief or behavioral dyscontrol) but otherwise avoided [75]. Flexibility is essential when assessing the need for targeted, symptom-based pharmacotherapy of BPD, which is supported by some evidence [76, 77] that antipsychotics and mood stabilizers (but not antidepressants) may help to control interpersonal problems, cognitive-perceptual symptoms, and affective/behavioral dysregulation. At the same time, frequent evaluation of a need to continue pharmacotherapy is necessary; only a short-term administration of medication at times of crisis and symptom exacerbation is indicated, and polypharmacotherapy must be avoided through a careful cost-benefit analysis for each medication, keeping in mind the patients' medical and mental status as well as their preferences and values [75, 78].

Then, patients are informed about the mechanisms of action, the doses, the duration and the side effects of antidepressants, mood stabilizers, antipsychotics, and benzodiazepines, as well their limited therapeutic use in BPD, thus establishing a context for using medication to address specific symptom groups defined above (affective instability, impulsive and self-destructive chronic behaviors, cognitive and perceptual symptoms).

They are also informed about the risks of sedative agents, which can be used cautiously during a crisis. The link between polypharmacy and the increased incidence of associated medication side effects is reinforced.

They are also informed about the risk of abuse of sedatives, which may be considered cautiously during a crisis, and about the fact that polypharmacotherapy is associated with an increased risk for multiple side effects.

This session ends with the information that the cornerstones of BPD treatment are empirically supported psychotherapy or structured interventions incorporating common effective elements from established psychotherapies for BPD. This topic will be reinforced in the following group meetings. Participants are also informed that nevertheless medications can also be used as an adjunctive symptom-targeted component of the treatment under some circumstances, e.g., for comorbid conditions, or one at a time, for limited time periods, to improve specific BPD symptom dimensions during periods of crisis. This information will prevent patients from developing unrealistic expectations about medications.

Sixth Meeting: Psychotherapy

The coordinators provide information about different forms of evidence-based psychotherapies for BPD, as the sole PD for which several treatment trials have been performed (see [79] for a meta-analytic review of the effectiveness of psychotherapies in BPD).

The research findings suggest benefits for six long-term, specialized, treatments for BPD: dialectical behavior therapy (DBT), mentalization-based treatment (MBT), transference-focused psychotherapy (TFP), schema-focused group therapy (SFT); systems training for emotional predictability and problem-solving (STEPPS) and general psychiatric management (GPM).

DBT [42] is specifically designed to target affective instability and to reduce impulsive behaviors, teaching patients alternative ways to manage emotion dysregulation. The program emphasizes the empathic role of the therapist providing "validation" for the inner experience of patients. Key to DBT is the development of skills to improve impulse control and affect regulation in particular as these impact suicidal and other self-destructive behaviors.

MBT, developed by Bateman and Fonagy [80, 81], is derived from the concept that patients with BPD show reduced capacities to "mentalize," i.e., to stand outside their feelings and accurately observe emotions in themselves and others. Patients are taught to observe their emotions, to learn how to tolerate them, and to handle them in more adaptive ways. The goal is to reduce mistrust and improve attachment security through an increase in mentalization.

TFP is a manualized [55], psychoanalytically oriented psychotherapy, based on Kernberg's conceptualization of BPO [82]. It focuses on the problematic interpersonal dynamics in the patient's life, which emerge in interactions with the therapist in the transference. These patients-therapist dynamics are examined to resolve the splits between good and bad representations of self and others that drive instabilities in affect and relationships. Key to TFP is the exploration of activated affectively charged interpersonal interactions with the therapist and other people in the patients' environment.

SFT [83], is a hybrid of cognitive-behavioral therapy and psychodynamic therapy that aims to modify maladaptive schema, patterns of thinking and behavior by deriving from adverse experiences in childhood.

STEPPS [84] is a group intervention that helps patients with BPD to develop better ways of dealing with emotions, teaching skills related to leisure, sleep, eating habits, and exercise.

Finally, GPM [85] closely followed the American Psychiatric Association guidelines for the treatment of BPD. It focuses on an interpersonal hypersensitivity model of BPD, and it is proposed as a flexible and practical model, which reflects the best general psychiatric treatment that could be used by generalist mental health clinicians with minimal additional training. It also has a psychoeducation component and emphasizes the goal to "get a life."

After the explanation of different evidence-based therapies, the patients are invited to consider that although the different methods employ distinct approaches to treating patients with BPD, the failure of comparative trials to find significant differences in outcome suggests that common factors are of critical importance.

The main, nonspecific, factors of these therapies are: (1) a clear, structured, treatment framework, which also involves a clear theoretical rationale for the treatment; (2) a focus on affect, with close attention to the emotional experience of the patient during sessions; (3) a focus on the relationship with the therapist, which is actively engaged in a collaborative working alliance with the patients; (4) the use of supportive interventions and exploratory interventions, aimed at encouraging reflection on the mind of self and of others and (5) change-oriented interventions, with a practical problem-solving approach and attention to functioning [86, 87].

Seventh Meeting: Transference-Focused Psychotherapy

In this meeting, the coordinators concentrate on TFP, defined as a highly structured, twice-weekly modified psychodynamic treatment aimed at promoting an enduring personality change through fostering identity integration (the concepts of identity diffusion and split-off dyads described in previous meetings will be recalled). However, in settings where standard TFP is not feasible, the coordinators will explain that TFP principles can serve as an organizing framework to structure existing "generalist" psychiatric treatments. This might be particularly useful because research has shown that, out of all the effective treatments for BPD only TFP leads to personality change as indicated by changes in attachment coherence, levels of personality organization, and reflective function [88–91]. By changing the structure underlying the personality disorder, TFP has the ambitious goal to improve three arenas of life: work and career, social and creative life outside work, and love and sex, with the exact aims tailored to each patient [88]. Applied-TFP initiatives may benefit from focusing on these "external reality" and "functional" outcomes.

The content of this meeting will differ according to the type of treatment that is actually available to the patient group in that particular country, mental health system, and setting. If the PE program is being delivered to patients who will be receiving standard TFP, the coordinators will describe the general features of such an individual psychotherapy (twice a week outpatient setting, free association, joint attention to internal world and external reality). If the PE program is being attended by patients seeking treatments that apply TFP principles across different treatment modalities (i.e., day hospital, inpatient units, community-based psychiatric services, group therapies), then the group coordinators will also explain the characteristics of those treatment contexts.

In all circumstances, this meeting will explain, using straightforward language, the main features of a TFP-oriented approach to treating patients suffering with BPD or another cluster B PD operating at a mid-low BPO level.

As was outlined in the preceding meetings of this PE program, individuals with BPD usually exhibit four areas of difficulties, which are all addressed by TFP or TFP-informed interventions:

1. Rapidly shifting emotional states, which can be challenging
2. Difficulties in relationships, often experienced as frustrating or disappointing because of a desperate need to be perfectly cared for by significant others
3. Acting out behaviors, which are often the symptoms that get attention, but that can be understood as maladaptive ways to cope with inner pain
4. Identity diffusion associated with inconsistent goals and values, reflecting the patient's lack of a solid identity foundation; this lack of identity consolidation is linked with episodic distress [56].

In TFP interventions, these areas of difficulty are consistently addressed by the therapist and other mental health professionals. This is done within a structured framework that allows both the patient and the clinicians to observe how these difficulties unfold in the patient's life. The clinician's first goal is to have the patient reflect on the difficulties listed above, rather than acting them out. The ultimate goal would be the patient's mastery of these challenges, thus promoting the capacity "to work and love." The group coordinators will discuss with the participants what is meant by "work and love" and will link this functional outcome and the concepts of integrated identity (as opposed to identity diffusion) that were addressed during the second meeting of the PE program, as well as with other concepts related to symptoms and etiology of BPD. This will clarify that TFP interventions aim at fostering successful psychosocial functioning through resolving identity diffusion. The coordinators may use a graphic illustration on the flip chart to illustrate this (Fig. 3.5).

The concept of recovery and progress toward recovery will therefore be addressed, using plain language. According to TFP, recovery is seen as establishing an integrated sense of self, which means being able to reflect upon aspects of one's own inner psychological world and to say, "that's part of me." This would allow individuals to eliminate extreme reactions. This would also imply accepting a lot of pain, feeling it, but not acting it out, or correcting negative reactions (mostly arising in individuals from perceived interpersonal threats) [57]. The group coordinators will clarify to the participants that learning more about themselves during TFP treatments will allow them to overcome painful things like "hating" themselves and feeling completely worthless. TFP will help them to consider that they don't have to meet unrealistic internal standards all the time to feel that they can deserve to exist.

On the practical level, the relationship with the therapist in standard TFP, as well as with other clinicians in "applied" TFP initiatives, is structured under controlled

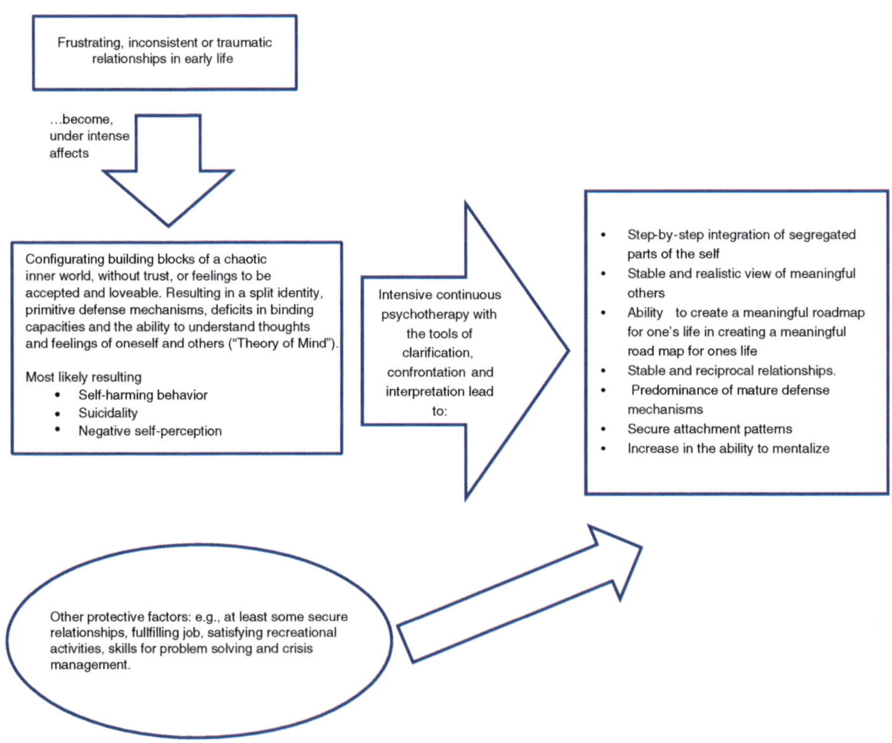

Fig. 3.5 TFP model of change

conditions, to allow patients to experience strong affects without destructive consequences for their lives. Therefore, structuring the treatment is central both in standard TFP and "applied" TFP. Common elements of this structure, or frame, are as follows:

1. Sharing the PD diagnosis with the patient and providing psychoeducation about it
2. Evaluating the level of PD severity
3. Timely contact with previous treaters and family members to gather information about potential obstacles to treatment
4. Establishing treatment goals
5. Establishing a treatment contract between the patient and the treating clinician(s). The contract will clearly outline patients' and clinicians' responsibilities during treatment and will anticipate potential obstacles to treatment, as they have emerged from the patient's previous history (i.e., drop-outs from previous treatments, uncontrolled substance abuse or eating disorder, suicide attempts, dependency on family or state). This will allow the clinician to collaboratively formulate a personalized plan with the patient that would ensure that these potential threats toward treatment will not eventually undermine the TFP interventions (i.e., plans to address non-attendance, to facilitate treatment for uncontrolled comorbid disorders, and to help limiting self-destructive behaviors, etc.). Typically, some patients would react to the contracting phase with anger and skepticism ("Don't you think that, if I could already do this all, I would not even be here?"). However, the contract also conveys to patients the message that they are responsible individuals with some difficulties, but also strengths, which they can use to change. Here, an aspect of paramount importance is the requirement in TFP interventions that the patients are involved in some form of meaningful activity. The coordinators will make clear to the group that psychiatric and psychotherapeutic help will work only if they have these activities in daily life. This requirement further conveys to the patients that change is indeed possible (and expected) and challenges their unconscious expectation that the clinicians are omnipotent others who will magically "fix" them. As such, the treatment contract provides a safe setting for the reactivation of the internalized self-other representations of the patients.

The TFP intervention will then start only if the patient and the clinician(s) have reached an agreement on the contract. In TFP interventions, the mechanism of change is the integration of the polarized concepts of self and others into a more complex, differentiated, and realistic perspective. This integration becomes possible through a process called analysis of "transference" in the therapeutic relationship(s). Transference means the patient's moment-to-moment experience of, and expression of feelings toward, the clinician. The patient's responses stem from the activation, in that particular moment, of their internal, polarized representations of self and others, rather than responses reflecting the "real" relationship with the treating clinician. The TFP clinician observes this experience, asks for clarification about it, and invites the patient to reflect upon it, to help to identify, understand, and modify their internal representations of self and others. The patient begins to reflect on what is going on in the present with the others, in light of these internalized paradigms and gradually becomes aware of the extent to which his or her perceptions are based more on internalized representations than on what is occurring now.

The integration of the split and polarized concepts of self and others helps to structure cognitively what at first seemed chaotic and allows for better modulation of affects. Indeed, the first signs of change are represented by a decrease in acting out behaviors: rather than putting into action an emotion or a feeling they can't bear so to get rid of it, the patient becomes able to feel emotions and contain them. Through the treatment, the patient learns a reflective process or "mentalization" abilities; they come to appreciate how a person can be so different at various points in time. This developing capacity to develop a more realistic acceptance of what is human, to think more flexibly, realistically, and benevolently, fosters a meaningful change of the patient's attitudes in work and relationships outside the treatment [57].

Eighth Meeting: Crisis Management

Patients with moderate to severe PD pathology, a category that includes patients with BPD, are well known to be at risk for crises of all kinds. This vulnerability to crises may be one factor that contributes to the widely described aversion to treating PD patients endorsed by clinicians of different backgrounds and in different locales. The objective of this part of the PE program outlined is to directly address this phenomenon of expectable crises in a way that helps both patients and clinicians appreciate those factors that contribute to crises and to develop strategies to minimize disruption to the patient's lives and their treatment.

In TFP as an extended, individual psychotherapy, part of the assessment process will include a thorough review of the patient's history that includes crises of different kinds. Obtaining parallel information from current and prior treaters and from family members is essential in this process. A discussion in advance of those crises that have impacted the patient's life and the patient's prior treatment experience will help the clinician in formulating details of the treatment contract that address in advance the possibility of similar crises going forward.

It is important to note that in TFP, the therapist will *expect* crises of different kinds. The goal is not to somehow forbid crises or punish patients when crises emerge, but rather to think together with the patient (and family, in some circumstances) about likely future crises and to explore this topic in a useful way.

In this meeting, the coordinators will begin by canvasing the group members about their experiences of crises and their understanding of what might have contributed to these crises and what might have helped them cope. The group is invited to clarify what they mean by the word "crisis." While group members share their subjective experiences of crises of different types, consensus generally emerges that a crisis occurs when a person is unable to cope with a situation, which causes acute anxiety and emotional suffering [92]. Typical crises described include periods of affective instability with associated impulsivity, self-injury, ruptured relationships, or transient paranoid thinking.

In general, patients in the group are reassured by this collective discussion of crises. Patients recognize in others' accounts aspects of their own history. This can be a source of relief, as patients feel they are not alone as others recount episodes of substance use or threats of suicide in the context of intense self-attack or sense of abandonment—all familiar narratives. The coordinators can explain how key elements of PD pathology, including identity diffusion, and the use of splitting-based defenses like denial, projection, and alternating idealization and devaluation, put patients at risk for disruptive, sometimes dangerous crises. Patients can recognize themselves in the coordinators' description of identity diffusion, for example. A patient may say: "Yes, I felt suicidal when I didn't get the job. I didn't feel I was worth anything, without the job, I didn't exist!" In a similar vein, the coordinators' explanation of the way alternating idealization/devaluation can predispose a patient to crises will be met with nods of recognition. As one patient in the group put it: "I was fine when I saw my new boyfriend as ideal; when I first saw something in him I didn't like, it moved me to despair and I started drinking and had a car accident."

The coordinators will explain the concept of "technical neutrality" in this part of the program. The therapist's goal in TFP of staying focused on exploration and avoiding coming down on one side or the other of a patient's internal conflict is explained as the process of maintaining technical neutrality. The coordinators will also explain how the therapist will deviate from technical neutrality in certain situations and share with the patient a very clear opinion, often associated with direct advice if the therapist feels that the patient may be engaging in some kind of clearly self-destructive act.

The patient in crisis may be moved to engage in destructive or self-destructive behavior that will require the therapist to deviate from usual practice. For example, a patient who is affectively overwhelmed by a break-up with his girlfriend, tells his therapist that he wants to impulsively withdraw from his competitive graduate school. While the therapist may at first try to engage the patient in exploration of this decision, if the patient persists in his destructive behavior, the therapist will give direct advice, in this case not to quit graduate school, and then at some point in the future, review with the patient the events that lead the therapist to move away from neutrality. In this part of the program explaining to patients the distinction between the TFP therapist's overarching goal of encouraging exploration, but with limits directly related a patient's destructiveness, will communicate a message to the patients in the PE group about basic parameters for TFP treatment.

Part of the coordinators' efforts include outlining those genuine crises that will require a change in the TFP approach and those familiar, expectable periods of turmoil that a patient may consider a crisis, but do not merit a change in how the TFP therapist conducts treatment. Crises that will alert the therapist to a need to alter course include the following: exacerbation of eating disorder symptoms that lead to medical compromise; escalation of substance use disorder symptoms that preclude the patient's ability to stay engaged; or a serious, life-threatening suicide attempt. In these cases, consideration of a higher level of care, transfer to an alternative treatment modality, or hospitalization, may be indicated.

In the next step information is gathered what may be helpful in solving a critical situation: Content could be:

- Concentrating on what had been helpful in the past
- Calling a friend or family member (most ideally there is a detailed plan put in place in advance for these kinds of crisis calls)
- Calling a public helpline
- Taking a crisis medication (as arranged with the treating psychiatrist)
- Seeing a psychiatrist, e.g., at the hospital emergency room

It is emphasized that a crisis should be addressed as central content at the next psychotherapeutic session or encounter with the treating clinician(s). The role of hospitalization may also be addressed, suggesting that there are situations, as referenced above, necessitating inpatient treatment. At the same time, the potential pitfalls of a psychiatric hospitalization are considered, as when the patient's desire to shed responsibilities through hospitalization, can disrupt studies, employment, or psychotherapy courses [1]. Therefore, hospitalizations in the context of emerging crises should usually be of short duration and restricted to focused problem solving and sometimes medication changes when indicated.

Ninth Meeting: Program Evaluation

The last meeting has several functions:

First, it can be useful to clarify with participants that material which remains unclear and to cover those additional topics that the participants identify as priorities that have not already been addressed.

Second, there is an opportunity for a general evaluation of the program as the coordinators ask whether the participants' expectations have been fulfilled and which goals have been achieved.

Finally, it is likely that the last session will have a significant emotional impact as the patients have had the opportunity to create strong bonds with each other and with the program therapists during the months of their engagement. Therefore, it is important for the coordinators to thank the participants and to convey a personal message to the group highlighting the investment of those involved and the quality of the interpersonal interactions observed.

Conclusion

This chapter has illustrated a TFP-oriented model of group psychoeducation for patients with BPD and other DSM-5 Cluster B presentations. This model can be flexibly incorporated in the pre-treatment phase of any TFP treatment program, either in the setting of a standard, twice-weekly outpatient individual psychotherapy or in various "applied" TFP interventions, as those described in the following chapters of this volume.

We have described how TFP principles can be used to convey to patients comprehensive and structured information about PD pathology. The program provides information about PD diagnoses (in terms of personality structure, symptoms, etiology, and course), what disorders can co-occur, what treatment options are available and which are the key elements of treatment according to TFP theory and practice. This model further aims to increase patients' motivation for treatment, particularly for TFP or any "applied" TFP intervention. As such, it may offer a guide for patients unfamiliar with psychotherapy but also offer to patients who may not be progressing as they would like in alternative treatment situations a different approach that provides hope and motivation. As noted, this chapter reflects a proposal for a TFP-informed PE program. Future objectives would include research projects that examine the benefits of this kind of PE program for both patients and clinicians. PE programs on their own have been found to help reduce symptom burden for BPD patients; other possible research questions include patient and clinician satisfaction, treatment drop-out risk, and treatment selection patterns.

References

1. Hersh RG, Caligor E, Yeomans FE. Fundamentals of transference-focused psychotherapy: applications in psychiatric and medical settings. Springer International Publishing; 2017. https://doi.org/10.1007/978-3-319-44091-0.
2. Hersh RG. Integration with transference-focused psychotherapy. In: Choi-Kain LW, Gunderson JG, editors. Applications of good psychiatric management for borderline personality disorder: a practical guide. American Psychiatric Association Publishing; 2018. p. 327–51.
3. Bäuml J, Froböse T, Kraemer S, Rentrop M, Pitschel-Walz G. Psychoeducation: a basic psychotherapeutic intervention for patients with schizophrenia and their families. Schizophr Bull. 2006;32(Suppl 1):S1–9. https://doi.org/10.1093/schbul/sbl017.
4. McFarlane WR, Dixon L, Lukens E, Lucksted A. Family psychoeducation and schizophrenia: a review of the literature. JMFT. 2003;29(2):223–45. https://doi.org/10.1111/j.1752-0606.2003.tb01202.x.
5. Colom F, Vieta E, Martinez-Aran A, Reinares M, Goikolea JM, Benabarre A, et al. A randomized trial on the efficacy of group psychoeducation in the prophylaxis of recurrences in bipolar patients whose disease is in remission. Arch Gen Psychiatry. 2003;60(4):402–7. https://doi.org/10.1001/archpsyc.60.4.402.
6. Colom F, Vieta E, Sanchez-Moreno J, Palomino-Otiniano R, Reinares M, Goikolea JM, et al. Group psychoeducation for stabilised bipolar disorders: 5-year outcome of a randomised clinical trial. Br J Psychiatry. 2009;194(3):260–5. https://doi.org/10.1192/bjp.bp.107.040485.
7. Miklowitz DJ, George EL, Richards JA, Simoneau TL, Suddath RL. A randomized study of family-focused psychoeducation and pharmacotherapy in the outpatient management of bipolar disorder. Arch Gen Psychiatry. 2003;60(9):904–12. https://doi.org/10.1001/archpsyc.60.9.904.
8. Dalgard OS. A randomized controlled trial of a psychoeducational group program for unipolar depression in adults in Norway (NCT00319540). Clin Pract Epidemiology Ment. 2006;2(1):1–8. https://doi.org/10.1186/1745-0179-2-15.
9. Katsuki F, Takeuchi H, Konishi M, Sasaki M, Murase Y, Naito A, et al. Pre-post changes in psychosocial functioning among relatives of patients with depressive disorders after Brief

Multifamily Psychoeducation: a pilot study. BMC Psychiatry. 2011;11:1–7. https://doi.org/10.1186/1471-244X-11-56.
10. Rocco PL, Ciano RP, Balestrieri M. Psychoeducation in the prevention of eating disorders: an experimental approach in adolescent schoolgirls. Br J Med Psychol. 2001;74(3):351–8. https://doi.org/10.1348/000711201161028.
11. Le Grange D, Binford R, Loeb KL. Manualized family-based treatment for anorexia nervosa: a case series. JAACAP. 2005;44(1):41–6. https://doi.org/10.1097/01.chi.0000145373.68863.85.
12. Zanarini MC, Frankenburg FR. A preliminary, randomized trial of psychoeducation for women with borderline personality disorder. J Pers Disord. 2008;22(3):284–90. https://doi.org/10.1521/pedi.2008.22.3.284.
13. Zanarini MC. Zanarini Rating Scale for Borderline Personality Disorder (ZAN-BPD): a continuous measure of DSM-IV borderline psychopathology. J Pers Disord. 2003;17(3):233–42. https://doi.org/10.1521/pedi.17.3.233.22147.
14. Zanarini MC, Conkey LC, Temes CM, Fitzmaurice GM. Randomized controlled trial of web-based psychoeducation for women with borderline personality disorder. J Clin Psychiatry. 2017;78(3):160–5. https://doi.org/10.4088/JCP.16m11153.
15. Ridolfi ME, Rossi R, Occhialini G, Gunderson JG. A clinical trial of a psychoeducation group intervention for patients with borderline personality disorder. J Clin Psychiatry. 2019;81(1):160–9. https://doi.org/10.4088/JCP.19m12753.
16. Black DW, Blum N, McCormick B, Allen J. Systems training for emotional predictability and problem solving (STEPPS) group treatment for offenders with borderline personality disorder. J Nerv Ment Dis. 2013;201(2):124–9. https://doi.org/10.1097/NMD.0b013e31827f6435.
17. Grenyer BF, Bailey RC, Lewis KL, Matthias M, Garretty T, Bickerton A. A randomized controlled trial of group psychoeducation for carers of persons with borderline personality disorder. J Pers Disord. 2019;33(2):214–28. https://doi.org/10.1521/pedi_2018_32_340.
18. Project Air Strategy for Personality Disorders. Staying connected: a family, partner and carer resource for improving relationships with people with a personality disorder [DVD, 30 min]. Wollongong: University of Wollongong, Illawarra Health and Medical Research Institute; 2012.
19. Project Air Strategy for Personality Disorders. Family, partner and carer intervention manual for personality disorders. Wollongong: University of Wollongong, Illawarra Health and Medical Research Institute; 2016. http://www.projectairstrategy.org
20. Hoffman PD, Fruzzetti AE, Buteau E, Neiditch ER, Penney D, Bruce ML, et al. Family connections: a program for relatives of persons with borderline personality disorder. Fam Process. 2005;44(2):217–25. https://doi.org/10.1111/j.1545-5300.2005.00055.x.
21. Hoffman PD, Fruzzetti AE, Buteau E. Understanding and engaging families: an education, skills and support program for relatives impacted by borderline personality disorder. J Ment Health. 2007;16(1):69–82. https://doi.org/10.1080/09638230601182052.
22. Pearce J, Jovev M, Hulbert C, McKechnie B, McCutcheon L, Betts J, et al. Evaluation of a psychoeducational group intervention for family and friends of youth with borderline personality disorder. Borderline Personal Disord Emot Dysregul. 2017;4(1):1–7. https://doi.org/10.1186/s40479-017-0056-6.
23. Betts J, Pearce J, McKechnie B, McCutcheon L, Cotton SM, Jovev M, et al. A psychoeducational group intervention for family and friends of youth with borderline personality disorder features: protocol for a randomised controlled trial. Borderline Personal Disord Emot Dysregul. 2018;5:1–7. https://doi.org/10.1186/s40479-018-0090-z.
24. Pitschel-Walz G, Spatzl A, Rentrop M. Psychoeducational groups for close relatives of patients with borderline personality disorder. Eur Arch Psychiatry Clin Neurosci. 2023;273(4):853–64. https://doi.org/10.1007/s00406-022-01395-8.
25. Leichsenring F, Heim N, Leweke F, Spitzer C, Steinert C, Kernberg OF. Borderline Personality Disorder: A Review. JAMA. 2023;329(8):670–9. https://doi.org/10.1001/jama.2023.0589.
26. Bohus M, Stoffers-Winterling J, Sharp C, Krause-Utz A, Schmahl C, Lieb K. Borderline personality disorder. Lancet. 2021;398(10310):1528–40. https://doi.org/10.1016/S0140-6736(21)00476-1.

27. Paris J. Why psychiatrists are reluctant to diagnose: borderline personality disorder. Psychiatry. 2007;4(1):35.
28. American Psychiatric Association. Diagnostic and statistical manual of mental disorders: DSM-5. Washington, DC: American Psychiatric Association; 2013.
29. Akiskal HS. The bipolar spectrum—the shaping of a new paradigm in psychiatry. Curr Psychiatry Rep. 2002;4(1):1–3. https://doi.org/10.1007/s11920-002-0001-1.
30. Paris J. The treatment of borderline personality disorder: implications of research on diagnosis, etiology, and outcome. Annu Rev Clin Psychol. 2009;5:277–90. https://doi.org/10.1146/annurev.clinpsy.032408.153457.
31. Chanen AM. Borderline personality disorder in young people: are we there yet? J Clin Psychol. 2015;71(8):778–91. https://doi.org/10.1002/jclp.22205.
32. Zanarini MC, Frankenburg FR, Hennen J, Reich DB, Silk KR. Prediction of the 10-year course of borderline personality disorder. Am J Psychiatry. 2006;163(5):827–32. https://doi.org/10.1176/ajp.2006.163.5.827.
33. Skodol AE, Gunderson JG, Shea MT, McGlashan TH, Morey LC, Sanislow CA, et al. The collaborative longitudinal personality disorders study (CLPS): overview and implications. J Pers Disord. 2005;19(5):487–504. https://doi.org/10.1521/pedi.2005.19.5.487.
34. Zanarini MC, Frankenburg FR, Reich DB, Fitzmaurice G. Time to attainment of recovery from borderline personality disorder and stability of recovery: a 10-year prospective follow-up study. Am J Psychiatry. 2010;167(6):663–7. https://doi.org/10.1176/appi.ajp.2009.09081130.
35. Biskin RS. The lifetime course of borderline personality disorder. Can J Psychiatry. 2015;60(7):303–8. https://doi.org/10.1177/0706743715060007.
36. Gunderson JG, Stout RL, McGlashan TH, Shea MT, Morey LC, Grilo CM, et al. Ten-year course of borderline personality disorder: psychopathology and function from the Collaborative Longitudinal Personality Disorders study. Arch Gen Psychiatry. 2011;68(8):827–37. https://doi.org/10.1001/archgenpsychiatry.2011.37.
37. American Psychiatric Association. Practice guideline for the treatment of patients with borderline personality disorder. American Psychiatric Association Publishing; 2010.
38. Project Air Strategy for Personality Disorders. Treatment guidelines for personality disorders. 2nd ed. Wollongong: University of Wollongong, Illawarra Health and Medical Research Institute; 2015. http://www.projectairstrategy.org
39. Barnicot K, Katsakou C, Marougka S, Priebe S. Treatment completion in psychotherapy for borderline personality disorder–a systematic review and meta-analysis. Acta Psychiatr Scand. 2011;123(5):327–38. https://doi.org/10.1111/j.1600-0447.2010.01652.x.
40. De Panfilis C, Marchesi C, Cabrino C, Monici A, Politi V, Rossi M, et al. Patient factors predicting early dropout from psychiatric outpatient care for borderline personality disorder. Psychiatry Res. 2012;200(2–3):422–9. https://doi.org/10.1016/j.psychres.2012.03.016.
41. Rentrop M, Reicherzer M, Bäuml J. Psychoedukation Borderline-Störung Manual zur Leitung von Patienten- und Angehörigengruppen. München: Urban & Fischer; 2007.
42. Linehan MM. Cognitive-behavioral treatment of borderline personality disorder. New York: Guilford; 1993.
43. Colom F. Keeping therapies simple: psychoeducation in the prevention of relapse in affective disorders. Br J Psychiatry. 2011;198(5):338–40. https://doi.org/10.1192/bjp.bp.110.090209.
44. King-Casas B, Sharp C, Lomax-Bream L, Lohrenz T, Fonagy P, Montague PR. The rupture and repair of cooperation in borderline personality disorder. Science. 2008;321(5890):806–10. https://doi.org/10.1126/science.1156902.
45. Unoka Z, Seres I, Áspán N, Bódi N, Kéri S. Trust game reveals restricted interpersonal transactions in patients with borderline personality disorder. J Personal Disord. 2009;23(4):399–409. https://doi.org/10.1521/pedi.2009.23.4.399.
46. Domsalla M, Koppe G, Niedtfeld I, Vollstädt-Klein S, Schmahl C, Bohus M, et al. Cerebral processing of social rejection in patients with borderline personality disorder. Soc Cogn Affect Neurosci. 2013;9(11):1789–97. https://doi.org/10.1093/scan/nst176.

47. De Panfilis C, Riva P, Preti E, Cabrino C, Marchesi C. When social inclusion is not enough: implicit expectations of extreme inclusion in borderline personality disorder. Pers Disord Theory Res Treat. 2015;6(4):301–9. https://doi.org/10.1037/per0000132.
48. Weinbrecht A, Niedeggen M, Roepke S, Renneberg B. Feeling excluded no matter what? Bias in the processing of social participation in borderline personality disorder. NeuroImage: Clin. 2018;19:343–50. https://doi.org/10.1016/j.nicl.2018.04.031.
49. Liebke L, Koppe G, Bungert M, Thome J, Hauschild S, Defiebre N. Difficulties with being socially accepted: an experimental study in borderline personality disorder. J Abnorm Psychol. 2018;127(7):670–82. https://doi.org/10.1037/abn0000373.
50. De Panfilis C, Schito G, Generali I, Gozzi LA, Ossola P, Marchesi C, et al. Emotions at the border: increased punishment behavior during fair interpersonal exchanges in borderline personality disorder. J Abnorm Psychol. 2019;128(2):162–72. https://doi.org/10.1037/abn0000404.
51. Gerra ML, Ardizzi M, Martorana S, Leoni V, Riva P, Preti E, et al. Autonomic vulnerability to biased perception of social inclusion in borderline personality disorder. Borderline Personal Disorder Emotion Dysregul. 2021;8(1):1–14. https://doi.org/10.1186/s40479-021-00169-3.
52. Yeomans F. Myths surrounding borderline personality disorder. 2013. https://www.youtube.com/watch?v=KvNoQDqwrc4. Accessed 30 Dec 2023.
53. Schneider K. Clinical psychopathology. Grune & Stratton; 1959.
54. Skodol AE, Morey LC, Bender DS, Oldham JM. The alternative DSM-5 model for personality disorders: a clinical application. Am J Psychiatry. 2015;172(7):606–13. https://doi.org/10.1176/appi.ajp.2015.14101220.
55. Yeomans FE, Clarkin J, Kernberg OK. Transference-focused psychotherapy for borderline personality disorder: a clinical guide. Arlington: American Psychiatric Publishing; 2015.
56. Yeomans F. What is personality (and personality disorder)? W/ narcissism example. 2019. https://www.youtube.com/watch?v=bM11wlL25-c. Accessed 30 Dec 2023.
57. Yeomans F. Understanding the BPD Mind. 2010. https://www.youtube.com/watch?v=B_%2D%2DSCmZ9Fc. Accessed 30 Dec 2023.
58. Paris J. Clinical features of borderline personality disorder. In: Livesley WJ, Larstone R, editors. Handbook of personality disorders: theory, research, and treatment. 2nd ed. The Guilford Press; 2018. p. (2)419.
59. Santangelo P, Reinhard I, Mussgay L, Steil R, Sawitzki G, Klein C, et al. Specificity of affective instability in patients with borderline personality disorder compared to posttraumatic stress disorder, bulimia nervosa, and healthy controls. J Abnorm Psychol. 2014;123(1):258. https://doi.org/10.1037/a0035619.
60. Zanarini MC, Frankenburg FR, Wedig MM, Fitzmaurice GM. Cognitive experiences reported by patients with borderline personality disorder and axis II comparison subjects: a 16-year prospective follow-up study. Am J Psychiatry. 2013;170(6):671–9. https://doi.org/10.1176/appi.ajp.2013.13010055.
61. Stern A. Psychoanalytic investigation and therapy in the borderline group of neuroses. Psychoanal Q. 1938;7(4):467–89. https://doi.org/10.1080/21674086.1938.11925367.
62. Paris J. Treatment of borderline personality disorder: a guide to evidence-based practice. The Guilford Press; 2008.
63. Sheehan L, Nieweglowski K, Corrigan P. The stigma of personality disorders. Curr Psychiatry Rep. 2016;18:1–7. https://doi.org/10.1007/s11920-015-0654-1.
64. Levy KN, Johnson BN, Clouthier TL, Scala J, Temes CM. An attachment theoretical framework for personality disorders. Can Psychol. 2015;56(2):197. https://doi.org/10.1037/cap0000025.
65. Bandelow B, Krause J, Wedekind D, Broocks A, Hajak G, Rüther E. Early traumatic life events, parental attitudes, family history, and birth risk factors in patients with borderline personality disorder and healthy controls. Psychiatry Res. 2005;134(2):169–79. https://doi.org/10.1016/j.psychres.2003.07.008.
66. Gunderson JG. Borderline personality disorder: a clinical guide. Washington, DC: American Psychiatric Press; 2001.
67. Yeomans F. BPD, trauma & integrating your own aggression. 2019. https://www.youtube.com/watch?v=hlANA7Ekwv0. Accessed 30 Dec 2023.

68. Yeomans F. ‘Fighting BPD stigma’ a little too hard. 2019. https://www.youtube.com/watch?v=EZvAbog3psY. Accessed 30 Dec 2023.
69. Skodol AE, Gunderson JG, Pfohl B, Widiger TA, Livesley WJ, Siever LJ. The borderline diagnosis I: psychopathology, comorbidity, and personality structure. Biol Psychiatry. 2002;51(12):936–50.
70. National Collaborating Centre for Mental Health. Borderline personality disorder: treatment and management. National Institute for Health and Clinical Excellence: Guidelines. Leicester: British Psychological Society; 2009.
71. National Health and Medical Research Council. Clinical practice guidelines for the management of borderline personality disorder. Melbourne: National Health and Medical Research Council; 2012.
72. Herpertz SC, Zanarini M, Schulz CS, Siever L, Lieb K, Möller HJ, et al. World Federation of Societies of Biological Psychiatry (WFSBP) guidelines for biological treatment of personality disorders. World J Biol Psychiatry. 2007;8(4):212–44. https://doi.org/10.1080/15622970701685224.
73. Simonsen S, Bateman A, Bohus M, Dalewijk HJ, Doering S, Kaera A, et al. European guidelines for personality disorders: past, present and future. Borderline Personal Disord Emot Dysregul. 2019;6(1):1–10. https://doi.org/10.1186/s40479-019-0106-3.
74. Bridler R, Häberle A, Müller ST, Cattapan K, Grohmann R, Toto S, et al. Psychopharmacological treatment of 2195 in-patients with borderline personality disorder: a comparison with other psychiatric disorders. Eur Neuropsychopharmacol. 2015;25(6):763–72. https://doi.org/10.1016/j.euroneuro.2015.03.017.
75. Starcevic V, Janca A. Pharmacotherapy of borderline personality disorder: replacing confusion with prudent pragmatism. Curr Opin Psychiatry. 2018;31(1):69–73. https://doi.org/10.1097/YCO.0000000000000373.
76. Stoffers-Winterling JM, Storebø OJ, Ribeiro JP, Kongerslev MT, Völlm BA, Mattivi JT, et al. Pharmacological interventions for people with borderline personality disorder. Cochrane Database Syst Rev. 2022;11 https://doi.org/10.1002/14651858.CD012956.pub2.
77. Stoffers J, Völlm BA, Rücker G, Timmer A, Huband N, Lieb K. Pharmacological interventions for borderline personality disorder. Cochrane Database Syst Rev. 2010:6. https://doi.org/10.1002/14651858.CD005653.pub2.
78. Fineberg SK, Gupta S, Leavitt J. Collaborative deprescribing in borderline personality disorder: a narrative review. Harv Rev Psychiatry. 2019;27(2):75–86. https://doi.org/10.1097/HRP.0000000000000200.
79. Stoffers-Winterling JM, Storebø OJ, Kongerslev MT, Faltinsen E, Todorovac A, Jørgensen MS, et al. Psychotherapies for borderline personality disorder: a focused systematic review and meta-analysis. Br J Psychiatry. 2022:1–15. https://doi.org/10.1192/bjp.2021.204.
80. Bateman AW, Fonagy P. Psychotherapy for borderline personality disorder: mentalization based treatment. Oxford: Oxford University Press; 2004.
81. Bateman AW, Fonagy P. Mentalization based treatment for borderline personality disorder: a practical guide. Oxford: Oxford University Press; 2006.
82. Kernberg OF. Severe personality disorders: psychotherapeutic strategies. New Haven: Yale University Press; 1984.
83. Young JE. Cognitive therapy for personality disorders: a schema-focused approach. Sarasota: Professional Resource Press; 1999.
84. Blum N, Pfohl B, John DS, Monahan P, Black DW. STEPPS: a cognitive-behavioral systems-based group treatment for outpatients with borderline personality disorder—a preliminary report. Compr Psychiatry. 2002;43(4):301–10. https://doi.org/10.1053/comp.2002.33497.
85. Gunderson JG. Handbook of good psychiatric management for borderline personality disorder. American Psychiatric Publishing; 2014.
86. Weinberg I, Ronningstam E, Goldblatt MJ, Schechter M, Maltsberger JT. Common factors in empirically supported treatments of borderline personality disorder. Curr Psychiatry Rep. 2011;13:60–8. https://doi.org/10.1007/s11920-010-0167-x.

87. Beatson J, Rao S. Psychotherapy for borderline personality disorder. Australas Psychiatry. 2014;22(6):529–32. https://doi.org/10.1177/1039856214555531.
88. Levy KN, Clarkin JF, Yeomans FE, Scott LN, Wasserman RH, Kernberg OF. The mechanisms of change in the treatment of borderline personality disorder with transference focused psychotherapy. J Clin Psychol. 2006;62(4):481–501. https://doi.org/10.1002/jclp.20239.
89. Doering S, Hörz S, Rentrop M, Fischer-Kern M, Schuster P, Benecke C, et al. Transference-focused psychotherapy versus treatment by community psychotherapists for borderline personality disorder: randomised controlled trial. Br J Psychiatry. 2010;196:389–95. https://doi.org/10.1192/bjp.bp.109.070177.
90. Fischer-Kern M, Doering S, Taubner S, Hörz S, Zimmermann J, Rentrop M, et al. Transference-focused psychotherapy for borderline personality disorder: change in reflective function. Br J Psychiatry. 2015;207:173–4. https://doi.org/10.1192/bjp.bp.113.143842.
91. Buchheim A, Hörz-Sagstetter S, Doering S, Rentrop M, Schuster P, Buchheim P, et al. Change of unresolved attachment in borderline personality disorder: RCT study of transference focused psychotherapy. Psychother Psychosom. 2017;86:314–6. https://doi.org/10.1159/000460257.
92. Sansone RA. Chronic suicidality and borderline personality. J Pers Disord. 2004;18(3):215–25. https://doi.org/10.1521/pedi.18.3.215.35444.

Part II

Transference-Focused Psychotherapy (TFP) Principles in Specific Mental Health Treatment Settings

Transference-Focused Psychotherapy (TFP) Informed Care within an Outpatient Community-Based Multi-professional Psychiatric Service

4

Chiara De Panfilis, Paolo Ampollini, Giulia Ciccone, Francesca Palombi, and Sergio Dazzi

Introduction

Patients with personality disorders (PD) pose unique challenges to the Italian psychiatric services, which are mainly tailored to the care of psychotic disorders. The goal of this chapter is to illustrate how multi-professional mental health teams working in Italian community-based outpatient psychiatric services can successfully learn and apply Transference-Focused Psychotherapy (TFP) principles in a coherent fashion to improve their standard of care of patients with PD.

Who Are the Clinicians?

Within the Italian National Health Service (INHS) psychiatric care for all citizens, including patients with PD, is provided by local, community-based Departments of Mental Health (DMH), which are in charge of planning and coordinating all mental

C. De Panfilis (✉)
Department of Medicine and Surgery, Unit of Neuroscience, University of Parma, Parma, Italy

Department of Mental Health, Parma Local Health Agency, Parma, Italy

Personality Disorders Lab, Parma, Italy
e-mail: chiara.depanfilis@unipr.it

P. Ampollini · F. Palombi
Department of Mental Health, Parma Local Health Agency, Parma, Italy
e-mail: pampollini@ausl.pr.it; fpalombi@ausl.pr.it

G. Ciccone
Department of Mental Health, Modena Local Health Agency, Modena, Italy
e-mail: g.ciccone@ausl.mo.it

S. Dazzi
Personality Disorders Lab, Parma, Italy
e-mail: sdazzi@dazzistudio.it

R. G. Hersh, C. De Panfilis (eds.), *Implementing Transference-Focused Psychotherapy Principles*, https://doi.org/10.1007/978-3-031-68062-5_4

health interventions provided to patients from a defined province or catchment area. At the outpatient level, aside from clinical psychiatric management, the DMH offers, when appropriate, different types of services provided by multidisciplinary teams (composed of child-adolescent and adult psychiatrists, psychologists, psychotherapists, nurses, social workers, educators, and personnel with specific training in psychosocial rehabilitation), which are articulated in an individually tailored, ongoing treatment plan. Partial or full-time psychiatric hospitalization can also be prescribed when considered clinically necessary; however, special emphasis is given to treating patients within their local community and specific milieu, on an outpatient basis, to prevent unnecessary hospital admissions and promote psychosocial rehabilitation [1]. When necessary, considerable efforts are directed toward ensuring smooth access to outpatient psychiatric care and integration in the local community for patients who may find it difficult to do that without any assistance, due to the deteriorating course of their illness. Examples include the full-day availability of the community psychiatric services, even in case of emergency; the direct delivery of medications to the patients by the DMH; the assignment of a dedicated psychiatric nurse to the patients to assist them in daily activities and foster treatment compliance; and the possibility of home visits by the mental health team; and the provision of sheltered jobs and financial and housing support.

The applied TFP initiative described in this chapter takes place in an outpatient community district of the DMH of the Province of Parma, Italy (Valli Taro e Ceno District). This district of the DMH comprises an adult mental health center (MHC), a child and adolescent psychiatry unit (CAPU), and service for pathological dependences (SerPD), including substance use, gambling, and other disorders. All three outpatient units are composed of distinct multidisciplinary teams that practice close collaboration. The collaboration among these teams ensures continuity of care, as with those adolescent patients moving into adulthood thus requiring different services, as well as coordination of care, as would be necessary for patients with co-occurring psychiatric and substance use disorders. Importantly, the various teams also include psychotherapists of various theoretical orientations and backgrounds (i.e., cognitive-behavioral, systemic, psychodynamic).

Who Are the Patients?

PD patients attending the Italian public psychiatric services are usually those regarded as suffering from severe personality disorder (SPD). The Valli Taro e Ceno mental health district is located in Emilia-Romagna, an Italian region that implemented regional "recommendation" guidance, largely drawn from the 2009 British National Institute for Health & Clinical Excellence (NICE) guidelines for Borderline PD (BPD) [2], to ameliorate the public, INHS-based standard of care for SPD (Linee di indirizzo RER per il trattamento dei Disturbi Gravi di Personalità, 2013) [3]. According to such guidance, SPD are defined as "conditions of psychiatric interest characterized by altered functioning in the areas of identity, self formation and stability, which manifest along the dimensions of impulsivity and antagonism.

These disorders particularly show impairments in interpersonal relationships and global functioning, causing a significant reduction in the individuals' capacity to adapt to their social role." [3]. This definition captures a patient population that, in object relations theory (ORT) terms, belongs to low-level borderline personality organization [4] and, in DSM terms, to Cluster B PD (with the exclusion of Antisocial PD). Comorbidity with other psychiatric disorders is usually the norm — as well as the main reason why these patients seek treatment. Comorbid conditions include mood disorders, substance use disorders, adjustment disorders, conduct disorders in adolescence, eating disorders, and a variety of social, vocational, and relational issues that pose unique challenges to the clinical and social systems of care.

Indeed, the international literature points out that SPD patients are common in mental-health settings [5], and tend to have a more complicated presentation, requiring higher levels of staff attention and resources, and more extensive risk assessment than do patients without PD [6]. Furthermore, SPDs are notoriously difficult to treat in standard, community-based mental-health settings [7]. With specific regard to the Italian context, research showed that PD patients are more likely to drop-out of psychiatric services, as opposed to, for instance, patients with psychotic disorders who exhibit high rates of treatment retention [8]. Among patients with BPD early drop-out rates from treatment (i.e., within 3 months) are as high as 33%, and early drop-out is particularly prevalent among patients with severe clinical presentations, as reflected by a prior history of suicide attempts [9]. Furthermore, a naturalistic 2-year follow-up on BPD patients attending public outpatient Italian psychiatric services found that 2-year remission rates for BPD were lower than those found among North American samples [10]. Finally, a recent multi-center Italian study showed that more experienced mental health team members report less caring attitudes toward BPD patients than unexperienced ones, especially in the absence of specific training for PD [11].

Taken together, on the one hand, these data indicate that the Italian psychiatric services are particularly committed to tackling the needs of patients with psychotic disorders. Indeed, the DMH were implemented after the 1978 reform law, which closed psychiatric hospitals offering long-term inpatient treatment to promote optimal community care and social rehabilitation for this severe patient population [1, 8]. On the other hand, this "disability model" of psychiatric illnesses on which the Italian psychiatric services were grounded might be detrimental when applied to the care of patients with PD, who might indeed show difficulties and limitations that can interfere with their psychosocial adjustment and behavior, but these limitations nonetheless do not prevent them from changing their behavior or learning how to do that. Thus, PD treatment requires a major modification of the traditional medical/psychiatric model of care [12].

What Is the Contemporary Standard of Care for Clinicians Treating These Patients?

The Emilia-Romagna regional guidance for SPD (2013) [3] was implemented to address the above-mentioned difficulties endorsed by mental health services in the treatment of patients with SPD. The overarching strategy was to encourage a shift from a treatment modality grounded on a disability model of pathology, to a modality that emphasizes (1) the active participation of patients in the search of solutions for their difficulties, even in crisis situations, (2) the ability of SPD patients to reflect upon potential choice options and their consequences, and (3) a clear and collaborative articulation of realistic short-term treatment goals, consistent with long-term ones, to show SPD patients that change is indeed possible, although it may take some time to occur.

For this aim, the guidance recommended the DMH provide SPD patients with a structured treatment, including a treatment contract and evidence-based psychotherapy interventions (i.e., dialectical behavior therapy (DBT), schema focused therapy (SFT), or TFP). Thus, starting in 2013 every local DMH in the Emilia-Romagna region promoted staff attendance to dedicated training programs aimed at spreading the contents of the regional guidance to all mental health professionals, and at implementing SPD treatment along these lines.

Specifically, the outpatient community mental health units of Valli Taro e Ceno District went through extensive regional training that lasted about 3 years (from 2014 to 2016) in order to: (a) create a district work group specialized in SPD management, (b) develop a specific and integrated care pathway for SPD inspired to the regional recommendations and based on the DBT treatment model, and (c) get full training in DBT for the psychologist of the team and a basic DBT Skills Training for all mental health workers composing the team.

Once the specific care pathway for SPD was released and fully operational, the mental health team professionals tried to approach SPD patients following the regional recommendations. Very soon, however, many relational issues emerged, either between practitioners and patients, or among the team members, or among different team units (i.e., the MHC, the CAPU and the SerPD units). What became clear was that the defense mechanisms used routinely by the patients (i.e., splitting, projective identification) were somehow "transferred" to the treatment team, and the team members began to act in often contrary and confusing ways (alternating caring/distancing or warm/cold attitudes) toward the patients, thus generating incoherent responses and team fragmentation. This might reflect the consequence of different training pathways of the various team members, different organization histories across the three diverse units, or the lack of an agreement upon a unique theoretical model of SPD psychopathology.

Thus, in spite of the introduction of some evidence-based interventions into the treatment plan of SPD patients (i.e., individual DBT provided by the team psychotherapist, and skills-training groups provided by other staff members), the team as a whole still lacked the necessary skills to implement a coherent and effective treatment. As Bateman and Tyrer (2004) pointed out [13], within community-based psychiatric services for PD all members must be able to communicate effectively, to get on well together, and to be clear about treatment boundaries and goals. This can be accomplished by systematically addressing the inconsistencies arising from splitting within teams. Notably, splitting is a representation of SPD patients' inner processes. Therefore, identifying the inner, unconscious mechanisms underlying SPD patients' chaotic behavior is necessary to promote coordinated treatment responses by all team members. Of note, this task is not solely a task for the psychotherapist, but for all staff, in line with a skills-shared model of care, where all members share the same view about PD pathology and each member is informed about the skills of other members, at least at a basic level [13].

What Are the Goals for Imparting to These Clinicians the Principles of TFP for Working with These Patients?

General Goals

To overcome the difficulties described above, the team members of the mental health outpatients' services of Valli Taro e Ceno district decided to initiate a specific TFP training/supervision program, with a certified TFP teacher and supervisor, in order to reach the main goals of (1) sharing a common model of the SPD pathology, informed by ORT and by TFP principles, within the whole team and (2) enabling all team professionals, regardless of their role, to recognize and share with other members which representation of the self and of the other the patient was enacting and which affect was involved in the relationship. Thus, the request to the TFP teacher and supervisor was *not* to train TFP therapists in order to perform standard TFP within the outpatient psychiatric service; rather, the request was to train all staff members in TFP principles to provide a coherent, TFP-oriented psychiatric management of SPD patients, which could also be integrated with other already existing interventions in the service (e.g., DBT interventions).

The team's other expectations following completion of the training/supervision program were to achieve: (a) a shared understanding of the clinical process of change, (b) a coherent fashion to respond to patients' communications, (c) a reduction of conflicts among team members as a result of an increased ability to recognize countertransference reactions, and (d) an increased ability to promote the integration of patients' split-off parts. These achievements, in turn, were expected to facilitate the relationships between team members and the patients as well as to promote, among SPD patients, a successful management of emotions and behaviors, an enhanced therapeutic alliance in rehabilitation and therapeutic programs, an improvement in social and intimate relationships and in working abilities, and finally an increased ability to acknowledge and contain emotional states without acting them out.

Specific Goals

This applied TFP initiative also included multiple, more specific goals.

- At the most superficial level, the aim was, through teaching, to change the global therapeutic vision of the psychiatric services staff, namely from "curing" to "treating". Generally speaking, in the usual clinical practice of the DMH work with patients with SPD there had been a risk that clinicians involved would enter into a process in which treatment is open-ended (chronic and endless) and devoid of specific goals related to personality change in the middle and long term. The ultimate goal, for these patients, of improving adaptation and fostering a more mature capacity to stay in intimate and social relations had remained implicit only, and therefore not meaningfully defined through intermediate treatment goals. In doing so, treatment would drift from lessening the level of involvement in periods of symptomatic quietness to an increasing activation —in terms of work hours and of number of staff members involved—in periods of crisis and acute impairment. TFP principles bring to the fore the dimension of "treatment through understanding" as opposed to "cure." In the TFP-oriented approach described here, the staff sets up, on the basis of the initial patient's evaluation, specific treatment goals in the short or middle term. The treatment is planned to come to a conclusion, be it positive or negative. In either case the TFP-oriented treatment ends, but that does not necessarily mean that the patient will then be discharged by the DMH. Rather, a treatment other than the TFP-oriented one can begin, which may be more supportive in nature or oriented specifically to foster social rehabilitation. This new treatment phase will be built on the evaluation of the failures or difficulties of the preceding one, with a new contract and a new definition of goals. This procedure aims at fostering the persistent "structuring" of treatment, although the more ambitious goals of the TFP-oriented approach may not be the focus of therapy anymore.
- The above-described aim needed to be supported by a deeper level of teaching that, consistent with TFP principles, involves a full assessment of the level of personality organization. This is accomplished by using the structural interview (SI) [14] provided by an expert clinician or by the structured interview of personality organization (STIPO) [15]. The SI focuses on assessment of identity formation, along with the associated domains of defensive operations, and reality testing, to characterize personality as organized at normal-neurotic versus borderline level of personality organization. Further refinement of the diagnosis along the spectrum of severity is provided by the assessment of the quality of object relations, moral functioning, aggression and affect integration. Importantly, in this interview, Kernberg connected the present functioning of the patient with the interaction of the patient with the interviewer. The SI follows a predetermined order, but the interviewer can pursue material as it emerges in the patient's self-representation and responses to the interviewer. Thus, the SI represents a cyclical process in which the interviewer is given the flexibility to return to important, perhaps contradictory elements, in order to delineate an increasingly

in-depth picture of the patient's internal and external functioning. For example, the interviewer could return to previously stated aspects in the description of a person that contradict the present description ("I notice that you are describing your partner in very negative words, but before you said he was the best partner you could imagine – how does that fit together?") [16]. As such, the SI is a sophisticated and valuable clinical tool to evaluate the level of personality organization. However, it relies on the interviewer's clinical judgment and inference to follow the patient's lead, thus requiring high clinical experience and familiarity with ORT. In addition, because the interview does not provide a structured sequence of questions, even with more experienced interviewers coverage of symptoms and domains of functioning might be uneven among interviewers, leading to varying levels of interrater reliability across settings and studies [16]. To overcome these limitations, Clarkin and colleagues (2004) developed the STIPO, a semi-structured version of the SI that allows a more rigorously standardized approach to structural assessment that is accessible to less experienced interviewers [15]. Similar to the SI, The STIPO and its revised, shorter version (STIPO-R) [17] evaluate patient's functioning across several domains, i.e., identity, object relations, defenses, aggression, and moral values. In doing so, however, the STIPO and STIPO-R provide standard questions, follow-up probes, and scoring guidelines to ensure a reliable assessment of the level of personality organization.

The use of such interviews is of paramount importance in the clinical practice of the DMH. A thorough evaluation, including a detailed personal history as well as the assessment of the level of functioning, when needed, of the social environment of the patient, will inform the definition of goals and of those aspects of the contract that stir up the prominent conflictual aspects in the patient. Importantly, the diagnostic evaluation needs to be shared with all team members.

– At an even deeper level, teaching TFP principles aimed at providing the mental health staff tools for understanding the patient's structural functioning and object relations. Staff members needed to acquire the capacity to maintain a therapeutic relationship with patients informed by the principles of contemporary ORT; familiarity with these concepts could not be taken for granted. Introducing TFP principles to the psychiatric services team meant proposing the acquisition of a completely new style of work, based on a new theory, rather than the accruing of a new tool in an already familiar way of collecting clinical data and planning a way to proceed. A view of personality pathology rooted in identity diffusion [4, 18] and related clinical phenomena and symptoms would undoubtedly compel staff members to move from a dominant view based on social adaptation and descriptive symptoms to one informed by observing interpersonal interactions. Thus, teaching TFP principles has implied inviting the staff to move from a stance aimed at changing a patient's dysfunctional behavior (basically a reactive, directive approach), to one based on a shared exploration with the patients of their difficulties. This shared exploration, i.e., thinking together with the patient about "what is going on" in the here-and-now of the treatment relationship, can provide a foundation for promoting meaningful change over time.

What Is the Source of Institutional or Government Support for This Initiative?

The TFP-informed training/supervision program of Valli Taro e Ceno mental health district was implemented under the institutional and financial support of the Province of Parma DMH, as part of the development of an integrated care pathway for SPD inspired by the regional guidance. At the regional level, most of the education initiatives that had been developed following the publication of the guidance focused on DBT, which was initially deemed the easiest to learn and to disseminate among the various evidence-based therapies for SPD. Importantly, however, the request for additional training on the conceptual model of ORT and TFP principles was a "bottom-up" initiative of staff members of the Valli Taro e Ceno District, who were not satisfied with their skills in dealing with splitting and relational issues, and were concerned about their inconsistent treatment responses to patients with SPD. This led them to request specific training and supervision aimed at overcoming these particular difficulties. The initiative was facilitated by the presence, at the local level, of certified TFP teachers and supervisors belonging to the Personality Disorders Lab, an association affiliated with the International Society for transference-focused psychotherapy (ISTFP).

What TFP Principles Might Be of Utility for The Clinicians Working with These Patients?

In this initiative, the teaching of TFP principles was informed by the level of clinical expertise of the staff, with efforts made to present the material using accessible and straightforward language.

In teaching the applied TFP model proposed here, it is useful to introduce TFP principles utilizing the framework provided by Gunderson's Good Psychiatric Management (GPM) for BPD [19].

GPM, considered a "generalist approach model for treating BPD," is a theoretically eclectic approach, an amalgam of psychodynamic, behavioral, and case management interventions. It pragmatically prioritizes what works to help patients get a life, an aspect that granted GPM a clear public health mission. TFP and GPM share some key elements —active therapist, open discussion of diagnosis, psychoeducation for patient and family, and a focus on meaningful activity (work, studies, social and creative life), among others. However, their approaches are clearly different [20]. For instance, while GPM was developed to provide various clinicians with a basic intervention approach toward BPD in particular, TFP also targets a broader spectrum of patients with PD pathology —namely, those showing a borderline personality organization. In addition, the goal of GPM is to provide a "good enough" treatment for patients with BPD, with the expectation that most of them will get better over time and with keen attention toward avoiding the risk of iatrogenically induced problems, possibly fostered by an excess of ineffective treatments. Conversely, TFP is a more purely psychodynamic intervention that focuses on the patient's experience of the treatment; at the same time, however, it pays extensive attention to the patients' functioning, in all spheres, outside the treatment. In addition, the basic tenet of GPM is to impart to the patient an appreciation of the role of interpersonal hypersensitivity as an underpinning for a variety of maladaptive behaviors and to do so with guidance, direction, and support. TFP rests on a more complex theoretical and psychodynamic background of pathological functioning. In TFP, the explicit goal is to help the patient move from a level of personality functioning characterized by splitting and identity diffusion to one characterized by identity integration. This goal is pursued through examining the constant splitting of thoughts, actions, and feelings enacted by the patients in their relationships with others and, particularly, with the therapist [20].

However, both GPM and TFP emphasize the need to extensively discuss with patients to define their own goals for treatment. Furthermore, both approaches are interested in clarifying the nature of change and the nature of the therapeutic approach in the treatment of personality pathology.

- First, in the TFP-applied initiative described in this chapter, TFP teaching described a theory about the nature of change for patients with SPD:
  1. *The nature of the pathology* is in the realm of "acting instead of thinking." The first step in introducing the TFP-informed treatment paradigm begins with teaching how acting is a defense against thinking in the patient with SPD. At the same time, it is stressed that for the staff, acting in place of exploration must be limited and, more importantly, must be considered a hindrance to change rather than a tool to provide change. With this aim, the clinical utilization of the first steps of TFP strategies [21] is introduced, namely understanding dyads, naming the actors, and tolerating the confusion. The focus of teaching stresses the validity and relevance of this process given the profound resistance among staff members to considering that "thinking about what is going on" is "real work," as their usual practice prioritized solving patients' problems as the only way to meet their needs (i.e., a "reactive" stance), while exploration of motivations ("proactive" stance) is experienced as a painful waste of time.
  2. *Exploration versus adaptation*: The challenges faced by patients with SPD can be approached with different overarching theoretical orientations. An approach stressing adaptation would promote support for the SPD patient's accommodation to chronically impaired functioning and limitation in autonomy. Within the community-based Italian psychiatric services, which often have to deal with a socially disadvantaged and severely ill population, this contributes to a prevailing view of "rehabilitation" as a key element of adaptation; this view has significant influence on the clinical attitude of the mental health staff. In contrast, TFP stresses active exploration. Implementing TFP [21] rests on basic concepts including the use of the treatment contract, limit

setting, and an expectation for an acceptable level of social productivity ensured by the meaningful activity requirement. Within this context, familiarity with TFP principles clarifies that the psychopathological core of SPD reveals itself in the socio-relational dimensions of life, and that successful adaptation can be achieved only by exploring and addressing SPD psychopathology.
3. *Corrective experiencing versus experiencing and understanding*. In the spirit of GPM [19], some sort of new (or corrective) emotional experience is essential for a good outcome and must be provided by a reliable, consistent, responsible, and flexible staff. In a TFP-oriented approach, this is made possible by the full exploration of the basic transference dispositions, or basic dyadic relationships invested with intense affective states of a positive (i.e., love) or negative (i.e., hate) nature, which are activated simultaneously toward different members of the staff. As a consequence, the clinicians' priority is the full understanding and clarification of these activations in the here-and-now. Only the persistent exploration and understanding of what has been activated in the ongoing exchange with a number of staff members, with different professional roles, offers the possibility for integrating the basic transference dispositions polarized around opposite affective states (i.e., love and hate). To put it simply, a good emotional experience is a prerequisite for changing, not a factor promoting change by itself.

- Second, TFP teaching describes the specific nature of the therapeutic approach:
  1. *The use of clarification* (a request for more detail when the patient's account is in any way unclear), and *confrontation* (a process of bringing to the patient's attention material or behaviors that are in some way contradictory) are critical interventions allowing the clinician to investigate how a patient organizes interactions with others in their world. The SPD patient will likely engage in repeated self-defeating or self-destructive behaviors that limit their flexibility in fundamental ways. As the patient better understands the pattern of reflexive responses in interpersonal situations, the less likely they will be condemned to repeat those maladaptive patterns that cause them distress.
  2. *Being active/not reactive versus being neutral*: the level of activity of the therapist is regarded as an important tool; specifically, TFP emphasizes the clinician's attitude of sustained curiosity about the patient's inner life and external reality. A major point is that the clinician's proactive stance can be consistent with a neutral and deliberate inquiry. As previously noted, the clinician using a TFP orientation will emphasize exploration over action, aiming not to correct the patient's reality, but rather encouraging reflection about how the patient perceives him/herself and others, with a focus on the dominant affective tone in evidence in relationships. In other words, staff members are encouraged to be curious about patient's external reality in order to help the patients to overcome the primitive, splitting-based defenses that lead them to act rather than to be curious and reflective about what's going on in their mind.
  3. *Being thoughtful:* While GPM stresses "thoughtfulness, reflectiveness and cautiousness", TFP would include these elements in the clinician's attitude

but also stress, through clarification and confrontation, the importance of the investigation of any vague and inconsistent aspects in the information shared by the patient. A major focus is the validation of the patient's viewpoint, through the process of "naming the actors," while at the same time tactfully identifying emerging contradictory dyads of an opposing nature. This process aims to stimulate the patient's reflection, rather than acting out their anxiety.

4. *Monitoring Countertransference:* TFP focuses on the clinician's appreciation of activated dyads; since staff members function as "participant observers," the concept of monitoring countertransference is of paramount importance. This intermingling of roles of participation and observation is particularly relevant in community-based psychiatric services, where many interactions take place outside a psychotherapy setting. Patients with SPD intuitively understand their impact on staff members and respond in kind to the staff members' response to that impact. The practitioners involved are keenly aware of their own subjective feelings (in "role responsiveness") to what has been projected and react in either a concordant or complementary way [22, 23]. Consequently, staff members need to be aware that their countertransference reactions require reflection, not reflexive action. Needless to say, this is the most delicate issue dealt with by the entire staff. This is what has been defined as the "regaining of patient authority" in the Austen Riggs model of treatment [24].
5. *To communicate that change is expected:* This TFP principle, also clearly delineated in GPM, is particularly difficult to implement within the Italian DMH standard of care. We previously referred to the distinction between "cure" and "treatment." In the former, we have observed that expectations for a "cure" can often lead to a treatment promising a general improvement but without any clear expectation for fundamental change. Conversely, the logic of "treatment" allows for expectations of change with more explicit markers. Importantly, longitudinal studies on PD course have pointed out that change and improvement are indeed possible [25–27]. Along this line, TFP includes expectations for change as a clinically evident dimension described in phases. Change does not only involve symptoms reduction but also implies an improvement in the capacity "to work and love", and foresees a structural change in personality organization. Therefore, TFP teaching is focused on the structural approach to SPD and on the step-by-step transition to a higher level of functioning (this will be described below).
6. *Accountability:* In GPM, the patients are held accountable for what they say and do, with a recognition that a patient's behavior, feelings, and thoughts have meaning and that the patient is capable of change over time. TFP adds to this perspective a focus on the patient's unconscious motivations, the idea the patient's behaviors, feelings, and thoughts might be impacted by motivations outside the patient's awareness. The goal of exploration rests on the expectation that bringing into the patient's awareness those elements can facilitate

meaningful change. By learning TFP concepts, the staff is introduced to this concept of unconscious motivation and internal conflicts, and to the potential benefit of exploring these phenomena from a position of technical neutrality.

7. *The attention on external reality:* All psychotherapeutic interventions for SPD require sustained attention to the patient's external reality. The application of TFP principles in the outpatient psychiatric care of Italian DMH rests on consideration of two critical concerns. The first concern is the well-recognized risk that patients' destructive behavior, acted out in their everyday life, threatens the outpatient treatment continuation within the DMH. The second concern relates to the risk that these aspects of the patient's psychopathology might be activated outside of the treatment milieu and, therefore, are not directly available for necessary exploration in the patient's interpersonal relations with staff members. The patient's destructive impulses, directly revealed to the treaters, or introduced only obliquely over time, are understood as useful subjects for investigation, as long as they do not fundamentally challenge the integrity of the treatment. Such destructive impulses are explored and contained, rather than becoming the subject of punitive responses.
8. *About being flexible, pragmatic, and eclectic:* Even in the context of a general psychiatric service, it is important to preserve the nature of the therapeutic attitude as described for standard TFP. The TFP-oriented clinician is not a coach, a counselor, or a crisis manager according to needs and circumstances. Rather, TFP-oriented clinicans try, as much as they can, to explore the meaning of behaviors, attitudes, and relationships. The contracting phase will aim at protecting neutrality, which will help the clinician to provide clarification and confrontation interventions. In the applied TFP initiative described here the maintenance of technical neutrality is even more challenging than in standard TFP, as attacks on the treatment contract will be notably strong and more frequent, particularly when the entire staff is involved and the patient's pathology is severe. It will be unavoidable, in some circumstances, with patients who behave and relate in a detached, withdrawn, or oppositional way, in the so-called out of contact mode [28, 29], that temporary suspension of the exploratory attitude will be required. Clinicians will be obliged to adjust to this circumstance for however long is necessary. The treatment will move back and forth between these two dimensions, maintaining technical neutrality and deviating from technical neutrality when necessary. The skillful clinician will accept that an exploratory attitude may not always be applicable and only a reactive, organizing, limit setting, and somewhat supportive attitude may be required in certain circumstances. What is most important to this approach is that the clinician appreciates that the possibility of trying to *understand* what is going on may have to be suspended because it is necessary to act on what is *actually* going on. In addition, this expectation for a deviation from technical neutrality has to be clearly communicated to the patient. Further, both parties need to fully accept that the possibility of acting

therapeutically may be temporarily suspended, but at the same time, they both aim at returning, as soon as possible, to the more exploratory stance.

What Are Possible Targets for Measurement to Gauge the Effectiveness of Instruction About Applications of TFP Principles?

The effectiveness of the training in TFP principles was assessed both at the staff level (i.e., staff satisfaction and attitudes toward SPD) and at the patients' level (i.e., SPD psychopathology). Staff members (N = 23) completed questionnaires evaluating the perception of organizational well-being and delivery of care and their attitudes toward BPD prior to the first step of the training, and after 6 and 12 months from its completion. Patients with SPD (N = 18) were assessed on DSM-5 level of personality functioning and reflective functioning at baseline, prior to the training, and again after 6 and 12 months. Staff reported a significant increase in their caring and empathic attitudes toward patients and in optimism about treatment, as well as a decrease in their negative emotional reactions. Patients showed significant improvements in the identity, empathy, and intimacy domains of personality functioning and a reduction in their level of uncertainty about mental states (i.e., hypermentalizing). Although limited by the small sample size and being preliminary in nature, these findings are particularly promising. Specifically, since the staff's goal and expectation from training were that of a reduction of splitting, relational difficulties, and conflicts within the team and between the team and SPD patients, these data support the effectiveness of TFP-oriented training for multi-professional mental health teams working in outpatient community psychiatric service in improving their sense of competency and their treatment attitudes toward SPD patients [30].

What Is the Format for Instruction of TFP Principles to This Audience?

The training consisted of five sessions, lasting 3.5 hours each, attended by the mental health teams of the Valli Taro e Ceno district during the period May–June 2017. The basic principles of the TFP model were taught by a TFP teacher and supervisor (SD) to the entire staff of the three units of the district (i.e., the MHC, the CAPU, and the SerPD units), in a group format. Every session covered a specific theme:

1. Personality organization and structural change over time
2. Therapeutic strategies and basic techniques
3. Structuring the treatment: the therapeutic contract in borderline personality organization
4. Building an alliance with patient and family
5. Transference and countertransference management by staff

All five points described above were addressed using clinical vignettes taken from real cases, who were treated in the outpatient units and discussed openly by the staff and the TFP teacher. Each member of the team (i.e., nurses, psychiatrists, psychologists, social workers, psychotherapists, educators) was encouraged to actively share with the supervisor their view of the patient. Based on the information provided by the staff members, the supervisor showed and collaboratively discussed with the entire staff, patients' diagnosis and level of functioning, patients' current major difficulties and predominant object relations patterns. Importantly, the discussion about the various clinical cases continued over time, in a longitudinal follow-up of the treatment process. This allowed for observation of the changes in patients' clinical picture and relational patterns with the team over time. Thus, the training made possible the collaborative delineation, by the mental health staff and the TFP teacher and supervisor, of a structured, TFP-oriented model of intervention to be applied within the context of community-based DMH that is articulated across phases of intervention. This multi-phase model is described below and is summarized in Table 4.1.

Furthermore, the training was followed by a supervision phase aimed at evaluating the effective application of TFP principles into the clinical practice of the outpatient psychiatric service. This phase took place during two consecutive years, April–September 2018, and May–October 2019, and consisted of five sessions per year, lasting 3.5 hours each. The goal was to follow-up and discuss with the supervisor three new SPD cases per year in which different professionals (psychiatrist, psychologist, nurse, social worker, educator) of all the three units (i.e., the MHC, the CAPU, and the SerPD units) were involved in the treatment plan, in order to verify the feasibility of application of TFP principles.

The TFP-oriented supervisions and clinical discussions then continued in an online format, due to the Italian Covid-19 prevention requirements. The staff of the mental health teams participated in four webinars, lasting 3.00 hours each, during the period October–December 2020. Three sessions were dedicated to discussion of specific issues for all professions involved in the care pathway: one session for the nurses, one for the therapists (psychiatrists and psychologists), and the last one for the socio-educational staff (i.e., social workers and educators). The fourth session involved the entire team and was dedicated to discussion with the supervisor of the capacity of the team as a whole to integrate in a structured and coherent fashion the various views and therapeutic stances of the different professionals.

All sessions during these 4 years were scheduled during the ordinary weekly team briefing, to facilitate regular attendance by all staff members.

A Model of TFP Oriented Approach for Severe Personality Disorders in Outpatient Italian Psychiatric Services

The proposed model is developmental in nature, as it deals with the most severe level of pathology at the beginning of treatment and proposes a sequence of phases to gradually integrate patients' split-off object relations. Albeit derived from standard TFP, it must not be conceptualized as a complete application of what goes on

Table 4.1 Phases of intervention with hierarchical goals

	Steps	Treatment phase	Clinical phenomena	Technical principles	Treatment priorities: where to intervene?
Admission to treatment (high severity)	1	Patient does not distinguish between "feeling subjectively better" and the previously agreed treatment aim (=change)	Chaos! Fast shifts in object relations Inflexible reactions and intense affects	Check contract adherence Management of contract ruptures Observation and cognitive containment of affect and behavior	Managing threats to treatment continuity Managing emergencies
	2	Increased verbalization Patient puts his/her experience into words Actions have an interpersonal meaning	Less acting out Observable dyads between patient and staff reflecting a range of defenses employed Interest in the meaning of actions—actions make sense	Use countertransference to understand dominant dyad relations Clarify what gets activated within the diverse relationships with staff members	Maintain integrity of the treatment structure Observe and clarify external relationships
Advanced treatment (low severity)	3	Some signs of integration observed in: meetings with patient/staff patient's increased valuing of psychotherapy	Clear object relations not dominated by splitting Intense affects are subjectively experienced and not acted out	Clarifying and interpreting all level of defenses observed in patient/staff relationships	Communicate and clarify object relations dyads between patient and staff Here-and-now AND external reality

in standard TFP, given the radical differences in settings. Nevertheless, since standard TFP aims at generating change across various stages or phases of treatment and this method has been manualized and empirically validated [21], other applied TFP forms of treatment may also benefit from such a step-by-step structure. In other words, even the simplest clinical application of TFP principles aims at activating a process of change in the structure of personality. In the model proposed here, we adapt the description of the sequence of phases of standard TFP to the specific setting of this outpatient Italian psychiatric service. Each stage is defined by the understanding of clinical phenomena in light of contemporary ORT and the related application of technical TFP principles.

The First Phase

The first phase starts, as in standard TFP, following the completion of the assessment process and the negotiation of a treatment contract that is accepted by both the patient and the clinician. In this applied TFP model, this initial phase poses significant challenges to the goal of fully applying TFP principles. Here, it is necessary to "tolerate the confusion and chaos" at this juncture, as mentioned in strategy 1 of the standard TFP manual [21]. The nature of PD pathology, its severity, and the concurrent social disadvantages experienced by the patient, will amplify the chaotic fluctuation in activated dyads. Of note, the frame of the treatment derived from the negotiated contract is attacked more aggressively in this applied TFP model than would be expected in standard TFP for outpatients. This more prominent attack on the treatment frame may reflect the patient's generally lower motivation for change in this context.

Three goals in this application of TFP are prioritized. First, the survival of the therapeutic relationship is paramount, as threats to the treatment are enacted and risk of dropout is increased. It remains of utmost important for the staff to maintain a focus on, and connection with, the patients in these situations. As in standard TFP, mental health professionals must avoid the exploration of transferential issues when the dominant affect conveyed by the patient relates to important developments in their external reality. This applied TFP model emphasizes the risk of addressing prematurely or excessively intensely internal object relations activated in the transference. Thus, the staff must accept the role imposed on them by the patient's behavior, specifically reacting, rather than exploring, when that behavior is marked by acting out as a primary defense.

At a deeper level, once the risk of dropping out is reasonably controlled, the staff has to face the risk of falling into a pattern of chronic reactivity; in this situation, the endless negotiations in response to interventions requested by the patient often become the only area of exchange between patient and staff. At this point, treatment can get overly rehabilitative, and in response to the defenses employed by the patient, opportunities for exploration will be destroyed. Examples include: the pressure on staff from the patient to deal with emergency situations (clinical as well as social); the patient's non-adherence to treatment conditions (impacted by the assertion that solutions to social problems must come first); and impasses marked by the patient's apparent misunderstanding of events or by the patient's manipulation of targeted figures in the staff, which can engender severe splitting within the mental health team.

In this fragile phase, the therapeutic task to be accomplished is the successful establishment of a treatment frame, as a set of rules, behaviors, and attitudes, introducing to the patient a new idea of treatment. Following this introduction, the protection of this treatment frame becomes the paramount priority. The frame requires protection from the expectable attacks from patients, expressed in their behaviors, fueled by expression of primitive defense mechanisms, all connected to the defensive operation of splitting, which is acted out with the entire staff. In this light, a patient's projections toward staff members would be understood as the activation of partial object relations, manifested as expressions of extremes of "good" or "bad" views of the diverse professionals within the team. The treatment frame must be identified as a "good object" in the staff's mindset, but it will be subject to contamination by the projections of patients. Some staff members will be moved to criticize the "rigidity" of the frame and the associated priority for exploration, as an excessive request for a weak and fragile patient who needs support. Other staff members will perceive the attack and aggression of the patient as the expression of his/her real "nature," requiring strict "limit setting". Notably, limit setting is not the same as maintenance of the treatment frame, but under the pressure of the patient's actions, the two may be conflated by staff members.

It is well known that conflict among staff members is routine, often reflecting different views of patient pathology and therefore contributing to different therapeutic attitudes [13, 31]. In this context, the cohesion of the mental health team will be undermined, and the implementation of treatment might be severely impacted. This phenomenon could be considered a variant of dropping out; while sometimes the patient is superficially allied with the implementation of treatment (i.e., he/she does not explicitly attack or threaten to destroy the treatment with repeated challenges), the staff themselves might abandon their expectation for a coherent, structured treatment. Conflicts among members will have a major destructive outcome, with members unconsciously sabotaging each other. This presumably reflects the projection of the patient's dissociated aggressive part onto the staff members; the staff members, in turn, identify with this projected aggression by devaluing and attacking colleagues.

The capacity for "containment" is one of the most effective interventions in standard TFP; in applied TFP, as in the program outlined here, learning how to master containment strategies can be even more challenging for clinicians than would be the case when learning standard TFP. Containing the patient's projections in order to promote the patient's capacity to think about mental states in self and others [32] is a fundamental step in promoting structural change. Building a solid frame of treatment is a prerequisite for effective containment of the patient's projections. Maintaining the treatment frame implies that the patient accepts, at least in part, that working on difficulties means discussing and talking about them and about relationships, instead of reflexively acting on them [4, 21]. However, in our model of an applied TFP approach, the treatment frame provided by the contract and by the patient's basic motivation to change are weaker and more vulnerable than in standard TFP. This phenomenon reflects the severity of pathology of the patients involved, the high number of staff members included in the therapeutic process, and the institutional mandate of the INHS community-based psychiatric service itself to handle emergencies. Nevertheless, some sort of frame is needed in order to allow the staff members to contain and reflect on SPD psychopathology. In this phase, the "case manager" has a central role in helping the whole team to maintain the treatment frame. The case manager is a member of the staff, ideally an expert in personality pathology, who has a supraordinate function to contain the container, i.e., to clarify to individual staff members the nature of the transference dispositions activated by the patient, as well as their countertransference reactions. Where this is not possible, involvement of an external consultant will be required. This same function could be implemented, in some cases, by the group itself, meaning that group members collectively can help contain the difficulties of the individual members of the staff, who might be overwhelmed by the strength of interpersonal pressure exerted by the patient's projections.

Clinical Case Illustration of Phase 1

Miss A is a young woman, with low level borderline functioning, with comorbid eating and substance use disorders. The plan of her long-term treatment at the MHC had basically been rehabilitative and supportive, given her socially disadvantaged environment. Among the staff members of the MHC, her deepest relationships were with a social worker and a nurse, who oversaw all plans aimed at fostering social adaptation. They built up a positive relationship, quite new in the patient's history, and the patient was committed in these strongly supportive relationships that provided emotional encouragement as well as intensive plans to help improve her social adaptation. In TFP terms, one would say that such an approach helped Miss A to contain her basic destructive tendencies in those activities and relationships she was involved in, while in the language of the rehabilitation-oriented view of the MHC, the rationale was to support an individual with significant deficits in learning how to develop a normal social life, by patiently strengthening positive experiences in real life. Over time, this approach adopted by the mental health professionals provided good results: the patient maintained positively invested relations with the staff—not to be given for granted, considering her past history of frequent drop-out from previous treatments—without any disruptive emergencies or severe pathological behavior. The staff's professional investment and long hours of involvement conveyed that Miss A was a "special patient," but the positive outcome of her involvement in the program appeared to justify the staff's behavior.

Despite the improvements observed during Miss A's initial participation in the program, in the last year the staff noted that Miss A's general response had reached a state of impasse. Miss A succeeded in symptom improvement, but her life felt by the staff to be just "a little better than miserable" [33]. *Specifically, a recurrent pattern of behavior was observed. The main objective of the therapeutic approach had been to help her find a stable job. The patient (who, in TFP terms, was fueled by the libidinal, or purely positive, idealized segment of the object relation activated with the staff) always complied without complaints. She consistently agreed to attend a new job position, where showed increasingly good social and relational skills and quickly learned to be productive. This proceeded to a point in which she was recognized for a promotion to a permanent work position. At that point she was insecure and depressed, loosing self-confidence and becoming stubbornly self-critical. At the same time, she exhibited some evidence of regression: minor acting out came to the fore and eventually she quit the job, which was a great source of frustration for the staff members.*

The staff grew frustrated but remained closely involved with the patient, willing to start again in trying to help her find a new, and maybe more suitable, job. During the TFP-oriented supervision, two aspects of the patient's internal world, and the associated impact of these elements on the staff, became clear. One aspect was reflected in the role the staff assumed of acting as a "good mother" to address the patient's fragility due to the many and severe traumatic experiences she had endured. They experienced gratitude when the patient conveyed how much she needed them. A second aspect was reflected more subtly in the staff dynamics, as several staff members became critical of the psychiatrist and her choice of medications, which did not yield the expected results. Simply put, in their critical stance, some staff members conveyed in their actions an identification with the patient's desire to find an ideal object, in this case, a prescriber whose choices would "perfectly" address the patient's distress. Their critical attitude suggested to others that only they could deeply understand the patient's vulnerabilities and what interventions would work best for her. One could say that their real job was to help the patient adapt to reality. This underscored the challenge in proposing the applied TFP approach: the therapeutic relationship aimed to provide concrete support, but it should have also helped the staff develop a comprehensive, integrated view of the patient's internal world. The staff members recognized the role they had acted out, and how they failed to contain the patient's rage, which was obscured by a superficial compliance and behavior associated with a "good" object relation. After a while, it seemed, she had to attack and deny what they had provided her. By acknowledging a sense of annoyance and disillusionment after every professional failure of Miss A, and their sense of hidden resentment toward the psychiatrist, both the social worker and the nurse got in touch with what they could not contain, namely their resentment toward the patient for not responding positively to their efforts and to the "goodness" they provided. They became also more confident about their reaction of unavoidable resentment that always followed, albeit undisguised, a phase in which they felt identified with a "totally caring parent" relating to "a grateful loving child" who, at some point, had to attack the "good mother"/staff members by destroying their efforts. This can be viewed, in an applied TFP context, as a form of negative therapeutic reaction.

At this point, the staff members did not change the focus of their work but started to approach it in a different way. It became central that the commitment to keep a job was a key prerequisite for treatment, not simply a way to recover. Slowly, but firmly, both the social worker and the nurse clarified that maintaining a job was a requirement for treatment to continue, and that quitting a job would be interpreted as breaking the treatment agreement. They did it in a straightforward way by explaining that the treatment agreement between patient and staff allowed for exploration of the patient's experience of self and others in real time. They stressed that the joint examination by the patient and staff of the patient's reactions to elements of the treatment agreement, including finding and keeping a job, allowed for useful exploration of personality traits.

The Second Phase

The successful management of the first phase brings up a scenario quite familiar to the clinician trained in TFP, with some meaningful aspects to focus on.

In this phase, what mainly affects the staff is that the patients now put thoughts into words and not only into actions. That does not mean that the picture is completely changed, as if the patients were fully capable of "mentalizing" their own experiences and those of others. Rather, some mental capacities of the patient (such as reflection and mentalizing) grow and gain space in the patients' relationship with the staff. The staff needs to closely monitor this change of mental attitude and the developing capacity of the patients to communicate their subjective experience.

Verbal exchanges about mental states increase, reflecting an increased awareness for the patient that "actions have a meaning", thereby decreasing actions discharged purely to address a need for immediate gratification. As the patient becomes more clearly represented in the mind of the staff members, as they "tolerate the confusion" and begin to identify emerging dominant object relations dynamics, the staff also becomes better able to use this information and to put it in words. This is the phase when the dominant affects expressed in relations with staff members will be more evident, and when it will be clearer how affects are polarized around extreme of good and bad, love and hate. The immediate consequence is that splitting, as the prevalent defense mechanism, will appear evident within the staff relational dynamics, both in relation to the patient (in experiencing deep involvement or rejection), and in relation to other staff members. This may become a major obstacle, but at the same time, a useful opportunity if correctly handled, in the general management of the clinical situation.

As the working alliance between the mental health team and the patients gets stronger and more evident, and the staff work becomes more proactive, slowly in the patient's mind the frame of treatment (and the treatment goals) starts to be differentiated from simply "getting better." The patients' increasingly nuanced appreciation of personal difficulties will challenge the clear and simple motivation for suffering (like the perceived flaws of their family, or their own chronic incapacity to organize a personal life), generating new questions and anxieties. It is striking that, while the staff feels more in touch with the patient, the patient can express more distress. "Being in touch" does not mean that the staff has a "good relation" with the patient and a smooth alliance in which they get along perfectly and in which the staff provides interpretations to a patient who gratefully feels cared for and understood. On the contrary, the staff members just better appreciate what the patient is subjectively experiencing and, at the same time, they feel involved in the clearly activated dyads, reflecting expectable patterns of splitting. At this point, the staff collectively must be able to contain and hold the various dyads into which individual members are, partly unconsciously, dragged into. The stereotyped picture is of staff members arguing one against the other, embracing conflicting views of the patient, all good or all bad, in the conviction of having understood the "real" patient. This inevitably results in splitting among the staff coming to the fore. But this is just the most apparent behavioral defense involving staff. At a deeper level, the staff can defensively respond by returning to a "reactive" stance, thus engaging in actions in order to influence the patient's external reality, rather than remaining focused on exploration. This is a countertransference resistance, as the containing attitude, meant to maintain psychological communication as the major channel for communication with the patient, has caused high levels of anxiety in the staff, reflecting both the heightened affective states of those involved and the high level of inner tension in the staff itself.

Individual staff members become aware of the specific and unique dyads activated in relation to the patient, as the focus of inquiry shifts from explicit behavior in the patient's external reality to the interactions with the psychiatric service in a more personal perspective. This is a meaningful moment of change (here meant in the working atmosphere more than in the patient's clinical state) in the present applied TFP approach, which can be defined as "the personalization of treatment." A very specific kind of personal interaction between the patient and each individual member of the mental health team develops, akin to what happens between the patient and the therapist in standard TFP. However, differently from standard TFP, the activation of the various split-off object relations and dyads will take place in a multi-faceted therapeutic setting, namely the psychiatric service context. As the main goal is the same, i.e., proceeding toward integration of dissociated aspects of personality in the patient, this diverse treatment setting shows advantages and disadvantages. Split-off relationships in the staff need to be integrated. This will be facilitated by continuous exchanges—sometimes in the form of arguments or conflicts among staff—that will promote a confrontation within the team. Having structured the treatment, in phase one, by defining the containing role of the staff as a "whole object", there may be situations that benefit from the guide of a case manager, or, in the most difficult cases, by the support of an external consultant. The goal would be for each staff member to be able to acknowledge complex, nuanced, evolving perspectives of the patient, informed by the patient's interaction with other staff members, as well as the observable interactions among staff themselves. In addition, the staff needs to repeatedly return to the basic concepts of ORT to fully understand the motivation for their therapeutic interventions, namely the powerful splitting-based defense mechanisms employed by the patient, e.g., projective identification. The staff will maintain coherence and integrity only if they fully acknowledge that individuals with SPD have the power to induce intense, specific emotional reactions. As previously noted, this phenomenon is likely to be stronger in a setting not as rigidly defined as in standard TFP. Only a strong adherence to this basic concept will allow staff to contain personal reactions, by observing and naming their personal reactions toward the patient, while at the same time observing their colleagues' reactions and neutrally giving a name to them as well. Thus, the capacity to observe the difference among alternative perspectives will facilitate the naming of the various split-off interactions. It is likely that the first step toward integration in the patient's mind comes through the capacity of the staff to fully observe the range of activated dyads between the patient and all staff members. As in standard TFP [32, 34, 35], this task is accomplished by the monitoring of countertransference, beginning with the clinician's affective response to the patient, and then locating it in the patient's narrative in that specific phase. This is the most prominent task involved in this phase of treatment.

Clinical Case Illustration of Phase 2

The social worker and psychiatric nurse, who were deeply invested in the maintenance of an idealized object representation and colluding with that impulse, kept to themselves feelings of disappointment in the patient's failure to grow professionally. They were aware that their personal reaction, which they tried to keep at bay, might be a threat to good clinical work; nevertheless, they failed to fully consider this reaction that could have been a source of important data in their exploration. Despite their feelings of disappointment toward the patient, they maintained that the patient had to be understood and appreciated in her efforts, and that the staff had to be patient in waiting for her functioning to improve. In sum, the negative countertransference reaction of the social worker and nurse had to be limited and contained. During the TFP-oriented clinical discussion, it emerged that perhaps this minimization of emerging negative countertransference elements was the "best" way to keep the patient's identification of her treaters as a "good object" alive.

At the beginning of this new treatment phase, supervision focused specifically on the splitting among the staff members. The psychiatrist as well as other staff members involved at various levels in the Ms A's treatment, brought a different view of the patient: she was detached, barely compliant, and exploitative, gaining a special role among the patient population. The supervision worked at two different levels. The first one focused on the so called "parallel process" often observed during standard TFP supervision: the therapist enacts with his own supervisor a relational dynamic similar to the one the patient enacts toward the therapist during treatment [35]. *In the applied TFP setting described here, a similar parallel process may emerge in the staff meetings and team interactions. The social worker and the nurse felt superficially rewarded by the staff for what they had accomplished with the patient, but just underneath they felt criticized for the limited results. Clarifying this helped them to gain an increased awareness that they, in fact, did feel criticized by the patient herself: they began to identify a dyad, in which the patient was an angry child expecting perfection by an omnipotent parent. Then, when confronted with their own critical view of the "frustrating" psychiatrist, it became clear how the negative dyad apparently acted by the psychiatrist was present in themselves too, as a deep resentment toward the patient, which had to be denied in order to maintain an idealized dyad alive. This helped the social worker and the nurse to start an integrative process in their minds, both understanding the parallel process as well as their own countertransference resistance.*

At this point, in which a consensus—or, better, cohesion—was reached in the group, the psychiatric service work moved to a second level. The patient was asked to jointly meet with the social worker, the nurse, and the psychiatrist. At first, the patient was confronted with one of the most common manifestations of splitting, namely that different professionals had in mind a different Miss A, all convinced that their respective perspective was accurate. The patient reacted angrily but benefiting from effective supervision, the social worker and the nurse were flexible and effective in their interventions. They helped the patient to observe that maybe she was not so grateful to them, that perhaps along with the positive alliance that had developed, there was also resentment felt toward them for not being the perfectly good, expected providers she might have hoped for. They raised the possibility that her way to express her negative feelings was to destroy, at some point, the rehabilitative project proposed. The social worker and nurse reflected that their increased appreciation of motivations that had not fully been in their awareness made it possible, for them, to be clearer with the patient and to connect in a different and meaningful way. This helped move the focus of their work from direct actions (finding a job, maintaining it, and so on) to reflection about the respective roles activated in the patient–provider interactions.

The Third Phase

In this phase, the capacity of the patient to initiate discussion of a problem and to understand the affective dominance of a specific issue at any given time can be observed. In the applied TFP model described here, it is expected that the patient, from the outset, will focus on aspects of his or her external reality, locating the source of their distress in their environment rather than relating their distress to problematic aspects of their own personality organization. During the initial phases of treatment, the SPD patient will be inclined to modify aspects of external reality, as opposed to develop greater self-understanding. This tendency usually leads the staff to be, at least partly, reactive. The transition to the more advanced phase of treatment will be marked by a decrease in this pattern of staff reactivity. In turn, the patient will be less likely to expect from staff input about direct modification of the patient's external world. Furthermore, the patient should develop a deeper appreciation of others' motivations and subjective experiences. The staff will likely notice that the patient talks less of others (i.e., "He did that to me.") and more of interactions with others ("Based on my evaluation, I did this to him and he answered doing that, and that stimulated me to do that because I thought that then he would have done.")

Clinical Case Illustration of Phase 3

At some point during the second phase, Miss A. decided to end treatment because she planned to move to another city to settle down with her boyfriend. Over time, she had idealized how she might be with him in a way consistent with a perfect bond, thereby denying her repeated tendency to submit to his subtle, mistreating attitude. As the patient lost touch with what had been a consistently negative aspect of her romantic relationship with her boyfriend, the staff increasingly feared the activation of a regressive sequence marked by phases of emotional crisis and severe, aggressive acting out against herself or her boyfriend.

The staff disagreed with the patient about this decision to move. The staff attempted to convey to the patient the defensive motivation of her decision, specifically the patient's wish for a new, "happy" life to replace what she experienced as disillusioning in her treatment. They described their impression that her experience of the staff as less than perfect led her to experience intolerable frustration. However, for the sake of the treatment and out of concern that the patient could lose the important social gains she had thus far achieved, they did not protest in a way that might have further alienated the patient. At the same time, mindful of external reality issues, the staff shared with the patient their understanding that a certain amount of personal growth was behind that decision. After many failures, this love relationship showed a stronger potential and the staff members agreed that a new capacity for love might be present. Simply put, staff did not know where regression ended and growth began, in other words, how much of the patient's behavior could be understood as reflecting elements of an emerging "depressive position" [36]. *They agreed with the patient to stay in touch, with a plan to intervene to help the patient identify local treaters if for some reason the patient's conditions were to deteriorate. After a few months, the romantic relationship ended, and Miss A came back to live in the catchment area of the psychiatric service. While she expected rejection and devaluation from the staff, at the same time, she showed implicit resentment because, on some level, she felt they did not protect her enough from her poor choice. However, these developments did not provoke any major regression in her behavior and subjective symptoms.*

The psychiatrist/case manager, the social worker, and the nurse set up a joint evaluation meeting with the patient. Among other topics the staff invited the patient to consider the motivations, conscious and unconscious, underlying her behavior. They offered a hypothesis about the patient's actions, suggesting that she was motivated by the urge to relate with an idealized object under her complete control (now a distorted view of the boyfriend) as a reaction of having been disillusioned by the treatment team. She deeply needed an omnipotently controlled loving and idealized object in order to subjectively experience a sense of self-worth and of being unconditionally loved. The professionals also clarified that they understood how, under the pressure of this need, the patient was limited in freely choosing and organizing her life. Miss A was able to appreciate these observations and reflected on how her actions might have threatened her improvement in functioning. At this point, Miss A was referred to a structured, individual psychotherapy, seen as an opportunity for her to continue exploration to build on the rehabilitation and support she had already received. Miss A had used the experience of applied TFP while working with the staff to move from a pattern of reflexive reactions to an increased capacity to put into words her experience.

Conclusion

The treatment of patients with SPD within Italian community-based, NHS-funded, general outpatient psychiatric services is often complicated by excessive reliance on a "disability model" view of personality pathology and by a related medical/psychiatric traditional approach to treatment. This may make it difficult for the multi-professional mental health teams to respond in a coherent and integrated fashion to the unfolding of SPD psychopathology and relational dynamics. In turn, the lack of a well-structured treatment environment and of a shared view of the core issues of personality pathology by the mental health professionals might prevent improvement over time and foster chronicity among patients with SPD. This chapter has described an applied TFP initiative aimed to overcome these difficulties in an Italian outpatient psychiatric service composed of multi-professional teams. Within this context, the introduction of TFP principles provided the staff with an increased and shared ability to understand SPD patients' chaotic behavior as a reflection of their inner world (i.e., splitting, identity diffusion) as well to reflectively and consistently respond to it. Furthermore, the appreciation of the nature of change for SPD based on TFP principles and ORT allowed for the delineation of a multi-phase approach to treatment that involved various professionals and can be applied to the practice of outpatient psychiatric services. While TFP principles are derived from standard, individual, twice-a-week TFP, their introduction proves useful even in the much different setting of a general outpatient psychiatric service. In this treatment setting, applying TFP principles can facilitatee structuring the treatment of SPD in a coherent fashion, ameliorate staff's attitudes and relational dynamics toward SPD, and ultimately improve SPD patients' psychosocial functioning by gradually fostering patients' ability to reflect on their inner world and issues with external reality.

References

1. Piccinelli M, Politi P, Barale F. Focus on psychiatry in Italy. Br J Psychiatry. 2002;181:538–44.
2. National Institute for Health & Clinical Excellence. Borderline personality disorder: treatment and management, National clinical practice guideline number 78. The British Psychological Society and the Royal College of Psychiatrists; 2009.
3. Regione Emilia-Romagna, Servizio Salute Mentale Dipendenze Patologiche Salute nelle Carceri. Linee di indirizzo per il trattamento dei Disturbi Gravi di Personalità 2013. https://salute.regione.emilia-romagna.it/salute-mentale/percorsi-di-cura/DGP
4. Caligor E, Kernberg O, Clarkin J, Yeomans F. Psychodynamic therapy for personality pathology. Washington, DC: APA Publishing; 2018.
5. Bender DS, Dolan RT, Skodol AE, Sanislow CA, Dyck IR, McGlashan TH, et al. Treatment utilization by patients with personality disorders. Am J Psychiatry. 2001;158:295–302.
6. Black DW, Blum N, Letuchy E, Doebbeling CC, Forman-Hoffman VL, Doebbeling BN. Borderline personality disorder and traits in veterans: psychiatric comorbidity, healthcare utilization, and quality of life along a continuum of severity. CNS Spectr. 2006;11:680–9.
7. National Institute for Mental Health in England. Personality disorders: no longer a diagnosis of exclusion. Policy implementation guidance for the implementation of services for people with personality disorder. 2003. https://personalitydisorder.org.uk
8. Percudani M, Belloni G, Contini A, Barbui C. Monitoring community psychiatric services in Italy: differences between patients who leave care and those who stay in treatment. Br J Psychiatry. 2002;180:254–9.
9. De Panfilis C, Marchesi C, Cabrino C, Monici A, Politi V, Rossi M, Maggini C. Patient factors predicting early dropout from psychiatric outpatient care for borderline personality disorder. Psychiatry Res. 2012;200:422–9.
10. De Panfilis C, Politi V, Fortunati R, Cazzolla R, Scaramuzzino M, Marchesi C, Maggini C. 2-year follow-up of borderline personality disorder patients in Italy: a preliminary report on prognosis and prediction of outcome. Int J Soc Psychiatry. 2011;57:528–37.
11. Lanfredi M, Ridolfi ME, Occhialini G, Pedrini L, Ferrari C, Lasalvia A, Gunderson JG, Black DW, Rossi R, The Italian BPD Attitudes Study Group. Attitudes of mental health staff toward patients with borderline personality disorder: an Italian cross-sectional Multisite study. J Pers Disord. 2019, on line ahead of print.
12. Gunderson JG. Borderline personality disorder: a clinical guide. American Psychiatric Publishing; 2001.
13. Bateman AW, Tyrer P. Services for personality disorder: organization for inclusion. Adv Psychiatr Treat. 2004;10:425–33.
14. Kernberg O. Structural interviewing. Psychiatr Clin North Am. 1981;4:169–95.
15. Clarkin JF, Caligor E, Stern BL, Kernberg OF. Structured interview of personality organization (STIPO). Unpublished manuscript, Personality Disorders Institute, Weill Medical College of Cornell University, New York, NY, 2004.

16. Horz-Sagstetter S, Caligor E, Preti E, Stern BL, De Panfilis C, Clarkin JF. Clinician-guided assessment of personality using the Structural Interview and the Structured Interview of Personality Organization (STIPO). J Pers Assess. 2018;100:30–42.
17. Clarkin JF, Caligor E, Stern BL, Kernberg OF. Structured Interview of Personality Organization - Revised (STIPO-R). Unpublished manuscript, Personality Disorders Institute, Weill Medical College of Cornell University, New York, NY, 2016.
18. Kernberg O. Severe personality disorders. New Haven: Yale University Press; 1984.
19. Gunderson JG. Handbook of good psychiatric management for borderline personality disorder. American Psychiatric Publishing; 2014. p. 15–20.
20. Hersh R. Integration with transference-focused psychotherapy. In: Choi-Kain LW, Gunderson JG, editors. Applications of good psychiatric management for borderline personality disorder. A practical guide. American Psychiatric Publishing; 2019. p. 327–51.
21. Yeomans F, Clarkin J, Kernberg O. Transference-focused psychotherapy for borderline personality disorders. Arlington: APA Publishing; 2015.
22. Sandler J, Sandler MA. Internal objects revisited. London: Karnac Books Ltd; 1998.
23. Kernberg O. Aggression in personality disorders and perversions. New Haven: Yale Univ. Press; 1992.
24. Plakun E. Treatment resistance and the patient authority. New York: Norton; 2011.
25. Zanarini MC, Frankenburg FR, Reich DB, et al. Attainment and stability of sustained symptomatic remission and recovery among patients with borderline personality disorder and Axis II comparison subject: a 16-year prospective follow-up study. Am J Psychiatry. 2012;169:476–83.
26. Stone M. The fate of borderline patients: successful outcome and psychiatric practice. New York: Guilford; 1990.
27. Stone M. Personality disordered patients: treatable and untreatable. Washington, DC: APA Publishing; 2006.
28. Transference JB. The total situation Int J Psychoanalysis. 1985;66:474–54.
29. Steiner J. Psychic retreats: pathological organisations in psychotic, neurotic, and borderline patients. London: Routledge; 1993.
30. Ciccone G, Dazzi S, Ampollini P, Palombi F, De Panfilis C. Treatment for patients with severe personality disorders in mental health services in Italy: a team approach based on object relations theory. Paper presented at the 48th congress of the Italian Society of Psychiatry. Turin, October 2018. Manuscript in preparation.
31. Kernberg O. Ideology, conflict and leadership in group and organizations. New Haven: Yale University Press; 1998.
32. Kernberg O. The inseparable nature of love and aggression. Washington, DC: APA Publishing; 2012.
33. Linehan MM. Cognitive-behavioral treatment of borderline personality disorder. New York: Guilford; 1993.
34. Carsky M. Managing countertransference in the treatment of personality disorders. Psychodyn Psychiatry. 2021;49:339–60.
35. Kernberg O. Psychoanalytic supervision: the supervisor's task. 2010. Psychoanal Q. 2010;79:603–27.
36. Klein M. Mourning at its relation to manic-depressive states. In: Contributions to psychoanalysis 1921–1945. London: Hogarth Press; 1948.

5 Using Transference-Focused Psychotherapy (TFP) Principles in the National Health Service (NHS) in the United Kingdom (UK)

Tennyson Lee and Jo-Anna Van den Bosch

Introduction

Overview of the National Health Service

The National Health Service (NHS) is the publicly funded health care system of the United Kingdom, made up of four semi-independent entities covering England, Scotland, Wales, and Northern Ireland. The NHS is part of the welfare state that emerged in 1945, created by the National Health Service Act of 1946, under Aneurin Bevan, of the Labour government.

Founding principles of the NHS include: (1) requiring funding by general taxation and National Insurance contributions, (2) ensuring that it is free at the point of use, with access based on clinical need, not an individual's ability to pay, (3) providing a comprehensive service, which puts patient care at the heart of everything it does, and (4) expecting that it works across organizational boundaries.

PD services for adults are arranged in tiers according to the increasing intensity of intervention. Tier 1 consists of primary care and the voluntary sector. Tier 2 refers to generic mental health care, customarily provided by a Community Mental Health Team (CMHT). Those with more severe difficulties require more specialist support, hence the need for tier 3 (local specialist treatment in the community) and tier 4 (regional or national specialist) services. The difficulties in smooth transition and referrals along the different tiers have been noted [1, 2].

T. Lee (✉)
DeanCross, Tower Hamlets Personality Disorder Service and Centre for Understanding Personality (CUSP), East London NHS Foundation Trust, London, UK
e-mail: tennyson.lee1@nhs.net

J.-A. Van den Bosch
Mental Health of Older Adults Services, South London and Maudsley NHS Trust, London, UK

R. G. Hersh, C. De Panfilis (eds.), *Implementing Transference-Focused Psychotherapy Principles*, https://doi.org/10.1007/978-3-031-68062-5_5

There are 54 Mental Health Trusts (MHT) in England that provide health and social care services for people with mental health disorders. A MHT provides clinical services to patients within a specific geographic catchment area. Within an MHT, the aforementioned CMHT is a group of clinicians who provide mental health care, including for those patients with PD pathology who are not deemed to require specialized services. Some MHTs will have distinct services under their auspices that will focus on defined patient subpopulations. We describe services designed specifically for patients with PD pathology, which also offer PD-related training and treatment not always available in other locales.

Who Are the Clinicians?

The clinicians involved in the mental health divisions of the NHS include representatives of different professional groups. These may include psychiatrists, psychologists, social workers, nurses, and psychotherapists. Together, these clinicians make up the multi-disciplinary CMHT, which are general psychiatric teams working on an outpatient basis. The programs focusing on the treatment of patients with personality disorder (PD) diagnoses, referred to as specialist services, will have a significant representation of clinicians trained in specific treatment modalities.

The NHS system of providing care operates as a team; this is distinct from a single or group practice of seeing patients in a private setting, as is also available in the UK and in other countries. This team approach is the backbone of the NHS system. Different services within the NHS are charged with making the best use of limited resources, which therefore informs thinking about the implementation of treatment modalities, including transference-focused psychotherapy (TFP).

Who Are the Patients?

As noted, the NHS guarantees medical care for all citizens of the UK. While there is a parallel, fee-for-service system that provides care for a small minority of UK residents, the NHS mental health services cover patients of all ages in a centralized, coordinated system.

The most attention within the system on patients with PD diagnoses has been on those patients with borderline personality disorder (BPD); this phenomenon is not exclusive to the NHS, as generally the vast majority of research on PD pathology has been focused on BPD. In our discussion, we will reference PD pathology generally, and in certain situations describe the particular subtypes of pathology as seen in NHS clinical services.

This chapter will focus on implementation of services for adults. The clinical illustration provided will highlight a novel program designed to provide treatment to the population of older adults with PD psychopathology.

As mentioned, the NHS is obligated to treat all patients eligible for participation. This obligation presents specific challenges that can include the necessity to accommodate the most symptomatic and complicated patients with PD diagnoses, without an option to refer these patients to other treatment systems. This phenomenon has earned the NHS a reputation for resourcefulness and flexibility as it provides a service for a subpopulation with severe PD psychopathology. That said, clinicians in the NHS can face the challenge of responding to patients who may feel entitled to receiving service without acknowledging the requirements for motivation and commitment they would need to allow meaningful treatment to occur.

What Is the Contemporary Standard of Care for Clinicians' Treatment of these Patients?

In 2002, the National Personality Disorder Development Program identified 11 pilot sites in England to develop specialist local (or Tier 3) PD services. These pilot projects demonstrated how different approaches with common principles could deliver cost-effective solutions [3]. Moving beyond specialist services, the policy implementation guide *Personality Disorder: No Longer a Diagnosis of Exclusion* [4] was a landmark document in the mainstreaming of management of PD patients within the rest of mental health services.

A workforce development guide, *Breaking the Cycle of Rejection: The Personality Disorders Capabilities Framework* [5], set the scene for the creation of a national training program (the Knowledge and Understanding Framework or KUF), which continues to be widely implemented to this day.

The coordinated aspect of the national program began in 2002, referenced above with 11 pilot sites, and was closed in 2011. Since then, ad-hoc service development has taken place. Considerable variation in availability and range of services exists, with little clinical strategy for the treatment of patients with PD diagnoses at the regional or national level.

The 2015 National Personality Disorder Service Survey [6] evaluated the availability and nature of services for people affected by PD. Of the 57 relevant English MHTs, 52 responded (response rate 91%) and of the 10 independent service providers approached 4 responded (response rate 40%). While 84% of organizations (hospitals, clinics) have at least one dedicated PD service, only 55% reported that patients had sufficient access to these services. Dedicated services commonly had good levels of patient participation and carer involvement, as well as engagement in education, research, and training. Table 5.1 shows the summary of evidence-based psychological interventions offered.

The survey concluded that while there has been a substantial increase in service provision for people affected by PD, continued variability in service availability persists and it remains unclear whether the quality of care has improved.

Key aspects of PD services in the UK are described below.

Diagnosis Use of the PD diagnosis remains variable. Ambivalence among professionals is paralleled by concerns, among some patient groups and others, that the diagnostic label itself can lead to stigma [7]. In general, there is a reluctance on the part of many clinicians to first make and then share, a PD diagnosis, even in circumstances when a clinical presentation would be best understood in this way. While there are some patient groups, as noted, who strongly feel that a PD diagnosis may be either inaccurate or stigmatizing, or both, there is also a PD advocacy movement within the UK that supports naming the disorder and thus empowering patients and families to make informed decisions about treatment options.

Medication Although no drug has a specific approval for the treatment of PD, 92% of patients with PD in the UK are prescribed psychotropic medications [8]. Although comorbidities are commonly cited as the reason for prescribing, the National Institute for Health and Care Excellence (NICE) discourages the use of medication specifically for BPD [9]. There is a well-documented trend toward polypharmacy and overuse of medication in this patient population [10].

Staff Needs Staff across all sectors report feeling insufficiently supported when working with patients with PD [4]. Feelings of inadequacy and hopelessness can be an inherent part of working with patients with PD. The diagnosis is considered by some staff to be stigmatizing, while at the same time, psychiatrists may have more critical and negative attitudes toward PD than other mental disorders [11, 12].

As shown in Table 5.1, TFP was not yet systematically introduced in the UK at the time of the survey. This is unsurprising as the first TFP training course within the UK occurred in 2012. As reflected in the 2017 survey referenced, over a third of

Table 5.1 Summary of interventions offered

	Dedicated service *n* (%)	Generic service *n* (%)
Biological interventions		
Medication management	42 (52)	45 (90)
Organic investigations	28 (35)	42 (82)
Physical healthcare interventions	27 (33)	44 (86)
MUS management	23 (28)	27 (53)
Psychological interventions, *n* (%)		
Psychoeducation	44 (54)	40 (78)
DBT	40 (49)	29 (57)
MBT	35 (43)	21 (41)
Psychodynamic	30 (37)	27 (53)
CBT	27 (33)	42 (82)
CAT	26 (32)	35 (69)
Art therapies	22 (27)	25 (49)
Therapeutic community	19 (23)	9 (18)
Family therapy	14 (17)	26 (51)
Motivational interviewing	14 (17)	22 (43)
SFT	10 (12)	23 (45)
STEPPS	8 (10)	8 (16)

CAT Cognitive analytic therapy, *CBT* Cognitive behavioral therapy, *DBT* Dialectical behavior therapy, *MBT* Mentalization-based therapy, *MUS* Medically unexplained symptoms, *SFT* Schema-focused therapy, *STEPPS* Systems training for emotional predictability and problem-solving [6]

dedicated services offer psychodynamic psychotherapy and these may be the services most amenable to adopting a TFP approach. At present, only three MHTs in the UK offer treatments by TFP practitioners accredited by the International Society for TFP (ISTFP).

Similar to MBT, TFP is listed in the British Psychoanalytic Council (BPC) as a "kite mark" training that is psychoanalytic in formulation but for which successful completion of the TFP didactic course does not itself lead to BPC registration. The BPC is the UK's leading professional association and accredited public register for psychoanalytic psychotherapy.

In the UK, TFP arrived at a time when there were several models of psychotherapy in use to provide treatment for patients with PDs. These models included: mentalization based therapy (MBT), cognitive analytic therapy (CAT), dialectical behavioral therapy (DBT), democratic therapeutic communities, and schema focused therapy (SFT). The UK has a history of publicly funding high-quality, evidence-based treatments for patients, including those with complex PD presentations. TFP is arguably the most purely psychoanalytic therapy of the empirically validated treatments for these disorders. The introduction of TFP in the UK follows a rich tradition of psychoanalytic theory and practice over many years; Freud spent the last year of his life in England; and Klein and Bion both worked for much of their careers in the UK. Of note, the Melanie Klein Trust continues to advance the work of object relations theory in contemporary practice.

Just as psychoanalytic thinkers in the UK generally have embraced a pluralistic approach, so too in work with patients with PD diagnoses, an openness to different treatment modalities now prevails, including the implementation of TFP.

What Are the Goals for Imparting to Clinicians the Principles of TFP for Working with These Patients?

When we focus on the goals of imparting to NHS clinicians the principles of TFP for their work with patients with BPD or other PD diagnoses, we examine two trends: (1) the application of TFP principles in treatment settings *other* than the extended, outpatient individual psychotherapy model, and (2) the adaptation of TFP as a once-weekly individual psychotherapy,

1. Lee and Hersh [13] outlined the benefits of integration of TFP principles in the work of NHS general psychiatry, distinct from recommendations for an exploratory psychotherapy. Using clinical vignettes related to familiar challenges in the work with patients with primary or co-occurring PD, they described practical use in crisis management and pharmacotherapy of core TFP concepts. Here, applied TFP for NHS personnel aimed to recast those principles as practical and common-sense, not inaccessible, or vague, as many psychoanalytic concepts are often experienced by clinicians in general practice. Establishing a treatment agreement, using countertransference, or monitoring the three channels of communication, were presented in this way as more easily mastered without

extensive training, and widely applicable in many areas of patient care for which NHS treatment teams assumed responsibility.

2. In contrast to standard TFP, which is offered twice a week, within the UK's NHS setting it is offered once a week. While a comparative study of once versus twice-a-week TFP therapy has not been done, anecdotally, TFP practitioners in the UK have felt confident in treating patients in a once-weekly modality. Clinicians have noted that the reasons for this confidence relate to the particular strengths of the model that include: (1) the focused use of the treatment frame, (2) the clear hierarchy of intervention, and (3) the higher level of therapist activity. Of note, the present group of TFP practitioners in the UK have a median of 17 years of clinical experience and this level of experience may also influence the successful implementation of once-weekly TFP. While once-weekly TFP does deviate from the standard format, the duration of TFP offered in the NHS, up to 18 months, may be an important factor. Research has emphasized the extended duration of an intervention required for the reconsolidation of unconscious patterns; the positive results observed anecdotally by NHS clinics offering once-weekly TFP may reflect the benefits of a more sustained intervention, albeit of less intensity. Thus, while UK practitioners are quite clear that the objective is structural psychic change, the degree of structural change that can occur may well be influenced by both intensity and by duration of therapy.

In a plenary address to the biennial meeting of the International Society for Transference-Focused Psychotherapy (ISTFP) in 2014, Frank Yeomans of Weill Cornell Medical College, the first author of the 2015 TFP manual *Transference-Focused Psychotherapy for Borderline Personality Disorder: A Clinical Guide,* outlined the many still unanswered questions about the determination of the recommendation for TFP as a twice-weekly modality [14]. This address aimed to examine the clinical, theoretical, research, and political or administrative implications of this debate.

British clinicians questioned the requirement for the twice-weekly requirement given their observations about useful weekly treatments conducted in the NHS. They raised provocative and informed questions about how to measure the benefits derived from TFP treatment, and where to locate in the treatment design those key areas that fostered both the lessening of standard BPD symptoms and the critical elements of identity consolidation and increased capacity for integrated experiences of self and others.

The British collective experience provided TFP therapists world-wide with a well-considered and thoughtful reconsideration of the treatment's design. In particular, the NHS experience is of great value to those systems that might not be sufficiently resourced to provide extended, twice-weekly treatment, but nevertheless find TFP's fundamental principles of use, including in the individual treatment setting.

What Is the Source of Institutional or Government Support for this Initiative?

TFP is at an early stage in the UK and there are few NHS sites offering TFP at present. We use (1) an established service, (2) a newly formed service, and (3) one at conceptual stage, to illustrate TFP development and thinking in the UK.

An Established Service: DeanCross

DeanCross is a specialist PD service in the East London NHS Foundation Trust. It is a multidisciplinary team, composed of psychiatrists, psychotherapists, and psychologists. The Royal College of Psychiatry, in awarding DeanCross Team of the year in 2019, recognized that one of the service's notable accomplishments was its early introduction of TFP in the UK. The recent position statement on PD by the Royal College of Psychiatry [11] identified the need for services that offer a range of specific, evidence-based interventions, and which are arranged in phases. The ability to draw on both MBT and TFP, with their predominantly deficit and conflict-based approaches respectively, facilitates this recommendation. DeanCross offers a coordinated package of treatment with each patient receiving both group and individual therapy.

The service currently serves as a TFP hub in the UK, through its treatment program, collaborative links with services starting TFP, training and supervision activities, and research via the Centre for the Understanding of Personality (CUSP), which is affiliated with academic psychiatry departments in Oxford and Queen Mary Universities.

DeanCross has recently introduced TFP to its existing MBT program. DeanCross identified the add-on value of TFP to its existent service as being both (1) "Applied TFP," i.e., application of its principles to the overall service, and (2) "Direct TFP," i.e., TFP treatment for narcissistic patients.

1. Applied TFP:
   a) Aiding the assessment process: Through its focus on the level of personality functioning, TFP enables a clearer assessment of personality dysfunction and more nuanced treatment strategies. TFP also enables a clearer mapping onto the new ICD-11 [15] diagnosis of Personality Disorder and alternative model of PD in the DSM-5 [16], particularly in relation to the emphasis on self and interpersonal relations and levels of severity of personality organization.
   b) Setting the treatment frame: The treatment contract, treatment frame, and treatment objectives are technical components, which have been particularly developed by TFP and can be used with great effectiveness as there is a greater ability to explore the *treatment relationship* in TFP due to its emphasis on the transference. Given the prominence of challenges in interpersonal relations that mark PD presentations, a treatment such as TFP that uncovers the individual's predominant mode of relating (by allowing a specific exploration of the patient's response to the treatment frame and structuring of the

relationship through the treatment contract) is an extremely useful contribution to the field.

c) Aiding the supervision process: Further training of its specialist staff in the management and technical use of the transference and countertransference, as informed by TFP principles, provides guidance in a critical aspect in working with patients with severe PD.

2. Direct TFP:

Patients with narcissistic personality Disorder (NPD) have consistently not done well in the program to date and there was a need for addressing this at a technical level, which TFP allows as it has a more developed approach to NPD [17]. Of note, this is of clinical use not only to patients with NPD but also to BPD patients with moderate to severe narcissistic traits. The service has a TFP group treatment for patients composed entirely of NPD patients diagnosed according to the Structured Clinical Interview for DSM-5 Personality Disorders (SCID-5-PD) [18]. Patients with a combination of BPD and narcissistic traits (either meeting full diagnostic criteria or subthreshold) are also slated to participate in a future TFP group.

Most importantly, in line with a guiding principle of the NHS as an accessible service based on clinical need, DeanCross believes it important that the most intensive and ambitious (for both patient and clinician) of evidence-based treatments for PD are available to patients in the public sector.

A Newly Formed Service: Lewisham PD Service

Lewisham's PD service was formed in 2021 and is in one of four boroughs in the South London and Maudsley NHS Trust (SLAM). The context for the new service was a reorganization of community services in the Trust following guidance from NHS England, with accompanying increased funding. There was recognition that provision for patients with a PD was inadequate when compared with services available for other conditions. The introduction of TFP was a "bottom-up" initiative by a group of Trust clinicians who had obtained charitable funding to train senior staff several years earlier. They arranged supervision from clinicians associated with the New York-based Personality Studies Institute (now TFPNY), as well as local senior-level British participation. They formed the TFP UK group, raising the profile of TFP in the Trust and nationally [19].

In 2020, the borough service director in Lewisham determined that the new Lewisham PD service would offer TFP, alongside MBT, which was already established across the Trust. The recognized evidence-base for TFP and its inclusion in the 2009 NICE Guidance [9] for BPD was crucial in this decision-making process. DBT would continue to be offered in the community mental health teams where it had been located for a decade.

As well as TFP and MBT, the Lewisham PD service also delivers Service User Network (SUN) groups. [20] These are 2.5-hour crisis and coping skills groups. Patients refer themselves and can attend up to three groups a week for as long as they wish. SUN offers containment to those at risk of suicide or self-harm. It reduces use of other services such as emergency rooms and other crisis services, tier 2 CMHTs, and general practitioners.

The PD Service also provides consultation to community teams (tier 2) and primary care staff (tier 1). Each team member is linked to a local CMHT to provide consultation on the suitability of referrals and advice on the management of patients. Consultation slots are weekly or every two weeks. There is also a plan to supervise CMHT staff delivering Structured Clinical Management (SCM) to patients with a PD [21].

The service has 11 clinicians equating to 9.5 full-time staff, as some staff work part-time. The team comprises psychologists and psychotherapists including a medical psychotherapist (a psychiatrist specializing in psychotherapy). The addition of a vocational advisor is also planned. Within the staff group, additional skills include psychiatric nursing, family therapy, social work, occupational and art therapy. Seven members of the team are training as TFP therapists under the head of service, an ISTFP teacher and supervisor, supplemented by external supervisors from New York and Barcelona.

Patients have a moderate or severe PD, predominantly BPD as well as other PDs such as NPD. They are referred from primary or secondary care teams, some via crisis and inpatient services. Patients have usually previously received therapies such as cognitive behavioral therapy (CBT) or CAT or have received standard psychiatric treatment from the CMHT, at the tier 2 level. Some have previously had a year of full DBT, or a seven-month DBT skills group.

The patients exhibiting the most severe acting-out, self-harm, and suicidal behavior are directed to DBT, which teaches means to control destructive impulses and to cope with emotional dysregulation. MBT is offered to patients organized at mid- and severe-borderline personality organizations (BPO) demonstrating significant deficits in mentalization. MBT's distinctive qualities include its support for emotionally reactive patients whilst making fewer demands than TFP in terms of contractual obligations and functioning in the world. However, TFP has influenced MBT in the service: MBT patients are expected to have day-time structure, work if they can manage it, and to stop or reduce self-destructive behavior such as cutting, drug-use or unhealthy drinking.

TFP emphasizes patients getting back to functioning in the world, as well as addressing underlying issues. TFP is offered to patients for whom there is a realistic prospect of achieving healthy vocational and interpersonal functioning. Patients are assessed over three to four sessions. The first session is a traditional clinical interview; the SCID-5-PD [18, 19] and Structured Interview of Personality Organization—Revised (STIPO-R) [22] are carried out in the second session, and a third session is for sharing the diagnostic impression and treatment planning. A fourth session involves meeting a family member with the patient. With advice from services in DeanCross, London, and from the Barcelona specialist services for BPD provided by the Trastorno limite de personalidad -TLP- Group, the Lewisham PD service designed a written treatment contract that emphasizes the importance of all patients exerting agency in pursuit of individually agreed aims.

Patients attend either the MBT or TFP programs, which are offered as weekly group therapy and weekly individual therapy. TFP group therapy follows Kernberg's model [23]. Those not yet able to exert sufficient control over parasuicidal or other self-harming behavior within these programs are directed toward DBT.

At Conceptual Stage: Belfast Self Harm Personality Disorder Service

The theory of TFP was introduced to Northern Ireland in 2013 when a member of the ISTFP conducted seminars to the Northern Ireland Psychoanalytic Society. The Belfast Self-Harm Personality Disorder service is largely an MBT service, made up of senior nursing and social work practitioners. A senior practitioner as well as the team leader and consultant psychiatrist have completed the foundation course in TFP and are progressing in training for certification as TFP therapists by offering individual therapy.

As with many NHS PD services, the Belfast service focuses on group treatment. However, for those patients who are unable to participate in a group modality, either because they are unwilling to do so, or likely to be disruptive to the group process, TFP, as a "close relation" to MBT, seemed a logical choice as an offering of an evidence-based intervention individual treatment for PD patients.

The service believes that the shared psychoanalytic/psychodynamic underpinnings of MBT and TFP allow for integration the two treatments within the one service in Belfast. The individual TFP is offered to patients who seem unable to make use of group treatments but are sufficiently psychologically minded to still have access to an evidence-based treatment for personality disorder. The goal in providing TFP within this service includes the recognition that while behavioral changes directly addressed in other therapies are of great importance, creating change in an individual's underlying personality structure requires a treatment that is influenced by psychodynamic techniques, with TFP offering a direct way of integrating this work within the service. The service also plans to use a TFP-informed approach in supervising psychiatry trainees in their psychodynamic training case.

What TFP Principles Might Be of Utility for the Clinicians Working in the UK NHS?

Assessment The diagnosis of PD is problematic for the clinician and for the patient, as has been referenced. Clinicians have difficulty in establishing a diagnosis of PD. TFP contributes through underlining the importance of a thorough assessment—particularly regarding depth and accuracy, including attention to the level of personality organization as described in Kernberg's structural interview [24].

TFP principles can help technically, as in guiding the clinician in the assessment process. In addition, TFP's focus on the psychological aspects of personality can help the clinician who may be daunted by the longstanding controversies about the

PD "label" or the relative validity of the PD diagnosis. TFP thus contributes usefully due to its particular emphasis on (1) identification of internal object relations and linking affect, and (2) on severity of PD pathology. In this way, TFP is very much in line with developments in ICD-11 and DSM-5. This approach is important firstly, as it is "clinically near" as the focus is on personality functioning through the prism of self or interpersonal (i.e., 'other') dysfunction. This is consistent with psychoanalytic theories of personality, in particular contemporary object relations theory with its emphasis on the individual's internal representation of self and others. Secondly, the dimensional nature of personality and PD pathology is reinforced by the focus on severity. This not only makes clinical sense but is also backed by research, for example, showing that generalized severity is the most important single predictor of current and prospective dysfunction [25]. The emphasis on the severity of personality organization and the focus on psychological aspects of personality, particularly identity diffusion, suggests that a TFP-informed approach to assessment is both clinically helpful and consistent with ICD-11 and DSM-5. Based on the above, a TFP-informed approach to assessment via the structural interview is of use to clinicians *even if they don't then offer* TFP.

Treatment Model TFP has operationalized and developed expertise in establishing the treatment contract as a critical element of the treatment frame. It has described how key psychoanalytic techniques, specifically the use of technical neutrality, active monitoring of transference and countertransference, and judicious interpretation, are relevant in psychotherapy and specialist PD services. The treatment model is thus usefully applied as a stand-alone model in some services, but equally important, these aspects of TFP, particularly its use of the treatment frame and treatment contract, can be applied in services using different approaches. In terms of direct treatment, the UK has accrued experience in developing TFP as a once-weekly treatment of one to one-and-a-half-year duration, through a careful application of the strategies, tactics, and techniques, rather than any specific modifications of standard TFP. In addition, Lee and Hersh [13], as referenced, described the key way that the introduction of TFP principles to clinicians in the NHS system can provide a set of useful, practical skills in managing primary or co-occurring PD pathology.

Application of TFP Principles in Different Settings The usefulness of the treatment frame, treatment contract, and of the operationalization of key psychoanalytic techniques, can be applied to different levels of care beyond psychotherapy settings, including within psychiatry, (as illustrated in the section to follow on old age and adult psychiatry) and within principle-informed supervision. Potential benefits of the dissemination of TFP principles within the NHS could include useful concepts for prescribers, inpatient psychiatry clinicians, and those medical providers seeing patients with identified PD pathology, or those simply identified as the "difficult patient" who may be demonstrating elements of PD pathology that have not been diagnosed.

Learning a Psychodynamic Treatment The characteristics of TFP, based on contemporary object relations theory, emphasizing key psychoanalytic techniques, and operationalized, means it has useful properties that could help clinicians who are learning how to undertake psychodynamic psychotherapy.

What Is the Format for Instruction of TFP Principles for this Audience?

TFP-Informed Supervision to Community Mental Health Teams Working with Older Adults

A pilot project of TFP-informed supervision for the CMHT of the SLAM Mental Health of Older Adults' service (Tier 2) offers an example of ways that applied TFP within the NHS can be assessed for effectiveness (see the Clinical Illustration below for more detailed information about this service). The use of TFP-informed supervision in this context grew organically from the needs observed by both patients and clinicians.

There is strong evidence that clinical supervision can lower emotional exhaustion and stress in clinicians [26]; the SLAM service developed a model using TFP as the frame to help the community teams think about this group of patients.

Key aspects of this TFP-informed supervision initiative are the following:

The Importance of Structuring the Treatment The strengths of the TFP model for this work is based on TFP's clear framework, which can protect clinicians against feeling overwhelmed. By describing some of the techniques of TFP, the supervision groups gave the clinicians a shared language to help them think about their patients, and an opportunity to explore and understand the strong feelings that were often evoked. Zerbo et al. [27] used a similar method when using TFP principles in a general psychiatric residency. When working with the multidisciplinary CMHT teams in a community setting it was often initially observed that in the treatment of patients with primary or co-occurring PD pathology, there was a feeling of chaos, compounded by the need of the clinicians to "do something." This need for action could mean feeling the need to pursue psychiatric admission, as clinicians did not feel effective or able to contain risk, or discharging a patient from the service entirely. Clinicians were vulnerable to developing problematic, and sometimes troubling, countertransference reactions with associated counterproductive actions; for example, concluding that patients were "manipulative" with the idea that the patient was purposely being difficult.

The Importance of Clarification Work with the CMHT informed by TFP principles focused on the importance of history taking in order to make sense of the behavior of the patient, together with an understanding that much of the behavior observed reflected unconscious processes, often learned as a defense against the abuse that some of the patients had suffered. Supervision helped the clinicians understand the need to ask for clarification about the patients' experience in order to directly address the patients' anxiety and to contain emerging affects by putting those affective states into words.

The Importance of Reflecting (as opposed to acting) The supervision encouraged staff to consider the emergence of expectable splitting behaviors exhibited by patients, approaching this pattern in an empathic manner, while providing modeling for the patient by creating a distance from intense affects and encouraging reflection rather than action, to promote thinking and understanding. The TFP techniques helped the clinician to tolerate confusion and to be able to step back think and pay attention to any countertransference currents. However, it is important to reinforce that this supervision was not developed with the goal of teaching these clinicians to be therapists, per se, but rather to help them understand the patients' experience in order to treat them more effectively and feel less overwhelmed in any number of clinical settings.

Part of the process was also to help clinicians understand the use of supervision. Supervision was framed as a space safe enough to talk about difficult feelings to ensure they did not get acted on. It was also deemed paramount that the clinicians did not feel judged.

The Importance of Monitoring the Three Channels of Communication This supervision also highlighted the three channels of communication: verbal, non-verbal, and countertransference. The communication patterns of PD patients were often observed to be rapidly developing, intense, unstable, and confusing. In the work with PD patients within the SLAM Trust, the staff's ability to think about the patient's inner world and communicate in a measured and deliberate way was frequently disrupted. Introducing staff to the concept of "technical neutrality" facilitated appreciation of the whole of the patient's experience that could then be examined, preventing the clinician from too rapidly taking sides with one part of the patient's story. It was important for the staff to understand the true nature of splitting and how it can manifest itself in a team, while also acknowledging that every team member is likely part of a split at some point.

The Importance of the Contract Setting The supervision stressed the use of a contract with the patient, but with the understanding that this was something collaborative that would provide an organizing framework to help consider some of the patient's more difficult behaviors. It was important to work with the idea that this was a contract that would likely be challenged but would also provide the frame to discuss expectations and contain threats to treatment such as non-engagement and suicidality.

These supervision sessions were also a place to think about the relevance and evidence of specific therapy models. However, the supervision also reinforced the awareness that treatment-resistant patients are also frequently part of a caseload and that clinicians needed support with their management to explore what could, or could not, reasonably be offered.

TFP Training to Young Psychiatrists

Training modules have been developed in a few trusts in the UK aimed at psychiatrists, at both trainee and consultant level. The premise of this training is that core principles and techniques of TFP can be used in general psychiatry to help in the management of patients with borderline PD (or other moderate to severe PDs) [13, 28].

The training focuses on: *knowledge* –appreciating how an understanding of object relations assists the clinician in assessment and treatment; *attitude*—developing a stance to managing the confusing and negative feelings that may arise in both clinician and patient; and *skills*—describing how the use of TFP techniques (the use of the treatment contract and technical neutrality, analyzing the transference and countertransference, and judicious use of interpretation) helps the clinician to continue thinking in the fraught clinical encounter.

Specifically, we describe one such training, developed in Tower Hamlet's East London NHS Foundation Trust (ELFT), which provides junior doctors working in psychiatry with a short series of teaching sessions on TFP theory and techniques aimed at providing a fundamental framework that trainees can apply when working with PD patients. Two cohorts of junior psychiatry trainees in ELFT received four teaching sessions, each of one-hour duration, on TFP theory and techniques. All four teaching sessions were given by a consultant psychiatrist, certified TFP teacher and supervisor. Sessions 1 and 2 described the theoretical and practical application of the strategy, tactics, and technique of TFP to the clinical encounter with a patient with PD, and sessions 3 and 4 demonstrated this by use of role plays.

The setting for the role-play was as follows: *Nina is a 34-year-old white Spanish woman. She moved to London 5 years ago following her boyfriend Raoul, who is in an on-off relationship with Nina.*

Nina has gone to the Emergency Room several times in the last year because of a strong urge to take an overdose of medication. She has previously been diagnosed as having a personality disorder.

Today, after an argument with Raoul, Nina has swallowed some of her sleeping tablets. Raoul has called for the ambulance to take her to hospital. After the hospital has checked that there are no serious medical complications from the overdose.

You are the psychiatrist meeting with Nina.

The lecturer and participants took turns taking the role of the psychiatrist. The actor who played the role of the patient is also a TFP-trained psychiatrist and in the debriefing gave feedback regarding the utility of different interventions. Importantly, the patient role necessitated statements demonstrating the pattern of oscillation in the interactions (in object relations terms, for example, the patient who alternates between the roles of victim and persecutor) and the confusion frequently arising in the encounter with a patient with PD. In this way, the training was intended to be highly applicable to clinical practice, allowing for live testing of the TFP teaching and the practice of new skills. The role-play was then followed by comments from all participants and direct feedback from the teacher on the understanding of TFP-based strategies, tactics, and techniques [29].

What Are the Possible Targets for Measurement to Gauge the Effectiveness of Instruction About Applications of TFP Principles?

TFP-Informed Supervision of Community Mental Health Teams

Research over a year, which was supported by pre- and post- measures both qualitative and quantitative, was conducted in the SLAM Mental Health of Older Adults' service. The results showed that supervision groups were found to be highly acceptable to the staff and there were high rates of satisfaction with the purpose, process, and impact of the supervision.

The common themes that emerged were (1) that the staff felt supported and gained confidence in working with service users with PDs, and (2) that staff felt they developed an understanding and skills in how to work with them. They felt better able to discharge patients safely and significant improvement was found in staff attitudes. While the response to this supervision for staff in their work with patients with PD diagnoses informed by TFP principles was generally favorable, particularly the nursing staff also conveyed feeling stressed about having to commit the time to supervision given their large caseloads. This concern about the additional time spent in supervision taking away from direct care highlighted the difference in culture between nurses and therapists and their respective attitudes about allocating time for supervision in this way.

These results helped the service managers to think about what was needed. Thus, regular supervision groups have been initiated throughout the service to support clinicians working in the community with this cohort of patients with PD pathology. Importantly, all members of the CMHT are encouraged to attend including psychiatrists, occupational therapists, nurses, and psychologists. The understanding of PDs in older adult services needs more research, but the clear evidence base and manualization of TFP provide a shared language for clinicians and TFP's roots in object relations and psychoanalytic thinking provide a system for learning to tolerate the very difficult emotions that surface in work with this population.

TFP Training for Young Psychiatrists

The East London NHS Foundation Trust training in TFP principles and techniques described above aims to improve the attitude and technical confidence among junior doctors working in psychiatry in the clinical encounter of a patient with a PD. The effectiveness of such a program is currently being evaluated in an ongoing pilot study. We report preliminary data from this study on 14 trainees, who completed 2 questionnaires, pre- and post-teaching, assessing clinicians' attitudes toward PD patients as well as their technical confidence in dealing with PD pathology:

- The Attitude to Personality Disorder Questionnaire (APDQ) [30] asks the responder to score from 1 to 6 on the frequency they experience certain feelings toward patients with PD. The individual statements are combined into scores for five themes measuring "Enjoyment/Loathing" (15 items), "Security/vulnerability" (10 items), "Acceptance/Rejection" (5 items), "Purpose/Futility" (3 items) and "Enthusiasm/Exhaustion" (2 items).
- In the absence of a suitable instrument, the ELFT research unit developed the Clinical Confidence with Personality Disorder Questionnaire (CCPDQ) [31]. This instrument consists of a set of 13 questions rated on a 6-point Likert scale addressing key issues identified in TFP including establishing and maintaining the treatment frame and in implementing the four main techniques, namely use of the transference, countertransference, technical neutrality, and interpretation.

Furthermore, a 1-hour focus group post-teaching was videorecorded, transcribed, and analyzed thematically [32].

On quantitative analysis, the Wilcoxon signed-rank test indicated statistically significant improvements in the total APDQ score ($P = 0.003$, $r = 0.81$), in Purpose/Futility ($P = 0.04$, $r = 0.53$) and Enthusiasm/Exhaustion ($P = 0.01$, $r = 0.70$), which indicate a large effect size.

The mean CCPDQ score at baseline was 2.58 (S.D. = 0.76) and it was 3.47 at T1 (S.D. = 0.71). A Wilcoxon signed-rank test indicated that there was a significant improvement in the questionnaire score ($P = 0.001$, $r = 0.88$), with a large effect size [33].

The thematic qualitative analysis showed an overall positive effect of the TFP teaching on their attitude and confidence: they felt it improved their understanding of the nature of personality disorder, their awareness and management of countertransference, awareness of object relations and relation dyads at play in the encounter. This is illustrated in one participant's response. *"I think understanding the object relations and the theory behind that and the affect that can be in the room...helps a lot, because it helps you name what's happening in an encounter and which can then reduce your own sort of feelings."*

Overall, these preliminary results indicate that, prior to the TFP-oriented training, trainees reported experiencing several difficulties in the clinical encounter with patients with a diagnosis of PD. They described a sense of helplessness, feeling out of control, unprepared and with a tendency not to set boundaries. Moreover, participants highlighted the necessity to get more teaching on PDs and how to manage this cohort of patients in different settings. The analysis of quantitative data from the APDQ and the CCPDQ questionnaires suggests that the TFP teaching gave rise to a positive change in trainee psychiatrists' attitudes toward people with a diagnosis of PD. Trainees reported an overall positive effect of the TFP teaching on their attitude and confidence: they felt that the TFP training improved their understanding of the nature of PD, their awareness and management of countertransference, awareness of object relations and relation dyads at play in their encounter of a patient with PD. Repetition of theory concepts and use of role-play was highly appreciated, according to the increasing literature on the methodological and evidence-based use of simulation in training [34, 35]. These findings, while needing replication in larger studies, match the international literature about the usefulness of TFP for psychiatry training purposes [28, 36–38].

Given the imbalance of expertise in PD and psychotherapy in different parts of the world, the contribution of teaching TFP abroad has significant potential, particularly in the light of this example being resource-light and delivered remotely.

Given the imbalance between the demand for services for patients with PD diagnoses and the relative dearth of trained clinicians, this four-session training method using TFP principles may have significant potential as one way to address this challenge. In particular, this training has the benefit of relative brevity; in addition, as with many supervising opportunities, experience from the years of the COVID-19 pandemic suggest that supervision delivered remotely can be effective.

Clinical Illustration: TFP-Oriented Supervision for CMHT Treating Older Adults with PD

Many countries and psychiatric organizations do not separate their services for older adults from those of working age. However, the SLAM Trust has a program for the mental health of older people, so those with mental health problems over the age of 65 are treated in a specialist service. Within this service, there are pathways covering all diagnoses, including PD presentations.

Diagnosing PD in the Elderly Even though the diagnosis of PD is no longer one of exclusion, there are still clinicians who struggle with its application. However, the publication of the ICD-11 has addressed this issue by underscoring the possibility that PD pathology can change over time. Moreover, the ICD-11 offers guidance about the treatment of older adults, pointing out that PD pathology can develop in later life, and this may be related to the loss of social support that has previously helped to compensate for personality disturbance [39].

The observation that clinicians appear to struggle to diagnose PDs in older adults can be linked to a broader resistance to diagnosing PDs in younger adults, together with a limited understanding of how the personality pathology of a younger adult can manifest differently in later years [40]. Therefore, there is a well-described risk of not making a proper diagnosis of a PD for patients given the high morbidity and mortality associated with that condition; clinical experience suggests that mental health providers can therefore lack the benefit of confidence in their diagnostic impression to then guide their interventions with this challenging patient population. The failure to deliberately elicit a patient's history that could support making a PD diagnosis can undermine the confidence of the clinician who can become confused and deskilled attempting to provide treatment for those patients with a primary or co-occurring PD diagnosis. It has also been widely observed that clinicians become anxious talking about such a PD diagnosis with patients, even when that diagnosis is reliably made [28, 29].

Clinical Presentations of PD Pathology Among the Elderly Older people with PD pathology may display self-harm behaviors less overtly. Beatson et al. [41] describe PD symptoms in the elderly as including: (1) the abuse and misuse of medication, including non-adherence to a medication regimen, especially those prescribed for serious physical conditions; (2) the sabotage of treatment, such as interfering with surgical wounds and catheters; (3) the refusal to engage in physical rehabilitation; and (4) the disordered eating behaviors in which patients violate or ignore prescribed diets and exercise advice, which could result in serious illness or death. Self-harming behaviors such as skin-picking and head-banging are also observed. Clinical experience would add that serious self-neglect can be seen in a patient's refusal to get out of bed and engage with any form of self-care. Emotional dysregulation can persist and there may be increased levels of depressive and somatic symptoms, and complaints.

Also observed among older people are greater manifestations of insecure attachments, which present as high levels of dependency on staff and carers, leading to excessive demands for medical care and somatic symptoms sometimes employed unconsciously to obtain closeness. Inpatient psychiatric admissions and challenges in the maintenance of continuity of care can contribute to an increase in needy or clinging behaviors, thus promoting intense anxieties among staff, and, at times, sabotaging discharge planning with associated concerning ramifications. Suicidality is something to be taken seriously in older adults as while there may be a reduction in the number of attempts, but they tend to be more successful when they occur. Harwood et al. [42] noted that along with depression, personality factors appear to have an important role in the suicide of older people.

It is also possible to see counter-dependent behaviors representing desperate attempts to deny emotional neediness. The result of the above makes caring and treating these patients very difficult, especially as they often arrive in the older adults' services without a helpful history and it can appear that a patient's PD symptoms have been in remission, as even dysfunctional relationships have added some level of support. Remission, of course, is not the equivalent of recovery, which becomes evident when that support is lost [43].

TFP for Older Patients with PD Within the Mental Health of Older Adults' service in SLAM, some individuals with PD diagnoses are treated with weekly TFP, over the course of a year to eighteen months. With its roots in psychoanalytic psychotherapy and contemporary object relations tailored to work with severe PD pathology, TFP not only focuses on relieving symptoms such as chronic suicidality, but as Kernberg [44] points out, it has the ambitious goal of personality integration and encourages people to re-engage with life, friendships, and creative and cultural pursuits.

Over the course of treatment, the SLAM clinicians witness patients working through dependency and chronically unstable relationships with family, and those around them, until they are able to tolerate intimacy in the therapeutic relationship and with others in their lives. Older adults often come with stories of the considerable neglect and abuse they have suffered, which they have retold many times, but through negotiating a working frame, or contract, with the therapist, followed by techniques of clarification and confrontation, and eventually interpretation, they can experience feeling heard and understood, albeit with periods of irritation, when they might feel interrupted by the clinician's exploration.

Case illustration: Mr. T. was a 74-year-old man who had been prescribed benzodiazepines from an early age by his father, a practicing physician, and was now buying high doses of these agents on the internet, which was having a paradoxical effect on his anxiety. A 2-month inpatient psychiatric admission allowed for a supervised medication reduction of benzodiazepine use with the support of the medical team. As the medication was reduced, he was engaged in CBT for anxiety symptoms, but elements of his mixed borderline and narcissistic PD pathology emerged. He was referred for TFP, which involved a standard assessment process aimed at clarifying the contribution of his PD pathology to his clear picture of longstanding benzodiazepine dependence. Previously he had sought psychiatric admissions for both depressive and alcohol use disorders, but learning about the contribution of PD pathology, even at this late date, provided the patient with a sense of relief, as he felt this information aided in his understanding of his struggles with meaningful relationships over the years. The local NHS services offered to support Mr. T. in 18 months of weekly TFP treatment, given their appreciation of his differential diagnosis and their assessment that such a commitment reflected a useful expenditure of resources.

At the outset of treatment, Mr. T. was invited by his therapist to reflect about how he communicated with those around him. He would tell long, digressive stories about his youth, which began to "anesthetize" his therapist. He was able to tolerate the therapist's repeated clarification questions, which slowly impacted his longstanding self-absorption, as he considered that the therapist had opinions that were different from his own. He became more forthcoming, in an affectively genuine way, that led him to be more able to consider in depth this relationship's history and the assumptions he made about what others were thinking. During periods of increased distress, Mr. T. wondered about using benzodiazepines again to help him with his difficult feelings, but through the therapist's reinforcement of the treatment contract, Mr. T. was able to explore his destructive impulses and stay focused on the reason he was in therapy. He explored his reemergence of feelings of anger, including with the therapist, whom he saw as preventing him from accessing the relief available through benzodiazepines, and he was able to tolerate his anxiety as the therapist contained this anger without retaliating. As he progressed, Mr. T. was able to consider the kind of parent he had been and come to terms with the fact that for certain reasons, such as his periodic drug and alcohol use, he was as emotionally absent from his children. This realization facilitated Mr. T.'s improved capacity to engage empathically with his adult children, something that had long eluded him.

Over time, Mr. T. was able to articulate and tolerate his feelings and to link his physical symptoms with anxiety. He saw how his anxiety was linked to aging and dependency. He realized that as he had lived as a lodger in someone else's house for many years; this had served to isolate him further, as he felt unable to engage with others in a comfortable, hospitable way. As treatment was ending, Mr. T. was able to identify a different, and more comfortable, living environment, that allowed him to connect with his children and his friends in a different and more gratifying way.

As reflected by this case material of Mr. T., PDs can be characterized by maladaptive features including affective dysregulation, problems with relationships, vulnerability to stress, and limitations in use of coping skills, all of which have a profound effect on others including the care professionals involved [43].

The implementation of this novel use of TFP in a patient population not usually offered this kind of exploratory intervention stemmed from a collective realization of the service involved regarding the needs of both patients and clinicians. Empowering clinicians with an organizing, grounding set of TFP principles helped to limit the familiar emotional exhaustion that often has led to negative attitudes about work with PD patients. This reluctance can sometimes translate into an avoidance of exploration with the patients of the details of their chief complaints and histories that might help confirm a PD diagnosis. Hersh et al. (2016) describe that despite being extremely experienced, many clinicians find themselves being drawn into "a maelstrom of confusion," which leaves them unable to treat the patient in their usually reliable way. This departure for many clinicians from their standard practice may result from an avoidance to first assess, and then name, past or active symptoms of PD pathology. Countertransference reactions such as guilt and anger can make thinking difficult in these periods of confusion, together with unexpected or bewildering reactions the clinicians experience to their interventions with the patient.

Conclusion

The NHS of the UK is a world-renowned system providing healthcare in a comprehensive, government-run organization. Providing care for patients with PD diagnoses is a significant challenge; the NHS simultaneously attempts to integrate contemporary empirically validated interventions for these patients while balancing a need to manage with limited resources. Into this mix, in recent years a group of highly motivated clinicians of different backgrounds have strongly supported the introduction of TFP as an individual and group psychotherapy, and its more generalizable principles, into the system.

The work of the NHS has provided those in the world of TFP with a real-time "experiment" in adapting TFP to a once-weekly format. This experience thus far has generated valuable anecdotal information about the treatment in this form, with the promise of a more rigorous evaluation of this adaptation. In addition, local branches of the NHS have on their own integrated TFP principles in a variety of applications, that too contribute to the burgeoning movement of applied TFP in clinical care, training, and clinician retention.

Acknowledgments We thank Jonathan Radcliffe (Lewisham Personality Disorders Service), Iain McDougall (Belfast Self Harm Personality Disorder Service), Harry Reid (Centre for Understanding Personality) and Arianna Sinisi (University of Modena and Reggio Emilia) for their useful contributions to this chapter.

References

1. Royal College of Psychiatrists. Services for people diagnosable with personality disorder: Position Statement; 2020:1–35.
2. Roughley M, Maguire A, Wood G, Lee T. Referral of patients with emotionally unstable personality disorder for specialist psychological therapy: why, when and how? BJPsych Bull. 2020;45(1):52–8.
3. Wilson L, Haigh R. Innovation in action. 2011. http://personalitydisorder.org.uk/wp-content/uploads/2015/06/Innovation-in-Action.pdf. Accessed 09 Apr 2022.
4. Department of Health, National Institute for Mental Health in England. Personality disorder: no longer a diagnosis of exclusion. London: Department of Health; 2003.
5. Department of Health, National Institute for Mental Health in England. Breaking the cycle of rejection: the personality disorder capabilities framework. London: Department of Health; 2003.
6. Dale O, Sethi F, Stanton C, Evans S, Barnicot K, Sedgwick R, et al. Personality disorder services in England: findings from a national survey. BJPsych Bull. 2017;41(5):247–53.
7. Lamb N, Sibbald S, Stirzacker A. Shining lights in dark corners of people's lives—The Consensus Statement for People with Complex Mental Health Difficulties who are diagnosed with a Personality Disorder. https://www.mind.org.uk/media-a/4408/consensus-statement-final.pdf. Accessed 09 Apr 2022.
8. Paton C, Crawford MJ, Bhatti SF, Patel MX, Barnes TRE. The use of psychotropic medication in patients with emotionally unstable personality disorder under the care of UK mental health services. J Clin Psychiatry. 2015;76(4):e512–8.
9. National Collaborating Centre for Mental Health UK. Borderline personality disorder: treatment and management. British Psychological Society; 2009.
10. Crawford MJ, Kakad S, Rendel C, Mansour NA, Crugel M, Liu KW, et al. Medication prescribed to people with personality disorder: the influence of patient factors and treatment setting. Acta Psychiatr Scand. 2011;124(5):396–402.
11. Lewis G, Appleby L. Personality disorder: the patients psychiatrists dislike. Br J Psychiatry. 1988;153(JULY):44–9.
12. Chartonas D, Kyratsous M, Dracass S, Lee T, Bhui K. Personality disorder: still the patients psychiatrists dislike? BJPsych Bull. 2017;41(1):12–7.
13. Lee T, Hersh G. Managing the clinical encounter with patients with borderline personality disorder in a general psychiatry setting: key contributions from transference-focused psychotherapy. BJPsych Advances. 2019;25(4):229–36.
14. Yeomans FE, Clarkin JF, Kernberg OF. Transference-focused psychotherapy for borderline personality disorder: a clinical guide. Washington, DC: American Psychiatric Association Publishing; 2015.
15. WHO ICD-11 Clinical Descriptions and Diagnostic Guidelines for Mental and Behavioural Disorders. 2018. https://gcp.network/en/private/icd-11-guidelines/disorders
16. American Psychiatric Association. Diagnostic and statistical manual of mental disorders. 5th ed. Washington, DC: American Psychiatric Association; 2013.
17. Diamond D, Yeomans F, Stern B, Kernberg O. Treating pathological narcissism with transference-focused psychotherapy. New York: Guildford Press; 2021.
18. First MB, Williams JBW, Smith BL. Structured clinical interview for DSM-5 personality disorders. Washington, DC: American Psychiatric Association; 2016.

19. Radcliffe J, Yeoman F. Transference-focused psychotherapy for patients with personality disorders: overview and case example with a focus on the use of contracting. Br J Psychother. 2019;35(1):4–23.
20. Miller S, Crawford MJ. Open access community support groups for people with personality disorder: attendance and impact on use of other services. Psychiatrist. 2010;34(5):177–81.
21. Bateman A. Structured clinical management: psychiatric care for personality disorder in general mental health services. Aust N Z J Psychiatry. 2017;51:16–7.
22. Clarkin JF, Caligor E, Stern B, Kernberg OF. The structured interview for personality organization-revised (STIPO-R). Weill Medical College of Cornell University, 2016. Available from: www.borderlinedisorders.com
23. Kernberg OF. A systems approach to priority setting of interventions in groups. Int J Group Psychother. 1975;25(3):251–75.
24. Kernberg OF. Structural interviewing. Psychiatr Clin North Am. 1981;4(1):169–95.
25. Hopwood CJ, Malone JC, Ansell EB, Sanislow CA, Grilo CM, McGlashan TH, et al. Personality assessment in DSM-5: empirical support for rating severity, style, and traits. J Personal Disord. 2011;25(3):305–20.
26. White E, Winstanley J. A randomised controlled trial of clinical supervision: selected findings from a novel Australian attempt to establish the evidence base for causal relationships with quality of care and patient outcomes, as an informed contribution to mental health nursing practice development. J Res Nurs. 2010;15(2):151–67.
27. Zerbo E, Cohen S, Bielska W, Caligor E. Transference-focused psychotherapy in the general psychiatry residency: a useful and applicable model for residents in acute clinical settings. Psychodyn Psychiatry. 2013;41(1):163–81.
28. Hersh RG, Caligor E, Yeomans FE. Fundamentals of transference-focused psychotherapy: applications in psychiatric and medical settings. Springer; 2016.
29. Sinisi A, Marchi M, Prior D, Lee T. The contribution of transference focused psychotherapy in improving psychiatry trainees' attitude and technical confidence towards patients with personality disorders. BJPsych Open. 2022;8(S1):S10–S11. https://doi.org/10.1192/bjo.2022.97.
30. Bowers L, Allan T. The attitude to personality disorder questionnaire: psychometric properties and results. J Personal Disord. 2006;20(3):281–93.
31. Reid H, Lee T. The clinical confidence with personality disorder questionnaire (CCPDQ) Centre for Understanding Personality. London; 2021.
32. Braun V, Clarke V. Using thematic analysis in psychology. Qual Res Psychol. 2006;3(2): 77–101.
33. Cohen J. Statistical power analysis for the Behavioral sciences. Routledge; 2013.
34. Kowalski C, Sathanandan S. The use of simulation to develop advanced communication skills relevant to psychiatry. BMJ Simulat Technol Enhanced Learning. 2015;1(1):29–32.
35. Neale J. What is the evidence for the use of simulation training to teach communication skills in psychiatry? Evid Based Ment Health. 2019;22(1):23–5.
36. Moscara M, Bergonzini E. Integrating the principles of transference-focused psychotherapy with psychiatric consultation for patients admitted to a general hospital: a clinical application of a psychotherapeutic tool. Int J Appl Psychoanal Stud. 2021;18(1):18–29.
37. Kanter Bax O, Nerantzis G, Lee T. Transference-focused psychotherapy as an aid to learning psychodynamic psychotherapy: qualitative analysis of UK psychiatry trainees' views. BJPsych Bull. 2022;46(1):57–63.
38. Bernstein J, Zimmerman M, Auchincloss EL. Transference-focused psychotherapy training during residency: an aide to learning psychodynamic psychotherapy. Psychodyn Psychiatry. 2015;43(2):201–21.
39. Bach B, First MB. Application of the ICD-11 classification of personality disorders. BMC Psychiatry. 2018;18(1):1–14.
40. Rosowsky E, Young AS, Malloy MC, Van Alphen SPJ, Ellison JM. A cross-validation Delphi method approach to the diagnosis and treatment of personality disorders in older adults. Aging Ment Heal. 2018;22(3):371–8.

41. Beatson J, Broadbear JH, Sivakumaran H, George K, Kotler E, Moss F, et al. Missed diagnosis: the emerging crisis of borderline personality disorder in older people. Aust N Z J Psychiatry. 2016;50(12):1139–45.
42. Harwood D, Hawton K, Hope T, Jacoby R. Psychiatric disorder and personality factors associated with suicide in older people: a descriptive and case-control study. Int J Geriatr Psychiatry. 2001;16(2):155–65.
43. Zanarini MC, Frankenburg FR, Reich DB, Fitzmaurice G. Time to attainment of recovery from borderline personality disorder and stability of recovery: a 10-year prospective follow-up study. Am J Psychiatry. 2010;167(6):663–7.
44. Kernberg OF. New developments in transference focused psychotherapy. Int J Psychoanal. 2016;97(2):385–407.

Using Transference-Focused Psychotherapy (TFP) Principles in Adult and Adolescent Day Hospital Settings

6

Eulàlia Ripoll, Maya Krischer, and Joan Vegué Grilló

TFP and the Theory of Object Relations

The work of the psychiatrist and psychoanalyst Otto Kernberg has enhanced the standard nosology of personality disorder pathology by introducing the concept of borderline personality organization (BPO), which describes a group of patients with defining elements of personality structure that include, but is not limited to, patients with borderline personality disorder (BPD). Patients with BPO are notable for the lack of integration of internal representations of the self and others, which leads to identity diffusion and to the use of primitive defense mechanisms, while reality testing is usually preserved [1, 2].

According to object relations theory (ORT), the internal world of patients with BPO is characterized by split-off self and other representations marked by positive and negative affects and, thus, by idealized and persecutory subjective experiences of interpersonal relationships. In ORT, such a split-off experience of the world is considered a normal phase of the early stages of an individual's maturation process. However, as the infant matures, the normal process consists of an integration of

E. Ripoll (✉)
Mental Health Center BPD program, Centre Psicoteràpia Barcelona – Serveis Salut Mental (CPB-SSM), Barcelona, Spain
e-mail: eripoll@cpbssm.org; eripoll@gruptlpbarcelona.org

M. Krischer
Department of Child and Adolescent Psychiatry, Psychotherapy and Psychosomatics at the University Clinic of Cologne, Cologne, Germany
e-mail: maya.krischer@uk-koeln.de

J. V. Grilló
Grup TLP Barcelona, Centre Psicoteràpia Barcelona – Serveis Salut Mental (CPB-SSM), Barcelona, Spain
e-mail: jvegue@gruptlpbarcelona.org; jvegue@cpbssm.org

R. G. Hersh, C. De Panfilis (eds.), *Implementing Transference-Focused Psychotherapy Principles*, https://doi.org/10.1007/978-3-031-68062-5_6

different, contradictory elements, which is possible because of a predominance of relationships marked by positive affect, which then allows for greater tolerance and neutralization of negative emotional experiences. Thus, the infant over time will integrate an experience of self and others that is "good enough", reaching the threshold for integration and stability. In the case of patients with BPO, this integration has not been possible because of the predominance of internalized relationships colored by negative affect. In this case, the individual will alternate between experiences of idealization and devaluation of both the self and of others. This split-off pattern of internal object relations represents the foundation of the patient's disturbed behavior, which is a source of problems and conflicts for the patient [2].

Transference-focused psychotherapy (TFP) is a modification of psychoanalytic therapy developed by Kernberg [2, 3]. It aims to foster a structural modification of personality that allows for the resolution of identity diffusion. This aim is achieved through the exploration of the splitting processes in such a way that the patient can integrate the polarized representations of self and others that are maintained in an idealized or persecutory mode [2, 4].

The goal of this chapter is to introduce two models that apply TFP principles in the day hospital (DH) setting for, respectively, adult and adolescent patients with BPO. The DH program for BPO patients, which is part of a BPO integrated care continuum program of the Centre Psicoteràpia Barcelona-Serveis Salut Mental (CPB-SSM) in Barcelona, treats adult patients aged 18 years of age. A description of the extensive integrated care continuum is provided in full in Chap. 9 of this volume. The DH program of the Department of Child and Adolescent Psychiatry, Psychotherapy, and Psychosomatic Medicine at the University Clinic of Cologne University is a specialized psychotherapeutic unit that treats adolescent patients meeting criteria for BPO.

The Day Hospital Program for Adult Patients with BPO of CPB-SSM in Barcelona

Who Are the Patients?

Indications for DH Treatment

The DH is indicated for patients with psychopathological decompensations who require continuous care without the need for full-time hospitalization, with the aim of achieving the optimal clinical intervention while at the same time avoiding separation from their usual environment during the period of treatment and recovery [5]. Specifically, the DH is indicated for the following patient populations:

- Patients meeting criteria for severe personality disorders; according to Kernberg's concept of BPO these patients would be described as having lower-level borderline organization.
- Patients requiring a more comprehensive and intensive care because of moderate to high clinical severity, who show severe symptomatology such as high levels of

impulsiveness and emotional deregulation, have serious mentalizing deficits, exhibit identity diffusion, and endorse high comorbidity with eating, affective, and substance abuse disorders.
- Patients who present frequently in crisis situations, requiring emergency care but without needing full-time psychiatric hospitalization. In these cases, the risk of harm to self or others is determined to be limited, and symptoms of frank depression that would preclude full participation in intensive outpatient treatment, as in the DH setting, are not in evidence.
- Patients needing to improve their level of functionality in daily life, in light of the critical interference that the disorder generates in their relationships and activities.

The patients described above will likely have needs for more specialized services than could be routinely provided by the mental health centers in the local Barcelona public system, where intensive outpatient treatment involving multiple visits per week with a team of clinicians is not generally available.

Diagnostic Process

An accurate diagnostic evaluation is necessary for appropriate guidance in recommending treatment. First, it is necessary to confirm a diagnosis consistent with BPO to enter the DH program. Second, it is also necessary to determine the patient's severity of illness; in assessing psychopathology along the continuum of BPO, factoring in a patient's level of functioning, capacity for insight, and risk for impulsivity or self-destructive behavior, will be critical. The process of evaluation will inform recommendations for treatments offered in the DH setting including dialectical behavioral therapy (DBT) [6], mentalization-based therapy (MBT) [7], or TFP [2, 4]. In addition to the assessment of personality structure, as reflected in the level of personality organization, the diagnostic process will also evaluate comorbidity with other often co-occurring disorders including eating disorders, substance use disorders, and mood disorders. These co-occurring disorders will be treated either before the patient enters the DH program, or simultaneously with entrance to the program, depending on their symptom severity.

When a patient is referred to the DH, a process of diagnostic assessment begins. As noted, the diagnostic process is initiated with the structural diagnostic interview by Otto Kernberg [1] to evaluate personality structure, level of functioning, and the presence of comorbid disorders. It continues with a battery of psychodiagnostic tests, which include the following:

- Structured diagnostic interview for borderline personality disorders revised (STIPO-R) [8]
- Semi-structured clinical interview for axis II of DSM-IV (SCID-II) [9]
- Personality inventory for DSM-V (PID-5) [10]
- Diagnostic interview for patients with borderline disorder—revised (DIB-R) [11]
- Barratt impulsiveness scale (BIS) [12]
- Childhood trauma questionnaire (CTQ) [13]
- Symptom checklist-90—revised (SCL-90-R) [14]

- Clinical global impression for patients with borderline personality disorder (CGI-BPD) [15]
- Reflective functioning questionnaire (RFQ) [16]
- The Borderline personality disorder checklist (BPD-CL) [17]

Who Are the Clinicians?

TFP has been recognized as an effective individual psychotherapy for patients with BPD [18]. Recent investigations have extended the utility of TFP to patients with BPO, who may present with other clinical manifestations than solely BPD [19, 20]. TFP has been used mainly for the treatment of patients in ambulatory settings; our integration of TFP in an institutional context in the DH is a novel application.

In the DH setting, we work in the frame of institutional therapy (IT) with a multidisciplinary team and with a multicomponent program (individual and group therapy, attention to social functioning, family involvement, health education, support for creativity, and work on activity planning) [5, 21]. This allows for a more intense and containing environment and the observation of different patterns in interpersonal relationships in situ, with both other patients and professionals, in different spaces. This environment can facilitate a better understanding of split dyadic relationships and of what happens in the patient's external reality.

In Barcelona, CPB-SSM developed a specific treatment program for patients with BPO in 2005. It was expanded and redesigned in 2009 and is still in full operation.

What Is the Contemporary Standard of Care for Clinicians Treating These Patients?

DH is a partial hospitalization service that is defined as an intensive, time-limited care resource. In our DH we have different programs of treatment (Fig. 6.1) coexisting with the BPO program. At the same time, the BPO program is included as part of an integrated continuum of care that involves other services where the patients are assisted depending on their progress in recovery. This is the Cross-Sectional Program for BPO. Elements of TFP-informed individual and group treatments were integrated into a pre-existing partial hospital program.

Once the diagnosis for BPO is confirmed, the patient enters the therapeutic program after agreeing on the therapeutic contract. Patients attend the DH three hours per day for about six months. The program includes both individual therapy and group therapy in the context of IT as a central axis, which we consider essential for the proper functioning of a DH treatment. This means that in addition to the psychopharmacological and psychotherapeutic interventions, interpersonal relationships established within the institutional community acquire a special therapeutic action and value. Each component has therapeutic purposes, working on all the relational dynamics that occur both in the groups and in the milieu, defined as the time of all

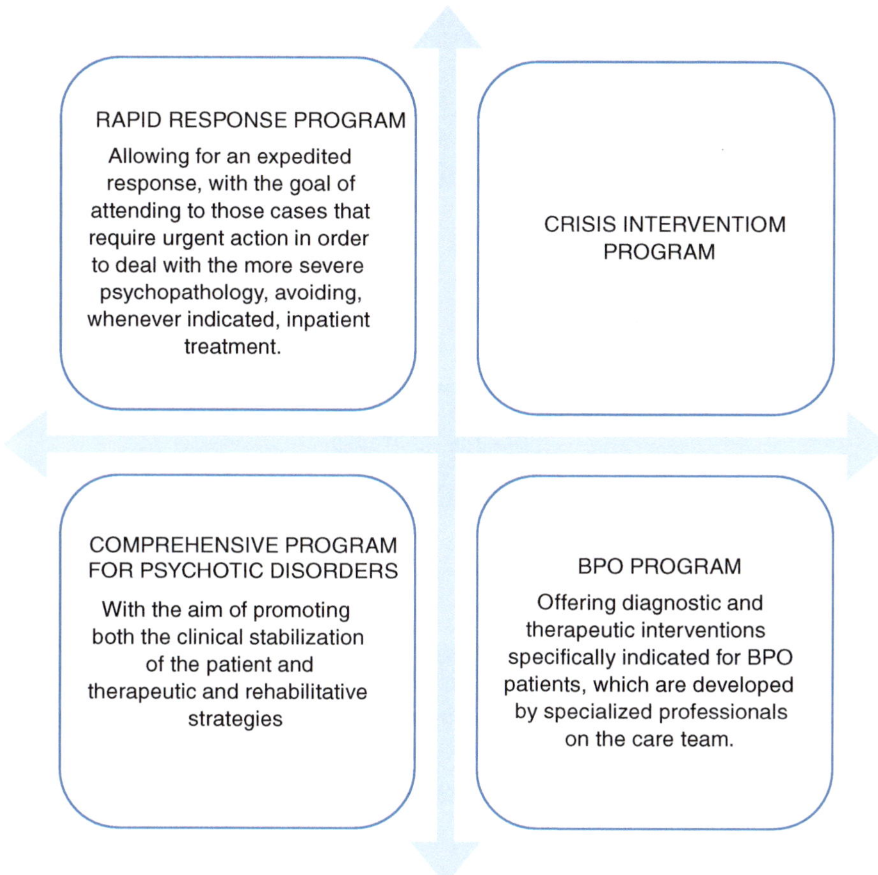

Fig. 6.1 Existing Programs within the Day Hospital of the Centre Psicoteràpia Barcelona – Serveis Salut Mental (CPB-SSM)

non-regulated activity, including time spent in common areas. For this aim, individual and collective activities, ranging from attention to daily needs to the expression of creative and recreational activities, are programmed to promote attitudes of adaptation and integration.

The characteristics of the program [5, 21] and its therapeutic components are illustrated in Figs. 6.2 and 6.3 and reported below:

- A multidisciplinary team that addresses individual, family, and community concerns.
- Treatment strategies that combine individual and group psychotherapy and psychopharmacology.
- Treatment planned in a hierarchical way, first addressing self-destructive, dysfunctional, and impulsive behaviors, and later working on increasing the

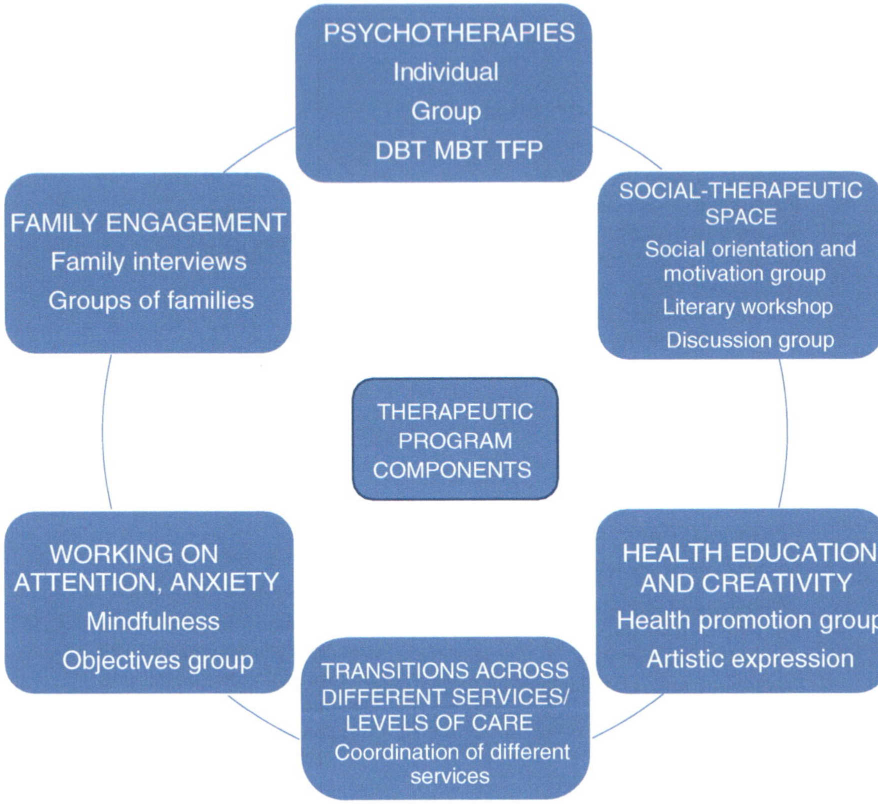

Fig. 6.2 Therapeutic components of the BPO DH Program of the CPB-SSM

reflective function or mentalization capacity and on decreasing the feeling of emptiness and identity diffusion.

What Are the Goals for Imparting to These Clinicians the Principles of TFP for Work with These Patients?

The DH applies TFP principles in general throughout treatment and also offers TFP as a specific individual psychotherapy modality.

The DH overarching design based on IT and the application of key principles of TFP aim to accomplish the following goals: (1) to allow staff and patients to develop a deep appreciation of dyadic patterns that emerge over time and (2) to facilitate observation in real time of the interactions among patients and between patient and

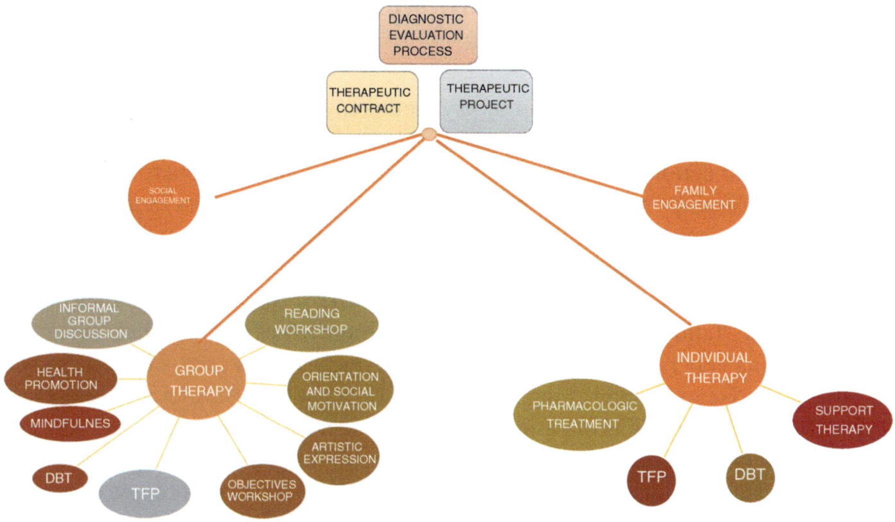

Fig. 6.3 Structure of the BPO DH Program Program of the CPB-SSM

staff. As with standard individual TFP, the main goal is to promote patients' process of identity integration. As recommended by TFP manuals [2, 4] we work with a therapeutic contract with anticipatory clauses, paying special attention to the idea that the patient must take responsibility for his treatment and has to commit to it together with the therapist. This key component of individual TFP, i.e., negotiating a treatment agreement at the outset with continued attention toward maintaining this agreement given expectable challenges over time, works in the DH setting much as it does in the individual, outpatient one.

In the DH setting, the choice of the modality of individual psychotherapy over the course of treatment includes the use of TFP at a specific time in the patient's treatment trajectory, and with specific goals that complement the use of DBT and MBT:

- *DBT* [6]: It is used in the initial phases of treatment for patients with self-destructive behavior, dysfunction, and marked impulsiveness.
- *MBT* [7]: It works in all institutional spaces, focusing on the analysis of relational aspects or emotional instability, to enhance the increase in reflective function or ability to mentalize.
- *TFP* [2, 4]: It is used in more advanced treatment phases, when the patient has developed sufficient impulse control and insight, to address aspects such as the feeling of emptiness and identity diffusion.

More recently, the program has also included eye movement desensitization and reprocessing (EMDR) [22] and systems training and problem-solving for BPD (STEPPS) [23, 24].

What TFP Principles Might Be of Utility for the Clinicians Working with These Patients?

Institutional Therapy (IT) is a form of psychotherapy in which the entire institution acts as a therapeutic agent, and the patient is an active part of the treatment milieu. The therapeutic action is in the environment, creating an atmosphere where interpersonal relationships reflect both what is happening for the patient in the here-and-now, and those aspects of the patient's past that inform present-day behavior [25]. The therapeutic process must encompass patients, family members, and team members, with a shared responsibility for treatment. The team behaves as a substitute and transition "family," which, through an environment of security and trust, promotes learning experiences that patients themselves could not carry out in their own families [26]. Hence, establishing an emotional atmosphere of tolerance and security within the institution is of paramount importance. Free communication between all members of the community and the expression of feelings and thoughts is essential. It makes it possible that the patient, despite his/her psychopathology, is considered a peer who interacts with the other members of the community and actively participates in the promotion of his/her own health [27, 28].

Individual TFP in the DH

After the diagnosis of BPO is confirmed, the therapist will share this diagnostic impression with the patient, and may recommend this treatment program, detailing the required therapeutic contract to be negotiated.

In this DH setting integrating the TFP model, individual therapy is one key element of the treatment, together with group therapy. The individual TFP treatment in the DH promotes the capacity to observe, explore, and finally integrate different object relations activated in the other parts of the DH program. Therefore, the exploration of the transference with the individual therapist will inevitably lead to exploring the patient's experience of the other members of the team and of the other patients in the program. When choosing the priority theme during an individual session, the therapist will thus consider the patient's interactions with the other patients and all team members. At the beginning of individual psychotherapy, the patient and the therapist determine the patient's overarching personal and treatment goals; the patient is therefore required to bring into the individual treatment the material related to those identified goals.

The observations of all team members are integrated into supervision and team meetings; this increases the staff's ability to identify the splitting in the patient's internal world, observe how it manifests in their interpersonal behavior, and appreciate how this might inform work in individual therapy. In this frame, we apply TFP principles with some modifications for the DH setting. Standard TFP interventions of clarification and confrontation are employed, as well as judicious interpretations that relate to observable splitting patterns. The variety of clinical situations within the DH allows for the observation of different roles.

TFP-Informed Group Therapy in the DH

The model we use in applying TFP in group therapy (Fig. 6.4) combines [29] the following:

- The consideration of Bion's basic assumptions operating in the group (i.e., considering the group as a whole) [30]
- The concepts of group analysis by Foulk and Anthony (i.e., considering the group as a social microcosm with fundamental interest in interpersonal functioning and interpreting group resistances but also individual ones) [31]
- The application of strategies, tactics, and techniques of TFP according to Kernberg [2, 4]: (1) countertransference monitoring, technical neutrality, interpretative process; (2) analysis of the dominant affects and dominant issues (by paying attention to the three channels of communication: verbal, non-verbal, countertransference); (3) facilitation of the activation of internalized and split-off object relations, with the goal of understanding the full range of the patient's affects and the different reactions of each member to that.

Specifically, in group TFP, each group member can observe and appreciate, in the same group session, different aspects of splitting, which in individual therapy could take much longer to be detected. The patient can identify the following:

- One's own behavior, reflecting one's own role or position in a conflict.
- How the other group members act, reflecting their different possible positions or roles in the same situation.
- How the other group members can act in different ways at different times, reflecting how their roles have been reversed within the group across the various sessions or even in the same session.
- The impact of one's own behavior on the other group members, which can help identify inappropriate behavior.

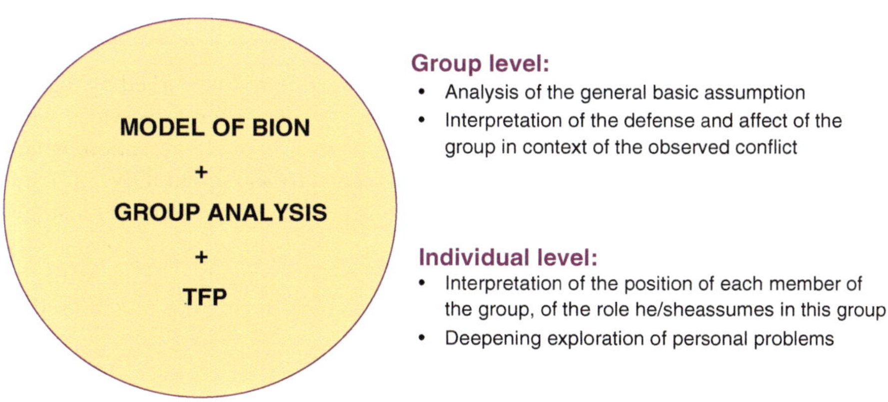

Fig. 6.4 Implementation of TFP principles in Group Therapy in the BPO DH Program Program of the CPB-SSM

Finally, once the different roles and the exchanges of roles have been detected, the reasons for one's own and others' splitting can begin to be interpreted (relation between dyads; defending dyads).

This TFP-based intervention applied to group therapy clarifies both patient-patient and patient-therapist interactions; this clarification, in turn, helps to foster behavioral change. Yalom defined eleven therapeutic factors operating in the interpersonal interactions in the group: installation of hope, universality, imparting information, altruism, the corrective recapitulation of the primary family group, development of socializing techniques, imitative behavior, interpersonal learning, group cohesiveness, catharsis, existential factors [32]. Group therapy is particularly helpful for BPO patients in the DH setting, as the feedback from the group is often more powerful than the feedback from one individual therapist.

General Principles of TFP and Specific Modifications for the DH

The DH setting has been implemented with the use of TFP strategies, techniques, and tactics, which are summarized in Fig. 6.5.

However, the application of TFP principles in the DH requires some modifications. Since the institutional frame of the DH implies a multidisciplinary team comprised of various professionals, patients relate to different professionals in different spaces. This point is the first and more relevant in making necessary modifications. The patient activates different internalized object relations in different spaces and in the different relationships with the various professionals who intervene in the treatment process. This understandably has both positive and negative implications; different staff members can develop conflicting ideas about the patient, depending on their own pattern of interaction with the patient. Relational patterns that may not initially appear in the patient-therapist interaction during individual therapy, and may take time to appear, can instead be observed at earlier stages of treatment in the

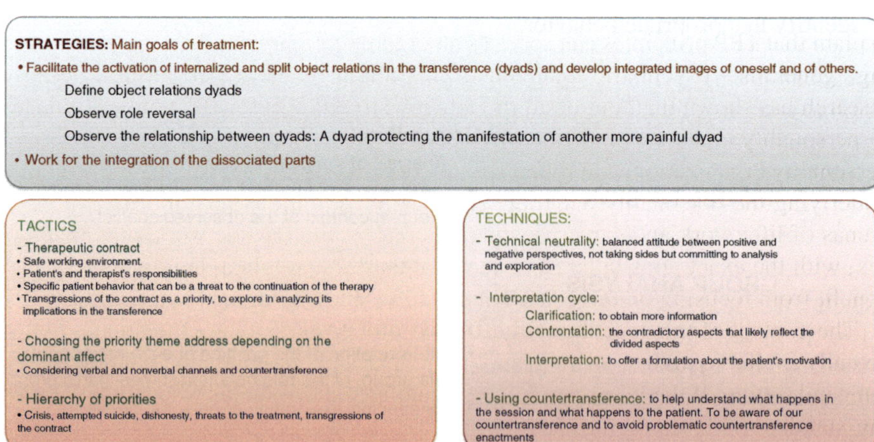

Fig. 6.5 TFP strategies, tactics and techniques that are employed in the BPO DH Program Program of the CPB-SSM

interactions between the patient and the other staff members of the DH. This process helps the clinician involved to better know the patient and to form a more nuanced idea of their inner world in less time. Notably, this process can be constructive as long as it facilitates the sharing of information and does not result in the creation of tensions within the team. For this reason, it is important that all the professionals of the team share the same treatment goals, have a similar appreciation of the internal dynamics of the patients, maintain the ability to monitor countertransference, and coordinate to share the information with the rest of the team. Therefore, an accurate coordination of the various therapeutic interventions is necessary, otherwise conflicts could arise within the team, and the information necessary to carry out intensive, multimodal therapeutical work would be lost. To make this possible, a regular supervision process is necessary to ensure team coordination, avoid splitting within the team, and eventually evaluate treatment progress and foster patient recovery. In addition, coordination with the other services of the local mental health network that will assume responsibility for the patient's care after discharge from the DH is also necessary. As described in Chap. 9, in the Barcelona catchment area these services include, along with the DH, outpatient units, inpatient facilities, and rehabilitation programs. Coordination between services is achieved by employing joint TFP-oriented supervision and careful planning, in advance, of the discharge from a service (i.e., the DH in this case) and of the consequent admission to a different level of care based on the individual patient's current clinical picture and unique needs. This provides continuity of care and shared treatment goals across the different levels of care.

Strategy Modifications

In TFP, strategies aim to promote changes in personality structure, in a way that fosters the development of a more consolidated identity, through the integration of the inner, split-off representations of self and others.

Given the limited duration of the treatment in the DH, completing this process is unlikely to be possible in such a setting. This limitation needs to be discussed with the patients from the early stages of treatment, with the aim of motivating them to continue treatment following discharge from the DH.

To work on this, various strategies of TFP are applied in both individual and group therapy. In the DH setting, the existence of different scenarios where the patient interacts with professionals and peers facilitates the appreciation of different dominant object relations, split dyads, and associated role reversals, which can be enacted by the patient throughout the day depending on the different people (peers or staff) she or he interacts with. The advantage of the DH is that this can be observed in less time than that taken in individual therapy. The referring individual therapist will then gather this information from the different staff members who observe the patient and will put it all together and use it in individual therapy. Thus, in the DH program individual therapy represents the axis of treatment, that is, the place where all the observations of the patient's behavior can be discussed with the patient and integrated: here, naming the actors of the various dyads, identifying role reversals, analyzing the motivations for the reversal and discussing with the patient if one of the dyads serves to protect him or her from a more painful other, will support the goal of promoting the integration of patient's split-off self and other representations. In another scenario, during group therapy, the different roles of the various dyads can be represented by a single patient during the same session or even across different sessions. In addition, the different roles of a dyad can be enacted by different patients at the same moment during a session. Pointing this out in the here-and-now of the group session can help the patient to understand the motivations of these differences and the motivations of the patient's own changes in roles. Here, the work will follow the principles of group dynamics as the main axis of intervention, and the individual involvement of each member of the group will be considered only in a second step. In turn, what happens in the group can also enrich individual therapy.

In sum, the DH team of individual and group clinicians aims to accomplish the following goals:

1. To enhance the patient's capacity for self-observation by examining the various interactions between the patient and both staff and other patients.
2. To facilitate the appreciation of the patient's pattern of roles enacted in different aspects of the milieu.
3. To link emerging roles with aspects of the patient's history.
4. To consider different patients' reactions to aspects of the milieu.
5. To increase patients' ability to reflect on their patterns of splitting, and to link this splitting with changes in affect and behavior.

Tactics Modifications

The Therapeutic Contract The negotiation of the therapeutic contract in the DH follows the general guidelines provided by standard TFP manuals [2, 4]. However, some additional aspects have to be considered in this specific setting:

- The patients are required to authorize the different members of the multi-professional team to share information about their clinical status, in order to enable the staff to provide an integrated treatment. The same applies with other professionals involved in the patient's treatment, i.e., those who have assisted the patients in the past or will do that in the future, following discharge from the DH.
- While it is not feasible to prevent patients attending the DH from having relationships among themselves outside of the DH milieu, patients have to assume the responsibility of bringing into therapy any problem or conflict that could arise from those interactions.
- The treatment frame applies not only to individual therapy but also to group therapy and the institution as a whole.
- Contract violations can occur outside of the patient's individual therapy, in the interactions with other professionals, or with peers. These violations then become material to be addressed during individual therapy.
- The therapeutic contract defines roles and responsibilities of therapists and patients in the same way as in individual therapy; what is generally allowed and what is not, and also specific aspects pertaining to each individual patient

depending on determined treatment objectives. It is necessary to emphasize the importance of controlling self-harming behavior and impulsiveness, and the patient's responsibility to ask for help when feeling unable to control destructive urges.

Choosing the Priority Theme Choosing the main topic to deal with at each moment will depend also on the dominant affect observed. Examples of these priorities are all kinds of acting out and deviations from therapeutic contract, and disruptive behaviors, as during individual therapy. Sharing information among the different professionals will allow the therapist to accurately choose the priority theme, to identify the splits in the patient's inner world and appreciate how they manifest in behavior, and ultimately to show these dynamics to the patient.

Techniques Modifications

In the same way as in individual therapy, the staff of the DH setting uses technical neutrality, transference analysis and countertransference monitoring together with the techniques of clarification, confrontation, and interpretation. Clarification and confrontation are particularly relevant in making the patients aware of the observed contradictions in their behavior determined by splitting mechanisms. Becoming aware of these contradictions facilitates, in the patient, an increased appreciation of the nature of the inner conflicts underlying the contradictions, and therefore a better understanding of the functioning of the patient's internal world. In any case, it is made clear to the patient that these steps of exploration are part of an extended process that will require long-term treatment after discharge from the DH setting.

Clarification and confrontation can be very useful and effective in group spaces, where patients, themselves, clarify and question each other; in these contexts, such techniques may be even more effective than when used solely by an individual therapist. Relational conflicts tend to occur in group therapy spaces, and this can be an opportunity for fruitful exploration.

The individual therapy, thus, can be further enhanced by the group work. The patient who shares experience with those group peers who are at a more advanced stage of treatment may find their guidance to be a source of hope and motivation for change.

Interpretation is also possible: the staff may offer potential explanations for the contradictory aspects that have been observed in the patient's here-and-now behavior across different spaces of the DH. The patient can play different roles depending on whether he/she is in an individual or group therapy space, in occupational activities, or in free time spaces when interacting with peers. These different self-representations can be pointed out and explored and the motivations that cause them can be interpreted. These changes in self-representation can signal the patient's different roles, their changing positions, and the motivations for these changes.

Every individual member of the treatment team needs to identify his or her own countertransference reactions to the patient's attitudes or behavior, which may greatly differ among staff members. These reactions will be shared with the other practitioners during daily meetings of professionals to assess incidents that require intervention, at weekly meetings to assess patients' progress and share the different views of the patient by the different professionals, and during clinical sessions and case supervision.

What Is the Source of Institutional or Government Support for this Initiative?

In 2006 we started to use the structural interview and we began to adapt and use TFP principles in the DH and, more broadly, within the whole Cross-Sectional Program for BPO of the CPB-SSM (see also Chap. 9 in this volume) and in the coordination/supervision work with the mental health teams of the various institutions. Furthermore, TFP has also been offered as individual therapy since 2012, and as a group therapy since 2013. Data on the evidence of efficacy of the Cross-Sectional Program for BPO, including the DH service (see below), have been reported annually to the government since 2006; this made it possible to deliver TFP-oriented interventions in the cross-sectional program within the local public network of mental health services.

What Are the Possible Targets for Measurement to Gauge the Effectiveness of Instruction About Applications of TFP Principles?

Using the assessment protocol before and after treatment, starting in 2006, we have begun evaluating if patients had benefited from their treatment in the DH as well as in the other services of the Cross-Sectional Program. Specifically, from 2006 to 2014 we assessed the efficacy of the DH program using several relevant outcome measures: suicide attempts, self-destructive behavior, paranoid symptoms, improvement of interpersonal relationships, fear of abandonment, identity, impulsivity, feelings of emptiness, dropouts, and psychosocial functioning. Results indicated the following data of patients discharged from the DH:

1. Patients had improved significantly in suicide attempts, self-destructive behavior, paranoid symptoms, interpersonal relationships, fear of abandonment, identity, impulsivity, and feelings of emptiness. A longer stay in the DH predicted greater improvement in BPO psychopathology [33].
2. Also, 28% of the patients in the sample prematurely ended their DH treatment; those patients showed the greatest impairment in functioning among this patient cohort [34].
3. The patients who did improve maintained their gains at a 5-year follow-up. This improvement was particularly robust for symptoms such as impulsivity, and less so for psychosocial functioning [5].

These results indicate that our DH treatment for BPO patients is effective in terms of clinical improvement in all of the core typical areas of BPO, and in most cases, it is associated with good treatment adherence. However, they also point out the need to develop effective therapeutic strategies to improve psychosocial functioning in the long term.

What Aare the Didactic Materials Required to Impart TFP Principles to this Target Group of Clinicians and What Is the Format for Instruction of TFP Principles to this Audience?

The didactic tools used to impart TFP principles to the clinicians working in the DH program for BPO patients of the CPB-SSM are the following:

- Training sessions included in the current annual institutional training program.
- Weekly supervision sessions for all the teams of the Cross-Sectional Program for BPO patients.
- Four supervision groups (every other week) on individual TFP therapy led by external TFP teachers and supervisors.
- Two supervision sessions focused on TFP group therapy (every other week) led by Dr. Otto Kernberg and two TFP teachers and supervisors of the institution.
- Annual meetings for all the teams of the Cross-Sectional Programs for BPO patients, where teams present cases that are analyzed and supervised using the institutional TFP model by a TFP teacher and supervisor.

Clinical Illustration

Ms. S. is a 25-year-old single woman who is participating in the DH program in the context of escalating difficulties in her studies and conflicts at home, marked by recurrent threats of suicide and periodic self-harm. Ms. S. frequently displays behaviors that suggest she is not able to control herself, easily becoming overwhelmed by angry feelings she cannot manage. These behaviors were manifested in the DH setting in her relationships with the staff and with other patients, marked by episodes of threat and verbal aggression. Ms. S.'s individual therapist in the DH was surprised by the fact that her attitude in their therapy sessions, usually cooperative and engaged, was different from the attitude she displayed with her peers in the program and with other DH professionals.

Indeed, while Ms. S. is generally collaborative with her individual therapist, in other interactions in the DH she is irascible and stubborn. She bluntly states that she cannot tolerate when something she wants is not possible. She explains that her parents let her do whatever she wanted because they were afraid of her. She acknowledges that there is a repeating pattern: she cannot accept when others do not bend to her whims and because of this she becomes overbearing and repetitive, as she is inclined to dominate others and impose her desires.

Ms. S.'s therapist shares with the treatment team that sometimes the patient conveys that her pattern of expressed rage should be avoided, but at other times she regards it as something that should be justified. When confronted about this, Ms. S. denies that she ever justifies her anger, but does so in a way that allows the therapist to comment on this phenomenon as they speak, noting "It seems you are doing so now." Ms. S. does not respond to this observation with increased reflection; rather, she continues to express her anger and accuses others of attacking her.

In this exchange, the therapist pointed out the aggression expressed in Ms. S.'s tendency toward wanting to impose her ideas and not accepting a response she felt to be invalidating. Ms. S. was surprised by this point, denied being aggressive, and expressed dismay at the therapist's reaction. She maintained that she reacted to others but never did that in an aggressive manner, describing herself as a "pacific" person. The therapist again invoked a recent meeting when the patient became antagonistic in response to the therapist's comment; at this juncture, the therapist considered that she was again involved with Ms. S. in a circular argument without likely resolution. The therapist pointed out to the patient this pattern of rejecting what was offered by the therapist, seemingly without trying to reflect on what was conveyed. The therapist focused on the exploration of aspects of the patient's paranoid transference, asking whether the patient experienced the therapist as harmful or attacking, and noting that the patient appeared to find it difficult to view the therapist as well-meaning or concerned.

T: "Before when you were talking, I stopped to listen to you, to think about what you were saying, with the goal of offering you a hypothesis about what was happening. You communicated that you did not feel that I could be of help to you, that I was incompetent or useless. This may be how you see me, and it would therefore make sense that you would be dismissive, or even experience me as harmful to you. On the other hand, there might be a scenario where you see me as trying to be helpful. For us to move together in a constructive way, it would be important to examine your reflexive negative feelings about me and what I contribute, as my guess is that this pattern repeats itself with your relationships with others in the DH program here and in your life outside of treatment."

Following this exchange, the patient appears to be listening to the therapist, her affect changes, and she begins to cry silently. The therapist offers an interpretation about the patient's sadness: she suggests that the patient's rage can cover feelings of pain that she only rarely shares. She suggests that the patient can become arrogant and controlling when she feels vulnerable. The patient confirmed this hypothesis and noted that being open about her sad feelings has often led to an intolerable sense of vulnerability, including with the therapist.

The University Hospital of Cologne Day Hospital Program for Adolescents with BPO

Who Are the Patients?

Diagnostic Process

Juvenile BPD can now officially be diagnosed from age 13 years up, based on the changes in DSM-5 and ICD-11. Nevertheless, given the longstanding controversy about whether it is appropriate to diagnose personality disorders in youth, and despite the recent essential changes in both classification systems DSM-5 and ICD-11, we suggest an especially thorough differential diagnostic process for adolescents with borderline personality pathology.

In recent years, we have observed an increasing number of juvenile patients with personality pathology who have sought treatment for a range of symptoms at child and adolescent psychiatric clinics in Germany [35, 36]. This has led to a cumulative interest in specialized treatment models for adolescents with personality disorders. We know that a basic level of functioning, coping, and defense strategies protects against an early breakdown in childhood. The gradual separation from the parents followed by the necessity to form a consolidated identity in adolescence leads—in juveniles with an early identity diffusion—to a seemingly sudden decompensation in adolescence, often marked by suicidal crises and severe self-mutilation [37, 38]. The increasing challenges of developing autonomy during this developmental stage, and the lack of ego-integration, are reflected in frequent affect swings, termination of friendships, and outbreaks of diverse symptoms [37, 39]. In clinical practice, adolescent patients with borderline personality pathology exhibit a variety of severe symptoms [38, 40]. These include recurring suicidal tendencies and suicide attempts, self-harm, episodes of severe depression, eating disorders, drug abuse, school absenteeism or school dropouts, psychosomatic symptoms, social anxiety, and recurring interpersonal disputes. Due to the severity of such symptoms, these adolescents make great use of the psychiatric care system without necessarily accepting consistent outpatient psychiatric or psychotherapeutic services. Instead, the therapeutic processes are characterized by frequent interruptions and relapses and -sometimes- tragic chronic developments.

After a long period of reluctance to label and therefore diagnose personality disorders in adolescence, solid empirical research has now led to the consensus that borderline personality pathology can be validly diagnosed from adolescence as early as 13 years of age [36, 41–43]. Nevertheless, in practice, there is a collective concern about falsely attributing the often crisis-prone aggravations in the symptoms of adolescents to a personality disorder instead of to an adolescent crisis [36, 44]. In order to distinguish reliably between an adolescent crisis and a personality disorder in adolescence, specialized diagnostics should be employed at the beginning of every treatment. In this regard, the concept of BPO according to Otto Kernberg [45] is particularly helpful in identifying primitive defense mechanisms and identity diffusion beyond an adolescent crisis [38, 46]. Kernberg's model of BPO distinguishes between patients with a structural deficit and those operating at a higher level with only circumscribed areas of conflict. Kernberg's model focuses less on behavioral and more on structural criteria, such as the nature of defense mechanisms, the formation of object relations, and affect regulation. To date, there is growing agreement that a diagnostic differentiation between adolescent crises and a personality disorder based on Kernberg's model of BPO is necessary before treatment [41, 47, 48].

The criteria for distinguishing between identity crisis and identity diffusion are well described [37, 39]. The sudden discrepancy between the changing physical self and psychological experiences might lead to a gap between self and object perception and thereby to a temporary identity crisis [46]. In contrast, Paulina Kernberg listed a number of criteria, which serve as indicators for an identity diffusion, such as a painful feeling of an incoherent self, the over-identification with groups or roles, an un-integrated super-ego and unstable fragmented self and object representations [49].

In order to establish a clear differential diagnosis for adolescent borderline patients, the Cologne DH program described here uses a number of diagnostic instruments either for adults modified for adolescents or well-validated instruments for juveniles. In doing so, we try to identify adolescent patients with BPO based on identity diffusion and primitive defense mechanisms. This battery of interviews and self-reports employed to establish a personality disorder diagnosis in adolescents includes the following measures:

- International personality disorder examination (IPDE) [50],: the existence of a probable diagnosis of a personality disorder (meaning a lower threshold or number of criteria that need to be met, e.g., four instead of five criteria) based on DSM-IV/DSM-5 Section II is sufficient for the adolescent diagnosis of a personality disorder and, in ORT terms, of BPO [51, 52]
- Structured interview for personality organization (STIPO) [53]
- Interview for the assessment of operationalized psychodynamic diagnostics in childhood and adolescence (OPD-KJ) [54]
- Dimensional assessment of personality pathology (DAPP) [55]
- Inventory of personality organization for Adolescents (IPO-A) [56]
- Youth self-report (YSR) [57], which assesses internalizing and externalizing symptoms and behavior.
- Overt aggression scale modified (OAS-M) [58], a short interview assessing aggression against self and others.
- Beck depression inventory II (BDI-II) [59]
- Inventory of interpersonal problems (IIP-D) [60]
- Questionnaire on self-mutilative behavior (FSSV) [61]

Who Are the Clinicians?

In the Cologne University Hospital, a day clinic program for adolescent BPO patients was implemented in 2014 as a specialized treatment program for juveniles aged 13 to 17 years based on applied (TFP) transference-focused psychotherapy for adolescents (TFP-A) principles [37, 38, 62]. The program is located at the Department for Child and Adolescent Psychiatry and Psychotherapy at the University Clinic of Cologne in Germany and lasts for 12 to 16 weeks and treats six juvenile patients at a time. The unit is set up as a secure environment with clear boundaries and rules, transparent relationships, and tasks. From our experience, most juvenile borderline patients come from disorganized family structures [63]. The structured program at the Cologne unit serves as a container for emotions and self and object representations among all given relationships: other patients as well as the treatment team and therapists.

All members of the treatment team have been trained in ORT and TFP-A strategies, tactics, and techniques by the international society for transference-focused psychotherapy (ISTFP) supervisors. The individual and the group psychotherapists are certified TFP-A therapists. The treatment team consists of the following:

- TFP A- certified psychotherapist
- TFP-A certified group psychotherapist
- Psychodynamically educated and TFP-A trained body-oriented movement therapist providing a group therapy intervention focusing on body sensation
- Four members of the treatment team (two nurses and two social workers) who have all been trained in the TFP-A theory
- TFP-A certified supervisor as director of the program

All members of the day clinic team receive ongoing TFP supervision by external ISTFP supervisors every other week.

Within the program, the daily routine of all six adolescent patients who are treated simultaneously is based on the acceptance of responsibilities and common rules of external reality; this means that they agree to give up self-destructive and self-damaging behavior such as school avoidance, social isolation, and self-mutilative behavior. As part of the individual agreement (of adolescent, parent/ caregiver, and DH team) every patient has to attend their home school for at least 4 up to 6 lessons every day, depending on the distance between their school and the clinic. The DH program rule is "As much school as possible, as little as necessary," as long as the DH program attendance can be assured. In the early afternoon patients have lunch with the treatment team and other patients. In the afternoon—until 5 p.m.—the patient has to attend different treatment appointments. These include psychotherapy with a certified TFP-A therapist twice a week, group therapy based on TFP-A principles twice a week, body-related psychodynamic treatment once a week, daily teatime with the treatment team, a skills group once a week, a unit group for organizing the weekly schedule, as well as daily household routine.

A psychopharmacological treatment (often with an SSRI, such as fluoxetine) is quite common for the adolescents entering the present DH program. The medication regimen is periodically reconsidered, reduced, or stopped completely during the day clinic program when it does not influence depressive symptoms or seems only to serve the argument that "nothing really helps."

Once the diagnosis of a personality disorder is confirmed and the patient shows sufficient treatment motivation, the treatment contract is negotiated with the adolescent and one or both parents (see the following description). After agreeing to the treatment contract, the adolescent patient enters the treatment program.

What Are the Goals for Imparting to These Clinicians the Principles of TFP-A for Work with These Patients?

The aim of the DH program is to provide access for juvenile patients to an effective, specialized outpatient treatment and thus to counteract the self-destructive "revolving door" pattern of repeated hospital stays and chronic crises, which are typical in adolescence. This means that the program aims at: (1) reducing self-destructive and impulsive behavior, (2) limiting secondary gain of the disorder, (3) strengthening the acceptance of responsibility, and (4) finally, preparing patients for long-term (outpatient) TFP-A treatment. As mentioned earlier, a large number of adolescents with borderline personality pathology only come in contact with the health care system after experiencing a complete breakdown of functioning in school and in social life (e.g., self-withdrawal from all juvenile tasks, school attendance and life parameters, such as hobbies, use of the public transportation system, or helping in the family house). Often, they end up in a psychiatric hospital after opening up about severe self-cutting, suicidal ideation, or suicide attempts. Some of them have a history of outpatient treatment trials that are terminated because of repeated, serious self-mutilation, recurring hospital stays, or a pronounced early non-adherence with treatment.

What TFP Principles Might Be of Utility for the Clinicians Working with These Patients?

As mentioned earlier, the applied TFP-A interventions largely correspond with the principles of standard TFP-A and provide for a number of strategies, tactics, and techniques that have already been described by Normandin et al. [40, 62], Krischer and Normandin [38], and Kehr and Koepp [39]. The major differences include involving the parents in the TFP treatment and modifying the interpretation process, meaning the greater use of clarification and confrontation, and in general, more interpretation of relationships outside the treatment before exploration of the transference with the therapist.

Strategies Modifications

In the DH program, individual therapy follows the principles of outpatient TFP-A psychotherapy. However, the use of TFP-A techniques in DH work is not solely the responsibility of the individual therapist but is also the responsibility of the entire treatment team, which also follows the strategic principle of defining and naming object relationship dyads (whenever possible and tactful) in everyday interactions with the adolescents and at the same time maintaining technical neutrality. The aim is to gradually make split-off aggression accessible and more ego-dystonic to the adolescent patient, and to facilitate integration. This can enhance the opportunity for reflection through constant confrontation with self and object representation transferences onto any relationship of the unit. Adolescents must gradually learn to take on responsibility for their future, which requires a disentanglement from their parents [39].

In accordance with the strategic principles of TFP-A, therapeutic work must always define those dominant object relations dyads that emerge, which are observed between the patient and the different therapists and co-therapists. These defined object relations dyads are then explored, with attention to any possible defensive function they might serve. The team remains sensitive to the superficial or most readily available material reflected by the dominant dyads, as well as the dyads less likely to be in the patient's awareness (i.e., defended against) that are then identified by the treaters involved. An essential element of the TFP-A-based day clinic program will be the observance of technical neutrality by the treaters; this refers to the goal of avoiding taking one side of the patient's inner conflict. This goal of technical neutrality is bolstered by the involvement of multiple members of the treatment team, thereby countering the risk that one member of the team might be overly identified with one specific part of a patient's inner conflict.

Kernberg, O. F. et al. [64, p. 675] wrote (with reference to Paulina Kernberg): The main modification of transference-focused psychotherapy for the treatment of adolescents consists in changing the frequency and length of some specific techniques (e.g., more clarification, more work on relationships outside of transference before moving directly to transference); the approach (e.g., the use of the involvement of the family during the diagnostic phase and in the time when the treatment agreement is established; the involvement of supportive interventions in the environment while maintaining the analytical attitude in the sessions), and strategies (e.g., the goal of removing blockages that stand in the way of normal identity integration development and not forced maturation [39, 64]).

The DH program focuses on the initial phase of treatment with adolescents with BPD and establishes the foundation for later standard, outpatient TFP-A. The goal is that TFP-A as an outpatient long-term treatment will be less likely endangered by persistent destructiveness against the treatment frame expressed through self-mutilation, repeated crises, and inpatient hospital stays. Actions such as self-harm, suicidal behavior or the use of addictive drugs are addressed during the DH stay. The major focus is the structural work before focusing on the underlying content. As Kehr and Köpp [39] pointed out about the beginning of a TFP-A outpatient treatment: "This applies in particular to the regulation of affects, to the holding and toleration of negative affects, to the development of a mental space through clarification, and to the improvement of self-perception." Based on the multiple relationship experiences in the DH program and the clear structure of the holding contract, we can offer an intense beginning phase. This involves constant interventions repeatedly addressing whether the patient follows the DH expectations and regulations or has a different agenda.

Tactics Modifications: Contract Setting

Tactical procedures include the agreement on a treatment contract, which includes the negotiation of how adolescents and their parents deal with behaviors that threatens the therapy. The agreement would outline the expectation that the adolescent patient acts responsibly in cases of acute suicidal tendencies by notifying family or other authority figures, refrain from self-injurious behavior if possible, or immediately report self-injury if it occurs. As the program continues for a duration of only 12–16 weeks, special emphasis is placed on a detailed pre-treatment diagnostic phase and on contracting before entering the program. The contract serves as an agreement between the juvenile patient, the day clinic team, and the parents, and sets the ground for exploring situations in which the adolescent acts out as a manifestation of a rigid and controlling internal world. The focus on expectable challenges to the treatment contract, and analysis of the emerging dominant self and object transferences in that context, will require extensive time and effort during the DH treatment. The treatment team supplements ego and super-ego functions by maintaining adherence to the agreed upon rules and agreements.

Mostly the acting out of the juvenile BPO patient serves the unconscious purpose of a defense against feelings of helplessness, rage, or resentment by controlling the parents. At a conscious level, however, the patient is often identified with the sense of a controlled child or victim of the parents.

Working with the contract agreement during the DH program is a way of stopping the powerful destructive cycle between juveniles and their parents; we have often observed parents repeatedly intervening as the adolescent patient stumbles from one crisis to the next.

Contract Between the Treatment Staff and Adolescent Patients

The DH team's focus on the adolescent patient's agreed upon treatment contract allows for a deliberate and systematic exploration of the emerging negative transference. As the patient challenges this agreement, as would be expected, the team can explore in a step-by-step way the patient's resentment about the agreement and ways that split-off, unconscious aggression is manifested in challenges to the contract. Often the patient and the team will need to re-contract when the patient's expression of destructiveness may change, as with the patient who initially presents with prominent self-injury, and then reveals a pattern of regular alcohol use.

In the Cologne DH program described here, a specific team member is assigned to work directly with every patient. This case manager helps to arrange daily matters such as school tasks or interface with family and teachers, as well as managing any emerging self-destructiveness. As part of the treatment agreement, any self-destructive behavior such as self-mutilation, suicidal ideation with active planning, or school absences, are considered challenges to the contract with the expectation that the patient would immediately report these developments to the assigned case manager. This material would then be the priority in the patient's next individual treatment session.

The contract determines that all patients need to address expectations and goals for the treatment on admission into the program. This approach highlights healthier ego capacities and aims at limiting regressive tendencies. These individual treatment goals need to be presented in group psychotherapy. Additionally, the group therapy follows the principles of a TFP-A-oriented psychodynamic group therapy, which has the goal of a "deep exploration of the complex cognitive and emotional processes of interactions in the here and now" [4] and focuses on the cognitive concept of self and others (TFP-A modified psychodynamic group therapy is described in detail in Chap. 10 of this volume). By insisting on individual treatment goals for each patient, we address the ambivalence and resistance of adolescents with borderline personality pathology to open up in psychotherapy. Failure to open up in a meaningful way can threaten the treatment, reflecting a common passive and resentful attitude of the adolescent, often associated with a prominent secondary gain. Diederichs-Paeschke [65] regards adolescence as the phase of life that is most marked by ambivalence and sees "staying or walking" as the main conflict of the adolescent, which is reflected accordingly in adherence to therapy [39]. Adolescent patients with BPO usually have very few reflective capacities available and identify with a child-like sense of self that cannot take on any kind of responsibility. Therefore, one of the aims of the DH treatment consists in exploring these aspects, lessening the inner resistance, and preparing the adolescent with increasing self-reflective capacities for regular TFP-A outpatient psychotherapy after finishing our program.

Therefore, in the contract phase at the beginning of the DH treatment we put a strong emphasis on ego capacities such as reinforcing the ability to attend school with the support of the day clinic structure. As explained in Chap. 10 of this book on group therapy, the peer patients as part of the group therapy and the DH program play an essential role for the adolescent in accepting rules and regulations, as well as confronting regressive tendencies and shame.

Contract Between the Treatment Staff and the Parents of the Adolescent Patients

The parents or other meaningful attachment figures (foster parents, etc.) are involved in drawing up the treatment contract, whereby they are also required to participate in the treatment of their adolescent child through regular parental co-sessions. Parental work is a core element of treatment with TFP-A in so far as working with adolescents without the support of parents usually leads to immense difficulties and possibly to the discontinuation of the treatment [see 46, 62]. The contract-drafting phase also serves to elucidate the psychodynamics of the parents who may act as an essential pathology-preserving component for the adolescent patient. For example, parents in highly conflictual relationships can deny young patients an inner space for reflection and meditation with little opportunity to develop independently and detach from their severely psychopathologically impaired parents. The process of drawing up and working with a treatment contract therefore also includes giving parents an understanding of the problems of adolescent patients. This may involve explaining the treatment approach and negotiating some acceptance and support in order to reduce undermining actions by the parents, which can include tolerance of the patient's secondary gain of illness.

By including a parent group as part of the treatment program, the Cologne DH program aims to facilitate an understanding of the adolescent diagnosis for parents in order to enhance their capacity to support the treatment of their children.

The parent group takes place once a month and at least one parent of each of the six juvenile patients has to participate. All parents agree to attend the parent group as part of the treatment contract; non-compliance can lead to termination of the DH treatment of their child. This rule is based on the experience that a high percentage of parents of BPO patients themselves have evidence of significant psychopathology [63] and are therefore inclined to "park" their child at the DH unit without being willing to participate in the treatment process. The parent treatment group is led by the director of the program and one member of the treatment team. In the beginning, the focus is on explaining the diagnosis of a juvenile BPO to the parents and emphasizing behavioral as well as symptomatic expression of BPO (such as regressive passivity and acting out in school and family matters) in detail. Moreover, the principles of the TFP-A treatment concept are explained. During the second part of the parent group, each participating parent has the opportunity to open up about the problematic behavior of their child and about typical patterns of interaction (reframed by the group leaders as an enactment of object relation dyads) between the parents and their child. Mutual discretion is agreed upon to protect patient and family confidentiality. The TFP-A therapist of the parent group uses psychoeducational techniques by explaining details of the contract as a way of "ego strengthening" for borderline adolescents. Based on the fact that most parents of BPO adolescents are chronically overburdened and frequently impaired in their parental function, one focus of the parent group is to strengthen the position of the parents. Furthermore, the therapist uses TFP-A principles by identifying typical object relation dyads between the parents and their child, which can sometimes reinforce a pathological family structure. This is explored and discussed with the parents within the group. In addition, the case manager on the unit has weekly phone calls with the parents focusing on daily matters of the juvenile at home and school.

Techniques Modifications

During the 12-week program, clarification is an essential technique of applied TFP-A treatment. The entire treatment team uses clarification and also confrontation in order to bring unconscious parts of object relation transference into the awareness of the juvenile patient. Through clarification, the predominant object relationship dyads are identified "as recurring patterns" and made aware to the adolescent. Contradictions are pointed out, cautiously but clearly, in the intervention of confrontation. In the DH treatment, there are lots of social contacts (school, new co-patient peers, daily contacts with treatment team members), which can be the focus of naming and exploration of object relationship dyads from the beginning. The aim is to capture the manifestations of the juvenile patient's internal world of object relations in experiences outside therapy and to make the adolescent aware of them. However, the DH therapists are more interested in observing the manifestations of the inner object world in interactions in real time with the DH staff than in interpreting them simultaneously in the patients' outside world [39].

In most cases interpersonal conflicts between the adolescent and the therapists or members of the therapeutic team concern the contractual agreements. This creates the opportunity to observe and gradually identify several typical object relation dyads in adolescent patients—such as a dyad with a perceived overly strict father figure and a helpless, passive victimized child, accompanied by an aggressive affect—early on in the DH treatment. The focus on interpreting such transferences is of great meaning during the DH treatment. In accordance with Kehr and Köpp [39], we consider it an additional technique in TFP-A to repeatedly address issues that have already been addressed in previous sessions and that can be related to current issues. The therapists act as "historians" referencing a collection of experienced object relationship dyads and associated emotions. This is especially transparent in a DH program where multiple relationship experiences take place. Through observation of these repetitions, the adolescent is first of all made aware of the connections between split experiences, before they are interpreted; they are initially offered as "interesting coincidences."

This stimulates self-reflection, encourages dialogue, helps to make self-mutilative behavior increasingly ego-dystonic, and strengthens confidence in the differentiation of self and object. In the first 6 weeks of treatment, the therapists and treatment team often experience great confusion and rapid shifts of complementary and concordant countertransference, reflecting opposing object relationship dyads with fragmented self- and object representations. Moreover, negative transference is often focused on one of the team members or therapists. The clinicians' initial confusion and the patients' frequent affect storms are often very strong and can lure staff into reactive acting out. Often, the opposing object relationship dyads and their rapid changes can be more easily observed in a treatment team with a variety of members. Consistent supervision is necessary to identify these transferences of idealization and devaluation and to protect the treatment team against problematic countertransference enactments.

What Is the Source of Institutional or Government Support for this Initiative?

The state health insurance pays for the DH program for adolescents in the Department for Child and Adolescent Psychiatry and Psychotherapy at the University Clinic of Cologne in Germany.

What Are Possible Targets for Measurement to Gauge the Effectiveness of Instruction About Applications of TFP Principles?

Possible targets for showing the effectiveness of instruction about applying TFP-A principles are the evidence of a reduced frequency of episodes of counter-acting by team members. This could be indicated by an increased capacity of the professionals to avoid focusing too strictly on each detail of the contract or an exaggerated compassion for the juvenile patient, being identified against the "evil" parent. With regard to the adolescent patient, the effectiveness of this DH program is reflected by the evidence of a substantial decrease of school absenteeism and of the number of inpatient admissions due to repeated suicidal crises.

What Are the Didactic Materials Required to Impart TFP Principles to this Target Group of Clinicians?

The whole DH staff became familiar with TFP principles by reading the manual for TFP for adults [4] and for adolescents [62] and the book on working with parents based on TFP-A [39].

What Is the Format for Instruction of TFP Principles to this Audience?

TFP principles were taught to the entire team of the DH staff by means of theoretical ORT seminars and role play in order to help identifying object relation dyads. The teaching program is led by TFP-A certified teachers and supervisors and directed to the entire staff of the DH.

Clinical Illustration

Dillan, a 15-year-old patient, introduced herself as a shy, tall, slightly obese girl of well-manicured, age-appropriate appearance at the beginning of the DH program. Her figure is hidden behind loose-fitting clothes. She reports symptoms of daily self-harming behavior during the past year, frequent mood swings, recurring suicidal ideation, multiple "panic attacks," repeated binge eating behavior, as well as social anxiety in school. Her hard-working parents of Russian descent hesitate to support Dillan's treatment at the DH program. They tend to see the cause of her problems as the onset of puberty and have great difficulty recognizing the severe structural personality psychopathology of their daughter. The parents report that Dillan, their oldest daughter (she has two younger brothers), has always been her father's favorite and is merely having "a rough time." Due to constant problems at home and in school they finally agree to allow Dillan to be treated at the DH and Dillan and her parents accept the BPD diagnosis and the treatment contract. The contract includes the agreement to reduce and stop self-mutilation, to report on any self-cutting behavior (despite agreeing on not doing so), to attend school on a daily basis, and to report any suicidal ideation.

Shortly after the beginning of the program, Dillan reports: "Actually, I want to change something right now, but on the other hand I have crazily become used to the fact that I am unhappy and now I am anxious about the prospect of being happy." The beginning of the DH treatment is marked by Dillan's resistance. She avoids in-depth thoughts and feelings and talks about day-to-day issues, which do not affect her emotionally. Her symptomatology increases and she tends to display passivity throughout all parts of treatment. Her tendency toward regression is apparent as she waits for the treatment team to approach her. When confronted with the fact, that by repeatedly self-mutilating and not reporting it, she is in breach of contract, she reacts with anger. Her dominant affect is usually boredom, with a monotonous voice as if nothing could affect her. After 3 weeks she asks to be treated with an antidepressant medication due to constant mood swings. At the same time, she does not really show any interest in exploring her inner thoughts and feelings.

As a result of the ongoing, consistent confrontation in the DH program Dillan stops her self-mutilative behavior after four weeks, but at the same time, she increasingly expresses psychosomatic symptoms, such as tinnitus and headaches. Her parents attend a parent group but participate in the program on an irregular basis, missing sessions or phone calls. It seems as if Dillan needs to present serious symptoms for her parents to pay attention to her. Confronted with this observation she reacts with denial and with the attitude of a helpless child who cannot take any active steps, switching between a clinging attitude toward the treatment team, which she idealizes and with whom she tries to prolong contact, and on the other hand, devaluing the therapists as not helpful and their contributions meaningless. In group therapy she seems to accept feedback only by her peer co-patients, but not the therapists.

Dillan is eventually diagnosed with avoidant personality disorder, as well as BPD, with associated narcissistic traits that do not meet criteria for narcissistic personality disorder. In ORT terms, she presents with BPO and narcissistic personality traits with predominant vulnerable manifestations, such as hypersensitivity to criticism or rejection, low mood, and feelings of helplessness. The dominant object relationship dyad is a demanding (or nerve-racking) child and uninterested mother (with a paranoid element), which defends against the split-off, idealized, libidinal dyad of a sick and well-cared-for child and a perfectly caring mother.

During the DH program, the patient is confronted with her regressive tendencies, her refusal to participate actively in the program, and her identification with the role of a sick child who cannot take responsibility. Based on the treatment contract and the repeated confrontation about her capacity to control her self-mutilative behavior, she finally reduces it (from daily to three episodes in three months) and attends school on a regular basis. In contrast to her resistance to stay in high school before treatment, at the end of the program she changes her mind and decides to pursue her high school diploma. Dillan completes the program on schedule and is transferred to an outpatient TFP-A therapist where she, despite multiple crises, manages to stay in treatment.

Conclusion

Principles of TFP may assist those clinicians working in settings such as the DH that are generally of higher acuity than a standard, outpatient setting. This chapter provided two examples of ongoing DH programs for adult and adolescent patients in two nationally diverse healthcare systems. These experiences demonstrate the applicability of standard TFP principles, although with some modifications, within DH settings. Specifically, this chapter highlighted the utility of applying to DH level of care several TFP elements, such as the structural interview to move beyond standard psychiatric nosology, psychoeducation for patients and family members, and a treatment agreement and ongoing attention to the details of that agreement throughout the treatment course. Major modifications of TFP principles included the following:

- The different nature of the treatment contact, as compared with the standard outpatient individual psychotherapy setting
- The focus on transference and countertransference dynamics between the individual patient and other patients as well as with the various staff clinicians

The two pilot DH programs described in this chapter hold promise for generalization to other healthcare systems that can look forward to implementing along with their usual treatment modalities specialized DH programs for both adolescent and adult patients with borderline pathology informed by TFP theory and practice.

References

1. Kernberg OF. Severe personality disorders: psychotherapeutic strategies. Yale University Press; 1984.
2. Clarkin JF, Yeomans FE, Kernberg OF. Psychotherapy for borderline personality: focusing on object relations. American Psychiatric Pub; 2007.
3. Yeomans FE, Levy KN, Caligor E. Transference-focused psychotherapy. Psychotherapy. 2013;50(3):449–53.
4. Yeomans F, Clarkin J, Kernberg OF. Transference-focused psychotherapy for borderline personality disorder: a clinical guide. Washington, DC: American Psychiatric Publishing; 2015.
5. Verdaguer E, Castillo JA, Plaza A. Efectividad del tratamiento y seguimiento longitudinal de pacientes con TLP tratados en Hospital de Día. Doctoral thesis. Universitat Ramon Llull. Barcelona; 2017.
6. Linehan M. Cognitive-behavioral treatment of borderline personality disorder. New York: Guilford Press; 1993.
7. Bateman A, Fonagy P. Psychotherapy for borderline personality disorder: mentalisation based treatment. Oxford: Oxford University Press; 2004.
8. Clarkin J, Caligor E, Stern B, Kernberg O. Structured interview of personality organization: STIPO-R. Personality Disorders Institute Weill Medical College of Cornell University; 2016.
9. First MB, Gibbon M, Spitzer RL, Williams JBW, Benjamin LS. Structured clinical interview for DSM-IV Axis II personality disorders (SCID-II). Washington, DC: American Psychiatric Press, Inc; 1997.
10. Krueger RF, Derringer J, Markon KE, Watson D, Skodol AE. The personality inventory for DSM-5 (PID-5)—adult. Medicapanamericana: American Psychiatric Association. Ed; 2014.
11. Zanarini M, Gunderson J, Frankenburg F, Chauncey D. The revised diagnostic interview for borderlines: discriminating BPD from other axis II disorders. J Personal Disord. 1989;3:10–8.

12. Patton JH, Stanford MS, Barratt ES. Factor structure of the barratt impulsiveness scale. J Clin Psychol. 1995;51(6):768–74.
13. Bernstein DP, Fink L, Handelsman L, Foote J. Childhood trauma questionnaire—PsycNET. APA PsycTests; 1994. https://psycnet.apa.org/doiLanding?doi=10.1037%2Ft02080-000
14. Derogatis L. SCL–90–R administration, scoring, and procedures manual. 3rd ed. Minneapolis: National Computer Systems; 1994.
15. Pérez V, Barrachina J, Soler J, Paascual J, Campins M, Puigdemont D, et al. Impresión clínica global para pacientes con trastorno límite de la personalidad (ICG-TLP): una escala sensible al cambio. Actas Españolas Psiquiatr. 2007;35:229–35.
16. Fonagy P, Luyten P, Moulton-Perkins A, Lee YW, Warren F, Howard S, et al. Development and validation of a self-report measure of mentalizing: the reflective functioning questionnaire. PLoS One. 2016;11(7)
17. Arntz A, Dreessen L. BPD checklist. Univ Maastricht Dep Med Clin Exp Psychol. 2001;
18. Doering S, Hörz S, Rentrop M, Fischer-Kern M, Schuster P, Benecke C, et al. Transference-focused psychotherapy v. treatment by community psychotherapists for borderline personality disorder: randomised controlled trial. Br J Psychiatry. 2010;196(5):389–95.
19. Caligor E, Kernberg O, Clarkin J, Yeomans F. Psychodynamic therapy for personality pathology: treating self and interpersonal functioning. American Psychiatric Association Publishing; 2018.
20. Diamond D, Yeomans F, Keefe J. Transference-focused psychotherapy for pathological narcissism and narcissistic personality disorder (TFP-N). Psychodyn Psychiatry Summer. 2021;49(2):244–72.
21. Rufat MJ. Programa TLP en los hospitales de día CPB: abordaje terapéutico multicomponente. Rev Psicopatología y Salud Ment del Niño y del Adolesc. 2011;3:37–9.
22. Shapiro F. Movement desensitization and reprocessing: basic principles, protocols, and procedures. 2nd ed. New York: Guilford Press; 2001.
23. Blum N, Bartels N, St. John D, Pfohl B. STEPPS: systems training for emotional predictability and problem solving: group treatment for borderline personality disorder. Coralville: Blum's Books; 2002.
24. Black D, Blum N, Pfohl B, St JD. The STEPPS group treatment program for outpatients with borderline personality disorder. J Contemp Psychother. 2004;34:193–210.
25. Sullivan HS. Socio-psychiatric research: its implications for the schizophrenia problem and for mental hygiene. Am J Psychiatry. 1930;10:977.
26. García BJ. Comunidad Terapéutica Psicoanalítica de Estructura Multifamiliar. Madrid: Tecnipublicaciones; 1990.
27. Mascaró MN. La Institución Psicoterapéutica. Av en Salud Ment Relac. 2013;12(2)
28. Jones M. Psiquiatría Social. Buenos Aires: Editorial Escuela; 1952.
29. Kernberg OF. Psicoterapia de grupo según el modelo de la TFP. In: Conferencia inaugural 14 de Septiembre 4ªs Jornadas anuales de Grup TLP Barcelona. 2013.
30. Bion W. Experiencias en grupos. Editorial Paidós; 1990.
31. Foulkes SH. Psicoterapia grupoanalítica. Barcelona: Gedisa Ed; 1981.
32. Yalom I, Leszcz M. The theory and practice of group psychotherapy. 5th ed. New York: Basic Books; 2005.
33. Rufat M, Barrachina J, Verdaguer E, Vegué J. Evaluación de la eficacia un Programa de tratamiento para el TLP en Hospital de Día (unpublished manuscript). 2014.
34. De Angel I. Estudio sobre la mejora de la funcionalidad en pacientes TLP tratados en Hospital de Día (unpublished manuscript). 2015.
35. Ponton-Rodriguez T, Krischer M. Prävalenz von Persönlichkeitsstörungen in einer psychiatrischen Inanspruchnahmepopulation Jugendlicher. Persönlichkeitsstörungen, Theorie und Therapie. 2018;77:186–95.
36. Kaess M, Brunner R, Chanen A. Borderline personality disorder in adolescence. Pediatrics. 2014;134(4):782–93.

37. Krischer M. Übertragungsfokussierte Psychotherapie für Adoleszente (Transference Focused Psychotherapy for Adolescents, TFP-A) mit Borderline-Persönlichkeitspathologie in der ambulanten und tagsklinischen Behandlung. Kinderanalyse. 2020;28(2):147–66.
38. Krischer M, Normandin L. Dayclinic treatment of adolescent borderline patients with techniques of the transference focused psychotherapy for adolescents (TFP-A): concept and first experiences. Persönlichkeitsstörungen, Theorie und Therapie. 2015;1:2–13.
39. Kehr G, Köpp W. Übertragungsfokussierte Psychotherapie für Jugendliche (TFP-A) mit Persönlichkeitsstörungen. Kinderanalyse. 2018;26(1):37–85.
40. Normandin L, Ensink K, Yeomans FE, Kernberg OF. Transference-focused psychotherapy for personality disorders in adolescents. In: Sharp C, Tackett C, editors. Handbook of borderline personality disorder in children and adolescents. New York: Springer Science & Business Media; 2014. p. 333–59.
41. Sharp C, Vanwoerden S, Wall K. Adolescence as a sensitive period for the development of personality disorder. Psychiatr Clin North Am. 2018;41(4):669–83.
42. Schmeck K. DSM-5: Das Konzept der Persönlichkeitsstörungen aus kinder- und jugendpsychiatrischer Sicht. Persönlichkeitsstörungen, Theorie und Therapie. 2014;18(1):6–15.
43. Sevecke K, Haid-Stecher N, Goth K, Bock A, Krischer MK. Zeit für etwas Neues? Paradigmenwechsel für die Persönlichkeitsstörung im ICD-11. Überblick und Chancen für das Jugendalter. Persönlichkeitsstörungen, Theorie und Therapie. 2019;23(4):299–309.
44. Streeck-Fischer A. Die Borderline-Persönlichkeit(entwicklung)sstörung im Jugendalter. Diagnostik, Behandlungsvoraussetzungen, Gestaltung des Rahmens, Phasen der Behandlung. Prax Kinderpsychol Kinderpsychiatr. 2008;57(8–9):693–717.
45. Kernberg OF. Neue Überlegungen zur Frage der Identität. In: Remmel A, Kernberg OF, Vollmoeller W, Strauß B, editors. Handbuch Körper und Persönlichkeit. Stuttgart: Schattauer; 2006. p. 3–21.
46. Sevecke K, Krischer M. Jugendliche Persönlichkeitsstörungen im psychodynamischen Diskurs. In: Resch F, Seiffge-Krenke I, editors. Psychodynamik Kompakt. Göttingen: Vandenhoeck & Ruprecht; 2016.
47. Krischer M, Ponton-Rodriguez T, Gooran GR, Bender S. Übertragungsfokussierte Psychotherapie von Borderline-Jugendlichen im tagesklinischen Setting. Prax Kinderpsychol Kinderpsychiatr. 2017;66(6):445–63.
48. Foelsch PA, Odom A, Arena H, Krischer M, Schmeck K, Schlüter-Müller S. The differentiation between identity crisis and identity diffusion and its impact on treatment. Prax Kinderpsychol Kinderpsychiatr. 2010;59:418–38.
49. Kernberg PF, Weiner A, Bardenstein K. Persönlichkeitsstörungen bei Kindern und Jugendlichen. 2nd ed. Stuttgart: Klett-Cotta; 2005.
50. Loranger AW, Sartorius N, Andreoli A, Berger P, Buchheim P, Channabasavanna SM, et al. The international personality disorder examination. The World Health Organization/alcohol, drug abuse, and mental health administration international pilot study of personality disorders. Arch Gen Psychiatry. 1994;51(3):215–24.
51. Fleischhaker C, Böhme R, Sixt B, Brück C, Schneider C, Schulz E. Dialectical behavioral therapy for adolescents (DBT-A): a clinical trial for patients with suicidal and self- injurious behavior and borderline symptoms with a one-year follow-up. Child Adolesc Psychiatry Ment Health. 2011;5(1):3.
52. Jahn C, Wieacker E, Bender S, Krischer M). Reduktion selbstverletzenden Verhaltens bei Jugendlichen mit Borderline Persönlichkeitsorganisation mittels der übertragungsfokussierten Psychotherapie. Prax Kinderpsychol Kinderpsychiatr. 2021;70:728–47.
53. Clarkin JF, Caligor E, Stern B, Kernberg OF. Structured interview of personality organization (STIPO). Weill Medical College of Cornell University; 2004.
54. OPD-CA-2 Task Force. Operationalized psychodynamic diagnosis in childhood and adolescence. Theoretical basis and user manual Hogrefe Publishing; 2017.
55. Livesley WJ, Jackson DN. Manual for the dimensional assessment of personality pathology. Port Huron: Sigma Press; 2001.

56. Biberdzic M, Ensink K, Normandin L, Clarkin JF. Empirical typology of adolescent personality organization. J Adolesc. 2018;66:31–48. https://doi.org/10.1016/j.adolescence.2018.04.004.
57. Achenbach TM. Manual for the youth self-report and 1991 profile. Burlington: Department of Psychiatry, University of Vermont; 1991.
58. Coccaro EF, Harvey PD, Kupsaw-Lawrence E, Herbert JL, Bernstein DP. Development of neuropsychopharmalogically based behavioral assessment of impulsive aggressive behavior. J Neuropsychiatry Clin Neurosci. 1991;3(2):S44–51.
59. Beck A, Steer R, Brown G. Beck depression inventory. In: BDI-2. München: Pearson; 1996.
60. Horowitz LM, Rosenberg SE, Baer BA, Ureño G, Villaseñor VS. Inventory of interpersonal problems: psychometric properties and clinical applications. J Consult Clin Psychol. 1988;56(6):885–92. https://doi.org/10.1037/0022-006x.56.6.885.
61. Reicherzer M, Brandl T. Der Fragebogen zum selbstverletzenden Verhalten (FSSV)—ein neues Erhebungsinstrument für die klinische Praxis. Psychother Psychiatrie, psychotherapeutischer Medizin und klinischer Psychologie. 2011;16:199.
62. Normandin L, Ensink K, Weiner A, Kernberg O. Transference-focused psychotherapy for adolescents with severe personality disorders. Washington, DC: American Psychiatric Association Publishing; 2021.
63. Kehr G, Gleiss I, Köpp W, Psychosozial-Verlag. Übertragungsfokussierte Psychotherapie mit schwer gestörten Jugendlichen: Therapiebegleitende Arbeit mit Eltern und Betreuungseinrichtungen; 2021.
64. Kernberg OF, Krischer M, Foelsch PA. Übertragungsfokussierte Psychotherapie für Jugendliche: Der vorläufige Stand. Prax Kinderpsychol Kinderpsychiatr. 2008;57(8):662–92.
65. Diederichs-Paeschke V. Abbruch—eine spezielle Beendigung psychoanalytischer Behandlung bei Jugendlichen. (unpublished manuscript); 2002.

Using Transference-Focused Psychotherapy (TFP) Principles in Short-Term and Extended Inpatient Psychotherapy Settings

7

Birger Dulz, Bernhard Grimmer, Mathias Lohmer, Olga Wlodarczyk, and Gerhard Dammann

Gerhard Dammann has died before the publication of this book.Introduction

Contemporary psychoanalytic approaches to inpatient treatment of patients with severe personality disorders can be traced back to the efforts of the first generation of psychoanalytically trained psychiatrists in Germany in the 1920s. In addition to providing intensive individual psychoanalytic treatment, the initial efforts were directed toward providing patients with a communal life with fellow patients through concrete tasks in the community designed to increase their general level of social functioning and adaptability—an early form of a therapeutic community approach [1].

This approach subsequently developed independently in various clinics in Great Britain and the United States and was used in a somewhat more modern form in the early programs of the Menninger Clinic in Topeka, Kansas, in the 1940s and 1950s. Otto Kernberg, as director of the C. F. Menninger Memorial Hospital, developed an integrative model for hospital treatment of severe personality disorders between

B. Dulz
German Society TFP (DGTFP)/TFP-Institute North (TIN), Hamburg, Germany
e-mail: kontakt@birger-dulz.de

B. Grimmer
Department for Psychotherapy, Psychiatric Clinic Münsterlingen, Münsterlingen, Switzerland
e-mail: bernhard.grimmer@stgag.ch

M. Lohmer
TFP-Institute Munich, Munich, Germany

O. Wlodarczyk (✉)
Department for Personality Disorders, Asklepios Clinic Nord Ochsenzoll, Hamburg, Germany
e-mail: o.wlodarczyk@asklepios.com

G. Dammann (Deceased)
Mental Health Services Thurgau, Münsterlingen, Switzerland

R. G. Hersh, C. De Panfilis (eds.), *Implementing Transference-Focused Psychotherapy Principles*, https://doi.org/10.1007/978-3-031-68062-5_7

1969 and 1973. In this hospital, he implemented a model based on psychoanalytic object-relations theory and utilized the analytic approaches to group and organizational functioning is elaborated by Tom Main and the Tavistock Clinic under the direction of Jack Sutherland (1952). He later developed these approaches further with his research groups at the New York State Psychiatric Institute (NYSPI) and then as Director of the Westchester Division of New York Hospital [1].

After a heyday of inpatient milieu therapeutic treatments in the 1960s and 1970s, psychodynamic treatment of personality disorders in the English-speaking world shifted largely to the outpatient setting from the 1980s and 1990s. This occurred primarily against the backdrop of shortened lengths of stay, increasing outpatient treatment in psychiatric planning, and cost pressures in the health care system [1].

Accordingly, transference-focused psychotherapy (TFP), as a disorder-specific, manualized, and evidence-based psychodynamic procedure for the treatment of personality disorder (PD) patients as we know it today, is designed for outpatient therapy [2]. At the heart of the treatment is the processing of internalized and, due to defense mechanisms such as splitting and projection, non-integrated self-object relational representations of the patients that were formed in early childhood and are actualized in the therapeutic relationship. In particular, the respective affectively dominant reenactments of the internalizations reflected in the here-and-now of the transference and countertransference relationships are the focus of the treatment [2]. Through the interventions of clarification, confrontation, and interpretation, they can be made conscious, understood, and subsequently better integrated by the patient. This process requires a therapeutic attitude of technical neutrality in order not to identify repeatedly with a part of the conflict and thus maintain the split. To reduce behavior that is dangerous to self, others, or the therapy, as is often the case with patients with a personality disorder (PD), appropriate therapy agreements or contracts are made. These clearly specify the patient's responsibilities and create a supportive and limiting framework.

The following is a brief overview of inpatient treatments for patients with PD as it is currently provided in the German-speaking D-A-CH countries (D = Germany, A = Austria, CH = Switzerland). Subsequently, it will be shown how TFP treatment principles can be modified and applied for inpatient treatments. For this purpose, a TFP inpatient treatment model lasting several months, as it is carried out today in German-speaking countries (e.g., in Hamburg/Germany, and Münsterlingen/Switzerland), is presented. Finally, some remarks on the application of TFP treatment principles for short-term crisis interventions or acute psychiatric treatments follow.

This article is essentially a condensation of the new German language manual on inpatient TFP treatment [1].

Who Are the Clinicians?

In the D-A-CH countries, inpatient treatments for patients with severe PD are provided by, among others, psychiatric hospitals within psychotherapy units (treating patients for up to several months) or acute units (treating patients from a few days to several weeks). The core staff of acute psychiatric wards and inpatient psychotherapy wards are nursing professionals, psychiatrists, psychologists, and social workers. Furthermore, in Germany, patients with PD are also treated in hospitals for psychosomatic medicine, which were founded after World War II and influenced by the idea of a holistic, humanistic, and psychoanalytically oriented inpatient treatment in contrast to the previous, largely biologically oriented, psychiatry tradition. The professional staff working in such inpatient psychotherapy units (located at universities and also provided by communal and private agencies) can include nurse practitioners, psychiatrists, psychologists, social workers, physicians, occupational therapists, sports therapists, movement therapists, art therapists, and physical therapists.

Who Are the Patients?

Primarily, the treatment of patients with PD diagnoses, generally, and borderline personality disorder (BPD), specifically, should take place on an outpatient basis [3, 4]. Therefore, the aim of any inpatient treatment should be that the patient is subsequently able to resume outpatient therapy. Ultimately, the severity of symptoms and the presence of comorbid mental disorders determine whether inpatient treatment is needed to effectively treat the disorder or at least prevent it from worsening. The severity of the disorder can be defined by persistent symptoms of illness, extensive use of the psychotherapeutic, psychiatric, or psychosocial illness system, as well as severe psychosocial dysfunction [5]. According to Häfner et al. [6], general criteria for inpatient admission are: crisis situations, suicide risk, crisis-like increase in anxiety and depression, worsening of symptoms, and medically related reasons (e.g., anorexia, bulimia). In some cases, the removal of the patient from a stressful living environment is a prerequisite for any psychotherapeutic benefit to become possible at all. In such cases, treatment in an inpatient setting is recommended [6]. While acute units primarily take patients in crisis, wards with inpatient psychotherapy take patients who are motivated and have a basic capacity for change. Additionally, more and more day clinics are being developed that work with a program similar to the ones offered by the inpatient units but that allow the patients to return to their homes in the evening.

What Is the Contemporary Standard of Care for Clinicians Treating These Patients?

The aim of treatment in acute inpatient psychiatric settings is mainly a basic stabilization of the patient using pharmacotherapy and supportive psychotherapy. By contrast, some of the specialized psychotherapy wards in psychiatric and psychosomatic settings treat patients with PD according to specific treatment models, like dialectical behavior therapy (DBT; [7]), mentalization-based treatment (MBT; [8]), TFP [2], or schema-focused therapy (SFT; [9]). The size of such a ward can have about 18–25 patients, depending on the hospital. Inpatient psychotherapy treatment involves many different components delivered by various professionals (for example, psychotherapists, psychiatrists, and nurses). The elements of psychotherapy may differ somewhat across the various specialized wards. The components of inpatient treatment may include individual therapy, group therapy, sessions with the primary nurse, contact with the nursing staff, nurse-led group services, social service involvement, occupational therapy, art therapy, movement therapy, and sports therapy.

What Are the Goals for Providing to These Clinicians with the Principles of TFP for Working with These Patients?

A specialized inpatient TFP setting can be implemented on wards in psychiatric as well as psychosomatic hospitals treating PD populations. The goal of inpatient TFP is to stabilize the patient symptomatically, motivate and prepare her/ him for outpatient therapy, and bring into her/his awareness dysfunctional, ineffective, inner (unconscious) patterns and conflictual object-relations issues that manifest themselves in the transference relationships during the inpatient treatment. A TFP-oriented therapy ward is populated with a broad mix of patients and staff. In this setting, the psychodynamics of the patients are staged as relationship patterns among themselves and in relation to the team. Simultaneously, the team dynamics, and transferences and countertransferences of the individual team members unfold. The different professional groups have different interactions with the patients due to different therapeutic or nursing tasks and roles, therefore stimulating accordingly different transference-countertransference processes. These are explored in team and case discussions in order to understand the often unconsciously activated self-object relationship patterns of the patients and to integrate them into a common understanding of the case and the illness. The treatment is thus always a group and team treatment.

The psychodynamic, TFP-oriented understanding of the illness shared by the treatment team makes it possible to appreciate what is happening around the patients, their behavior and experiences, and their mobilized interpersonal conflicts with fellow patients and the treatment team. It forms the basis for an integrated treatment plan that ensures that all treatment team members adopt a unified therapeutic stance and are guided by a common treatment focus. In this way, the structural psychological problems of the patients, which are manifested in various symptoms, can be understood.

Indication for Inpatient TFP

An indication for a referral for inpatient TFP is based on the professional's assessment of the patient's life situation, need for treatment, severity of the disorder, and current environmental and intrapsychic possibilities for improving his or her psychopathology [10]. It has been suggested that TFP can be used for patients with PD at both higher and lower levels of borderline organization, with TFP proving particularly effective for patients belonging to DSM-5 Cluster B PD (or, in ICD-10 terms, patients with borderline-type emotionally unstable, histrionic, narcissistic, impulsive, and treatable antisocial personality disorder) [11, 12]. A study by Hörz et al. [13] examined the relationship between structural level and clinical severity of BPD in a multicenter randomized-controlled psychotherapy study. Comorbid cluster B PD traits were found to correlate highly with the traits of identity diffusion, aggression, and primitive defenses [13]. The results are in line with Kernberg's theoretical concept, which describes identity diffusion as a central structural limitation at the core of borderline personality organization (BPO).

Against this background, outpatient TFP is indicated in the following cases:

- A severe identity disorder, which manifests itself primarily through pronounced difficulties in relationships, e.g., through impairments in professional life, in love relationships and partnerships, in sexual life, as well as in social "functioning".
- Pronounced aggression, mainly self-directed, in the form of suicidal and self-injurious behavior, especially in the context of "toxic relationships", or extensive use of primitive defenses, such as projection, splitting, or projective identification.

In the context of outpatient TFP, an individual psychotherapy contract aims to secure the treatment framework, which includes all aspects that may jeopardize outpatient therapy according to a dynamic checklist of priorities [14]. If the patient is repeatedly unable to adhere to the therapeutic framework in outpatient treatment, a referral to a day clinic or full inpatient setting seems sensible; both an outpatient and a day program setting presuppose a reliable ability on the part of the patient to comply with an agreement. Severe behavioral disturbances or an insufficient capacity for collaboration with outpatient psychotherapists may be an indication for a full inpatient setting.

Comorbid mental disorders are not an exclusion criterion for inpatient TFP treatment. On the contrary, a treatment focusing on BPD usually also leads to an improvement in comorbid mental disorders [15]. The extent of comorbid disorders (labeled in prior iterations of the DSM (DSM-IV) as Axis I) must be examined in this context and hierarchized accordingly in treatment [5]. If the comorbid disorder (e.g., severe substance dependence or an excessively low BMI in the case of anorexia nervosa) is so prominent that the treatment of the PD appears to be especially difficult or even impossible, the treatment of that disorder should be prioritized.

In addition to reducing symptoms, inpatient TFP—in contrast to the type of treatment delivered by general psychiatric wards—focuses primarily on working on internalized dysfunctional object-relationship patterns. The opportunity in an inpatient treatment setting lies in the fact that pathological relationship patterns can often be recognized more quickly and worked on in the relationships with the team and the patient community. A prerequisite for this is the development of the patient's motivation, however ambivalent, to enter into a therapeutic relationship in the course of treatment—although the ability to do so initially is often limited. Severe antisocial behavior represents a challenge with regard to the development of a therapeutic relationship; thus, the indication for inpatient TFP should be weighed and assessed on a case-by-case basis. However, in cases of severe delinquency, a structured setting in a more controllable environment would be required. In addition, the patient should have a certain degree of reflective capacity as well as motivation and the capacity for introspection. In addition to sufficient stability, which in the context of TFP includes some ability to deal with conflict, the patient must be sufficiently intelligent. Treating highly intelligent patients, however, who are accustomed to intellectualizing and rationalizing at the highest level, can prove particularly challenging, as focusing on relational aspects and emotions in the frame is often made difficult in the therapeutic relationship. Not uncommon and usually challenging are treatments of patients who themselves work in a helping profession; here the problem of role confusion must always be considered and addressed both at the beginning and in the course of treatment.

Ultimately, the indication also depends on the therapy goal. Therapeutic work on pathological relationship patterns, which are typical for borderline patients, requires a significantly longer treatment period than the reduction of acutely exacerbated symptoms and should therefore take place within the framework of a TFP-informed inpatient treatment. In addition, the treatment of severe pathology with correspondingly complex symptom formation for those patients with prominent identity diffusion functioning at a lower level of personality organization usually requires a multifaceted treatment of verbal and non-verbal therapy modalities, such as the combination of individual and group therapy with occupational therapy and movement therapy (a psychodynamically-oriented body therapy method), which can be offered in an inpatient setting [10].

What TFP Principles Might Be Useful for Clinicians Working with These Patients?

The TFP principles can be applied within the patient's individual therapy, in creative therapies, but especially in intensive group therapies [16–18]. The patient's varying experiences (with the individual therapist, nursing caregiver, other therapists, and fellow patients) are used in order to explore and understand unconscious and conflictual object-relation issues. The great strength of inpatient TFP-oriented psychotherapy as a special setting for BPD patients lies in the opportunity to initiate a learning process in a defined setting. When the patient in question has a pattern of severe relationship disorders, this inpatient setting facilitates intensive feedback on the patient's effect on his social environment, and the testing of new behaviors. Specifically, several TFP principles might be of utility in the above-described inpatient settings.

Establishing a Containment Function of Inpatient Hospitalization

The identity diffusion of borderline patients and the predominance of primitive defense mechanisms, as well as the activation of non-integrated object relation patterns under the stress of a group situation, will usually engender a temporary exacerbation of the patients' psychological functioning, which allows for a sound diagnosis of their psychopathology and their specific object relation patterns.

Therefore, it is important for a therapeutic team to see splitting not as a "bad habit" or as something intentional, but as an act of defense and attempt at protection that occurs within individual patients and patient groups [19].

The lack of integration of these splitting impulses, often amplified in moments of love and aggression, can have a profound impact on behavior that is disproportionately stronger than the affects observed in neurotic or even psychotic patients. The setting of inpatient psychotherapy can be understood here in terms of a containment system [20]. In each case, a superordinate system helps the subordinate subsystem to process, understand, and integrate emotional experience. The individual therapists thus support the patient's and the patient group's ability to process emerging affects and behaviors. The team holds, supports, and "contains" the individual therapists. And the next hierarchical level of senior physicians and the head physician in turn holds, regulates, and supports the team in this function.

There are critical aspects required for inpatient clinicians to successfully perform a containment function for patients:

- An awareness of the inevitability of these aforementioned splitting processes
- A shared therapeutic approach, as offered by TFP
- An encouragement to openly examine the countertransference
- A willingness to give each other feedback and to confront tactfully
- Communication and cohesion within the team, across all professions
- Open and respectful communication between team members and patients
- Clearly defined responsibilities across professional groups
- A shared knowledge of the patients across all team members
- Competent expertise across all team members
- Good internal and external supervision

This is how a team succeeds in being open and at the same time stable, flexible, and structured.

Structuring the Treatment: Therapy Phases: Sequence of an Inpatient TFP Hospitalization

Inpatient TFP-informed psychotherapy represents a short phase in the expected longer-lasting outpatient TFP treatment process for a personality disorder. The duration of treatment on a TFP-informed psychotherapy unit for personality disorders can last from about 12 weeks to a maximum of 6 months in some cases.

A special feature of inpatient therapy is a heightened risk of therapeutic regression, which is likely to be stronger than in outpatient therapy and which should be used constructively and must be distinguished from pathological or malignant regression. It is important to keep in mind that regressive impulses will emerge in the therapeutic relationship in this setting that can be addressed effectively in the treatment. Great difficulties can arise in the inpatient treatment of patients with borderline disorders if the therapist becomes involved unwittingly with a destructive aspect of the patient's attachment disorder. In that case, the therapist might act on the urge to provide emotional relief to the patient by fulfilling certain projected relational desires. Treatment, therefore, could be compromised by the therapist's reinforcement of the patient's pathological relationship patterns [21, 22]. In order to limit pathological regression associated with inpatient treatment, the discharge date is often already determined and communicated to the patient on the day of admission. In this way, therapy is geared to the end of the inpatient treatment phase from the very beginning.

A TFP-oriented psychotherapy unit should also be able to treat unstable and "complex" borderline patients. If the psychotherapy ward has too high a threshold in terms of admission requirements, there is a danger that a large group of borderline patients will continue to be treated only in acute wards. Longer-term treatment of borderline patients should not take place in general psychiatric or acute wards, because the disadvantages there are further exaggerated by inappropriate and mostly psychosis-oriented approaches of the team. Informed by the principles outlined in the manual for outpatient TFP, a TFP-oriented inpatient treatment follows the following phases [23]:

1. Preliminary phase/preliminary talks
2. Extended diagnostic phase
3. Therapy contract phase
4. Initial phase and focus formation
5. Mid-phase
6. Termination phase, optional extension
7. Transitional phase and outpatient coordination

The transitions between the different phases of inpatient treatment should not be understood as rigid, but rather as flexible. Although the different therapy phases tend to build on the previous one, it is often useful to address specific aspects from later treatment phases at the beginning of the inpatient treatment, such as details of further outpatient treatment.

Initial Phase

The aim of the initial phase is to assess whether an inpatient stay seems reasonable for the patient, which should be the result of joint communication between the patient, the referring clinician (if available) and the ward staff. In addition to the (preliminary) diagnosis, the patient's motivation for treatment, cooperation, and commitment should be examined during a preliminary discussion. This should help determine whether a TFP-oriented psychotherapeutic approach can be chosen or whether an (initially) more purely supportive intervention, for example, a social service consultation, is necessary. Occasionally, if, for example, the patient is very ambivalent or the treatment team is uncertain about the indication, a trial phase can be agreed upon; here, too, it is important that the exact duration and further steps are clearly defined and communicated to the patient.

In principle, the admission of a patient to a TFP-oriented ward should take place after a preliminary discussion and a visit to the ward. These appointments should take place promptly so that the impression is not created that a TFP-informed treatment is too high-threshold or that patients must bridge the waiting time in acute wards. In addition, patients' motivation can fluctuate, not least because they are afraid of the therapy and supposed reasons for withdrawing a request for admission may become "convenient" for them in an effort to avoid what they might fear.

Only highly experienced inpatient teams should consider deviating from standard procedures when determining the conditions of hospitalization. Some possible exceptions to the standard expectations of a continuous three-month commitment to inpatient treatment might include: (1) an agreement to authorize a shorter treatment at the outset because the patient in question has a long-planned trip abroad, or (2) an expedited inpatient treatment for a patient who already has a treatment place in a day program available for follow-up care. In general, it is advisable to avoid creating situations where certain patients are given "special status" on the inpatient service. At the beginning of treatment, contact should be made (usually by telephone) with the patient's outpatient therapist. Establishing contact with the outpatient therapist should be a framework condition for inpatient treatment as part of the therapy contract. This requires a written release of confidentiality. The value of involving and appropriately informing the pre- and post-treatment therapist is often underestimated.

Extended Diagnostic Phase

The planned admission of a patient for inpatient TFP only occurs with corresponding diagnoses from prior treatments or from the outpatient preliminary interviews. Nevertheless, the performance of an in-depth diagnosis by specially trained physicians or psychologists is recommended, since successful inpatient therapy is based on a detailed diagnosis and enables specific adaptation of the treatment [24, 25]. From a TFP-oriented point of view, it is relevant for the prognosis to explore how previous attempts at therapy went, whether a person is motivated to make amends after harm he or she has done, and whether he or she seeks trusting relationships or rejects them (for example, as an expression of weakness).

Applying a TFP approach to the diagnosis of PD will enable clinicians to evaluate the following aspects:

- Phenomenology (psychopathology)
- Relative comorbidity (such as addiction, depression, eating disorders)
- History, especially suicidality/suicide attempts
- Biography
- Prior treatment, in particular reasons for success or failure
- Structural level (informed by Kernberg's structural interview or by the Operationalized Psychodynamic Diagnostic)
- Social functioning (education, work, debt, etc.)

It would be desirable to conduct a diagnostic assessment of PD using standardized clinical interviews based on current ICD-10/ICD-11 or DSM-5 classification systems, e.g., using the structured clinical interview for DSM-5 disorders (SCID-5-PD; [26]).

In particular, the diagnosis of the structural level is of fundamental importance for treatment planning and can be carried out by means of the following procedures:

- Operationalized psychodynamic diagnostic [27]
- Structural interview [28]
- Structured personality organization interview—revised (STIPO-R, [29])

Since the structural level of a patient has a direct impact on the course of treatment, structural diagnostics provide essential information for treatment planning. Different treatment priorities are set according to the structural level. In one case, for example, the aim may be to develop an initial understanding of the illness, while in another, it may be to limit symptom excesses or behavior that poses a threat to self and therapy.

Therapy Contract Phase

In order to consolidate the treatment framework, a therapy contract is made with the patient before the therapeutic work begins, consistent with the approach in outpatient TFP.

In terms of content, the contract consists of both general and individualized points of consensus, which, in line with the outpatient treatment setting, sets limits and responsibilities where destructive behavior endangers the patient's life or the continuation of therapy.

Since, according to the TFP-informed concept of PD, the reactivation of destructive parts of the self is expected in the course of treatment, and the patient's structural problems can only be worked on if they occur within the framework of relationship dyads reactivated in the here-and-now; the aim of a therapy agreement is not, in principle, to prevent dysfunctional behavior. Rather, the development of a therapy contract is an attempt to secure the framework of the treatment and to limit the threat of destructive behavior. To achieve a mutual commitment, no prefabricated therapy contract is used, but the agreements are worked out and brought together in a discussion between patient and therapist. The therapy contract should be formulated neither too rigidly nor too arbitrarily. Excessive rigidity (perceived by the patient as a "dictatorship") can be counterproductive, just as a contract too lax or incomplete can present a different kind of complication. Furthermore, in the therapy agreement process, care should be taken that the patient does not merely consent to treatment but engages with the clinician through the negotiation of the contract in a sustainable way.

In terms of content, the therapy contract is based on the principles of outpatient TFP for borderline patients [23]. The general points of agreement include, on the part of the patient, the regular and on time attendance of therapy sessions, which may include individual therapy, group therapies, work with the primary nurse, and special therapies. If the patient is unable to attend an appointment, they must sign out in person with the respective therapist or nurse. However, regular attendance at therapies is an essential basis for therapeutic cooperation. Failure to provide this foundation may indicate that treatment cannot continue at that time, which could ultimately lead to the patient's discharge. Decisions regarding a possible discharge of a patient should always be made together as a team.

Furthermore, it is part of the patient's responsibility to present feelings and thoughts as uncensored as possible and to actively participate in the therapy by making an effort to reflect on the therapists' and caregivers' contributions, as well as his or her own, contributions and behavior.

On the part of the therapists and nurses, one of the responsibilities is to help the patient understand himself better through joint conversations in individual and group settings. For that, it is essential that the therapists and the nursing staff concentrate on the three channels of communication, similarly to what is done in outpatient TFP: what the patient says, the patient's behavior, and the clinicians' countertransference in the sessions or during the appointments. This is complemented by the observation of the patient's behavior on the ward, in the relationship with fellow patients and the team. This helps all to avoid slipping into general and unfocused psychodynamic speculations.

Just as with the patient, a TFP-oriented therapeutic agreement also clarifies that the team is obliged to attend appointments regularly and on time. The frequency of appointments for the respective therapeutic program is discussed precisely with the patient. A specific aspect of inpatient treatment is the continuous presence and responsiveness of the nursing staff as well as the greater availability of the therapeutic and medical staff. It should be clearly discussed with the patient whether and under which conditions, for example, therapeutic brief contacts can take place outside the regular session appointments. The form of this agreement differs depending on the interpersonal dynamics as well as the severity of the pathology. For example, in the case of a severely suicidal patient, it may make sense to offer crisis contacts for a limited period of time in addition to individual sessions, or in the case of a patient with frequent conflictual entanglements, to hold therapeutic/nursing social therapeutic conflict clarification discussions in addition to individual and group sessions. The design of contact with the care team can also vary; this can be left to the patient's own responsibility or arranged in a supportive and structured way with fixed appointments.

Careful attention must be paid to the fact that despite the rapid, deep, and immediate establishment of relationships by borderline patients, there can be no "exclusive" or secretive therapeutic relationships, something often desired by patients. Instead of having a focus on the two-person patient-therapist relationship like in individual outpatient treatment, in inpatient psychotherapy, all the individual perspectives of the different staff members are brought together in the team conferences. The goal of this approach is to counteract splitting mechanisms, with the specific task for the individual therapist of conveying to the patient the total transference situation observed by the team. In addition to the general therapy agreements, which are obligatory for all, individualized agreements are made with the patient to reduce resistance to exploratory work. By limiting therapy threats through specific agreements, the continuation of inpatient treatment is secured at the same time. In TFP, resistances and threats to treatment include [23] the following:

- Suicidal and serious self-destructive behaviors
- Homicidal threats, gestures, or attempts, including threats to therapists or fellow patients
- Lying or concealing information
- Substance dependence and substance abuse
- Disordered eating behavior
- Moderately self-destructive behaviors (scratching as opposed to cutting).
- Irregular attendance at meetings
- Attempts to intrude into the lives of the staff
- Creating circumstances that make payment for treatment impossible (e.g., unclear health insurance status)
- Creation of problems outside therapy that make it difficult to continue treatment
- Adherence to a chronically passive lifestyle that increases the secondary gain of illness

In the following, single exemplary points of the individualized agreements will be briefly discussed.

Suicidal Behavior A distinction must be made between:

- *Suicidality in the context of major depression*: In addition to acute forms of suicidality, for example, in the context of crises and adjustment disorders, borderline patients may also experience suicidality in the context of major depression (with typical symptoms such as anhedonia, low mood, and hopelessness). In these cases, acute suicidality should be treated according to the rules of crisis intervention and general psychiatry. Only sometimes does short-term treatment in an acute ward become necessary.
- *Chronic suicidality:* More complicated are cases in which there is chronic suicidality, even with numerous suicide attempts in the patient's past. In these cases, a

depressive, low mood syndrome is not necessarily present. Chronic suicidality can often be found in patients with certain narcissistic disorders [30], and a pattern of chronic suicidality is widely considered a "signature" of BPD pathology [31].

- In these cases, chronic suicidality is not an expression of crisis instability but, on the contrary, serves to stabilize. It is necessary to understand the function of chronic suicidality in these cases, which protects the patient from an even worse outcome, namely the experience of a kind of inner death (e.g., protection from being overwhelmed, acting out, and self-esteem issues).
- In these cases, it seems necessary to address this point, which prioritizes the intrapsychic function and dynamics of chronic suicidality, even when the patient is focusing on other aspects of his/her condition and minimizing the suicidality.
- *Acute suicidal tendencies:* In most cases, a transfer to an acute ward is the result of purely protective behavior, which makes a subsequent relationship-oriented psychotherapeutic treatment difficult or even impossible. If there is really no capacity for consultation and the therapeutic relationships are therefore not sufficiently sustainable, a transfer for the shortest possible period of time is carried out by necessity. Above all, it must be examined whether an acute suicidal tendency really exists.
- *Parasuicidality*: this must not be dealt with in terms of its psychodynamic significance alone, but also its real risks. This also applies to (provocative) suicidal behavior.

Particularly difficult are situations where the patient has lied to the team by concealing suicidal tendencies or where medication prescribed on the ward has been taken with (pseudo) suicidal intent. Again, the patient in this scenario is discharged, again with an offer of readmission. The expectation for honesty is extended to the unit staff as well; any example of lying to a patient by a team member is considered equally unacceptable [32].

In general, the effectiveness of an anti-suicide contract is minimal at best if this is not embedded in a good therapeutic relationship. By no means does such a contract replace a good therapeutic relationship; on the contrary, a contract without a therapeutically stable foundation can be experienced as repressive and leading to exactly what it is supposed to prevent—suicidal behavior or completed suicide. However, individually negotiated agreements, as are common in TFP for setting out the therapeutic framework and for forming a stable therapeutic relationship, can be very helpful. For example, a patient who may have felt neglected by his parents responds positively to the therapist's negotiation of a treatment agreement; the therapist conveys in a nuanced way that he genuinely cares about the patient's fate.

Self-Injuring Behavior In the preliminary interview and on admission, precise questions are asked about the patient's history of self-injury and possible manifestations of this pattern to be expected during inpatient treatment. As a rule, self-injuring behavior is not a sign of suicidality but, according to Sachsse [33], the opposite:

- A "pressure valve" for stress reduction
- A way of coping with dysphoric affects
- A sign of self-directed aggression and self-punishment
- A remedy for hyperarousal
- An antidote to dissociative states
- A behavior for regulating fluctuations in self-esteem

On an interpersonal level, it is to be understood as

- A non-verbal communication
- An expression of projective identification
- An escape from perceived excessive demands

According to the therapy agreement, the patient is expected to report self-injuring behavior and to be bandaged if necessary. The trigger of self-injuring behavior should be discussed and analyzed with the patient. It should be taken into account that many patients may be relieved, on the one hand, after self-injuring behavior, but, on the other hand, others may be extremely ashamed and thus burdened again.

Crisis talks after self-injurious behavior should be as short as possible, but also as long as necessary. It should be determined whether the self-injurious behavior was used to initiate a conversation. If so, the patient is referred to the regular interview appointment.

Sometimes self-injurious behavior may also be a sign of provocation. Then a very clear limitation regarding provocative self-injurious behavior is required. Those who injure themselves in the face or neck will be discharged. Such non-concealable injuries trigger fellow patients, and this must be avoided. Patients who are discharged for violating the therapeutic agreement because of self-injury are usually given another chance to be admitted. In the case of a severe violation of the therapeutic agreement, a consultation with the patient before readmission is required.

Dealing with Addictive Substances Borderline patients have high rates of comorbid substance use disorders and often exhibit a pattern of misuse of multiple substances. A precise addiction history at the beginning of therapy as part of the diagnosis is therefore of great importance. It should already be agreed with the patient in the preliminary discussions that a sustained abstinence from addictive substances such as drugs or alcohol and refraining from misuse of medications is essential.

Even though chronic severe addiction is rare, borderline patients often resort to addictive substances in order to situationally influence their emotional lives and states of tension. Substance abuse must consequently be considered a symptom of BPO, like other symptoms, e.g., self-injury, eating disorders, and parasuicidal acts. As part of the treatment agreement, the patient should commit to responsibly reporting relapses on his or her own, doing a behavioral analysis of them, and focusing on the behavior. Concealing relapses can lead to discharge, whereas reported and processed relapses can be tolerated in therapy as long as the patient is serious about working on the problem. The reduction of relapses during the course of therapy would also be an important signal of progress.

So, while we advocate for a flexible approach to relapse, there are clear limits when such activity reflects anti-social behavior. The patient who sells drugs for financial gain or takes alcohol onto the ward would face dismissal from the unit, although readmission under certain circumstances could be negotiated. In general, the basic dialectic of borderline patients applies especially in dealing with addictive behavior: firmness and flexibility have to be balanced against each other. An unclear attitude of the therapeutic team regarding addiction problems automatically leads to entanglements with the patient community. It would be dangerous if the treatment community had a nominal shared commitment to abstinence, while simultaneously a subculture of substance use was either suspected or tolerated.

General Therapy Contract In most cases, the therapy agreement is supplemented by general ward rules that organize the coexistence of patients on the ward and apply to all patients. The general ward rules described in the following are based on our experience from working on TFP-oriented wards.

Ward rules may include generally applicable agreements on the following topics:

- The design of the daily structure
- Body hygiene and the wearing of appropriate clothing
- Order and hygiene in patient rooms, common rooms, ward kitchens
- Rules on reciprocal visits of patients to each other's rooms
- Rules for dealing with external visitors
- Use of television, computer games, mobile phones
- Participation in common mealtimes, activities, patient general meetings, morning and evening rounds, and patient services
- Rules regarding the time spent outside the ward help to orient new patients at the ward
- Dealing with addictive substances
- Dealing with self-harm and suicidality
- Dealing with confidentiality and data protection
- Dealing with sex among patients, how to deal with partnerships

In any case, it should be kept in mind that setting rules too rigidly may severely impair the investigation of relationship dynamics and transference events. At the same time, this orientation toward rules and frameworks represents an important protection of the community against transgressions by individual patients. Therapeutic procedure and general safety also compete with each other here. The demand for more and more new rules points to primarily custodial and thus non-therapeutic team processes.

Only those rules that are retained and reinforced through actions by all team members should endure. Otherwise, there is a danger that the patient will receive different messages from different members of staff, which creates ideal conditions for the manifestation of divisions. In difficult phases, the call for more rules easily arises, although these phases are usually not to be "regulated" at all, but should be psychodynamically worked through (if necessary, in the context of supervision). Apodictic formulations of ward rules such as "If the patient does this, he will be discharged" should be avoided. In such a case, the team would no longer have any room for compromises if it does not want to "lose face." Formulations such as "If the patient does this, discharge *may* follow" sound quite clear, but allow room for compromises and thus make it possible to react appropriately to the situation. Likewise, the distribution of several notices of rule infractions (after "violations") should be avoided since inpatient psychotherapy represents a joint search for identifying solutions and ultimately the entire team should decide on how to deal with rule violations. This also refers to the simple "counting" of violations, with subsequent automatic dismissal ("after the third relapse there is dismissal").

In contrast to outpatient therapy, the set of rules in a ward is more present and, above all, more complex than the framework in outpatient psychotherapy. The rules also repeatedly become a topic of inpatient psychotherapy because—as already described by Ermann [34]—the resistance of patients in inpatient psychotherapy mainly expresses itself as resistance against the framework and takes the form of acting out. Typical boundary violations are violations of abstinence commandments (alcohol, drugs, and smoking), punctuality (keeping the peace at night, participating in therapies), violence, and erotic boundary transgressions.

Sexuality and love relationships: Dealing with sexuality and love relationships in inpatient settings is similarly fraught with complications as is dealing with addictive substances (see various articles on this in: Dulz et al. [35]). The position is generally shared that the threshold for a love relationship or a sexual relationship in everyday inpatient life must be high because the formation of a couple nullifies the central therapeutic experience in the inpatient milieu; the couple in the joint couple "shell" stabilizes itself artificially, seals itself off from the outside, and avoids the experience of crisis and self-reflection. In many cases, then, acted-out infatuation can be seen as a resistance to therapy. Sexuality is used here to evade the emotionality of the therapeutic process. To require patients to refrain from a new love relationship for three months during a hospitalization seems to be a reasonable condition—at least in theory.

A relativizing position on this is that infatuation cannot be "consciously" avoided and also reflects something that cannot be postponed. Since relationship pathology is the central problem of these patients, attempts at rapprochement should not be ignored. In some circumstances, the expression of infatuation and closeness in the protected setting of the ward can also be something progressive. It follows from this that love relationships are not desirable but must be dealt with when they occur; they must be addressed and cannot be forbidden by dismissal or decree. On the contrary, dealing with pathological "current" love relationship patterns holds a great opportunity with regard to a more satisfactory love life for patients in the future. Prohibitions here can only lead to concealment of corresponding feelings and relationship attempts, but also of sexual problems that should be included in therapy. Rigidity also corresponds to the behavior of many primary caregivers of borderline patients who avoid topics related to romance and intimacy.

Religiosity and Political Attitude Personal belief systems such as spirituality, religion, and world views require a neutral approach by the therapeutic team. However, there can be no neutrality toward racist, sexist, and similar attitudes and behaviors, e.g., toward clothes representing neo-Nazi codes, but also T-shirts with cannabis motifs or drinking slogans. Here the therapeutic neutrality must change into a clearly evaluative and confrontational attitude. A borderline area here is the attraction of some patients to satanism; such an interest could reflect a genuine religious or spiritual motive, or it could be a more concerning expression of antisocial tendencies.

Initial Phase

One focus in the initial phase is on limiting self-harming behavior and socially harmful relationship patterns, which can usually manifest themselves relatively early on in the ward. It is made clear to the patient that the ward is a reflection of the patient's social reality, and the patient will likely have relationships on the ward that are similar to the patient's relationship in his or her life outside of the hospital.

One possible method of treatment would be to place every patient in a psychotherapy group from the outset (first day). In contrast, however, it may also be appropriate to assign a patient to specific group therapies only after a detailed diagnostic assessment has been completed.

The patient's treatment plan is determined individually and should not be overloaded. If the therapy plan is too extensive, there is a danger that the patient will no longer have time to deal with his or her state of mind or real relationships with fellow patients; in this case, therapy participation can be described as an avoidance strategy or even "addictive." Apart from this, a beneficial therapy plan usually contains fixed building blocks that are valid for all and individually agreed upon. For example, a ritual to start the week together or to begin the weekend on Friday afternoon is recommended as an external structure, but also as a community experience. It is important to have enough time set aside so that the patients can experience certain day-to-day aspects of living together on the ward. Joint activities on the ward such as cooking, eating, cleaning, and game evenings afford the opportunity to experience oneself in the group. In the spirit of a therapeutic community approach, it is advisable to provide for certain tasks or roles on the ward, e.g., leadership of the ward group, patient committee participation, and cooking assignments. Especially for borderline patients, it is important to also experience themselves as competent, effective, deliberate, and comfortable in both leadership and followership roles. The patient's self-perception and assessment of his or her abilities can shift rapidly from overestimation to underestimation. Overestimation and underestimation can sometimes prevent a realistic assessment of one's own abilities. In this context, occupational therapy in which patients work in a concrete planning way or do something for the common life on the ward can be quite effective.

Determining the Treatment Focus After completion of the in-depth diagnostics and the negotiation of the therapy contract, it is important to review the patient in the whole team in order to develop a common understanding about the patient. The case presentation (approximately 45 minutes per patient) takes place in the ward about three weeks after admission. The individual therapist in charge—who, in the DACH system is also the administrator for the patient, responsible for all decisions concerning his stay and treatment—collects all information about the patient; it is important that the therapist has a sufficiently good knowledge of the case history and biography. The team members supplement with their observations and countertransference comments, including, for example, the supplementary therapists. These are: movement therapist (working with body movements, sometimes dance, helping the patients to experience bodily sensations and deal with boundaries to their fellow patients in groups); music therapists (using playing instruments in group or individual settings to foster the non-verbal expression of patients); art therapists (using painting and sculpting to foster the non-verbal and symbolic expression of inner images); occupational therapists (helping patients to strengthen their ego functions like planning, frustration tolerance but also to experience success when completing a piece of work). The goal of the case presentation is a deeper understanding of the patient's identity diffusion by identifying the dominant object-relations dyads. The overarching aim of the treatment is to integrate the dominant object-relations dyads into more nuanced and realistic representations of self and others which lead to an overall improved personality functioning [36].

Therefore, it is very important that all team members are able to identify and understand the dominant object-relations dyads that the patient experiences or acts upon in the social interactions of the different therapy offerings and in the milieu of the patient community. This approach is central to the TFP-oriented inpatient treatment. To formulate the dominant object-relations dyads and pull together the different perspectives provided, it is extremely important to gather comprehensive information from all therapy services and everyday life on the ward within the framework of a case presentation. In contrast to outpatient TFP, observations of the whole team regarding the verbal and non-verbal communication of the patient, as well as perceptions from transference and countertransference events, are important here. Despite the rapidly changing transference patterns in borderline patients, a limited number of the patient's assumptions about self and others map on to dominant object relations dyads [23]. Possible object-relations dyads that may change in various and numerous interactions between the patient and the team, as well as the patient community, include, for example, the unwanted child and the unloving, selfish mother or the kind, submissive self and the idolatrously admiring mother [23]. The dominant object relations dyads should be described individually and as accurately as possible.

The dominant object relations dyads are correlated with those elements elucidated in the structural interview that explain the patient's difficulties in, for example, intimate relationships, work, or studies. In this respect, a *twofold treatment focus* is aimed for: *one focus* is on the d*ominant object-relations dyads a*s they emerge during the inpatient treatment, the *other focus* is directed toward the major symptomatic areas of BPO—e.g., suicidality or self-mutilation. This symptom-oriented focus is related directly to further specific *treatment aims*, as for example degree of symptomatic burden and improvement of functioning in individual domains. The treatment focus is also an important part of the therapy contract agreed upon by the patient and the treatment team. The treatment focus, which is discussed together with the patient, represents a kind of operationalized condensation of the treatment aims. The overarching goal of engagement with the patient about the *treatment aims* is to prioritize those target symptoms to be addressed during hospitalization, thereby facilitating the patient's eventual transition to follow-up outpatient treatment as given below:

- The choice of treatment focus follows the consideration of certain aspects of the personality organization (severity of illness).
- The focus should be identifiable in both interpersonal relationships on the unit and in the transference relationship.
- The processing/awareness should on the one hand lead to sufficient stabilization for the patient, but on the other hand, also be "strenuous" for him or her.
- The chosen treatment focus should lead most likely to a progressive development of the patient.
- The focus can be a conflict, but it can also be about pointing out a non-integrated object relationship issue (e.g., experiences of dysfunctional early relationships) that is showing up in the relationship.
- Occasionally, the perspectives of the team and the patient differ regarding the focus of treatment (for example, the team defines the primary treatment focus as chronic suicidality while the patient would rather focus on his or her experiences of sexual abuse).

To ensure free reflection of the team, e.g., the possibility of formulating negative feelings about a patient, to find a patient "disgusting" for example, the patient is not always present at the case presentation. This may change over time, at the discretion of the team. This process described may contradict the orientation common in social psychiatry nowadays [37]. The treatment focus chosen according to the dominant object-relations dyads is at the heart of inpatient therapy. The focus is now also considered in the joint weekly meetings where clinicians involved in individual treatment, group treatment, nursing, and other types of therapy, assemble to review the progress of patients.

The TFP treatment focus also provides an important basis for dealing with the patient in various challenging situations. These situations can include: (1) the patient's symptomatic, dysfunctional behavior; (2) the staff's intense positive as well as negative countertransference feelings; (3) the staff's experience of the patient's active splitting process; (4) the patient's observed expressions of devaluation and idealization; and (5) the staff's experiences of phenomena of projective identification. The focus also represents what has been absorbed and digested by the treatment team [23] in order to make it possible for the patient to integrate this understanding.

Since the focus is formulated for the treatment team and the patients alike, the patients are often initially unfamiliar and occasionally overwhelmed with the unusual vocabulary that is new to them. Therefore, the treatment team is effortful in communicating with patients using straightforward, accessible language. At the same time, patients often feel valued by the team's efforts to understand them and the effort made to reduce their symptomatology [18].

Mid-phase

In the middle phase of treatment, the focus is on processing the relationship dyads between the patients and the different members of the multi-professional team of the ward. In particular, the different transference relationships are explored, for example with individual therapists, nursing caregivers, social workers, and therapists of other types of therapy (for example, occupational-, art-, music- or movement-therapy). Often patients are experienced very differently in different relationship contexts. This focus is achieved through working with the patient in both individual and group psychotherapy.

Individual Inpatient TFP Ideally, two sessions of individual therapy are delivered per week. In individual therapy, the dynamics from various interactions are considered together with the patient, processed, and increasingly integrated with the help of technical neutrality, concentration on transference and countertransference events, and the techniques of clarification, confrontation, and interpretation. In doing so, it is necessary to repeatedly work through the dominant object-relations dyads within the complex web of relationships.

As a rule, the patient's inner object-relationship patterns manifest themselves in the inpatient setting through manifold conflicts, alliances, and expressions of sympathy and antipathy. However, it can hardly be avoided in the context of inpatient therapy that the patient has repeated experiences of inner and interpersonal conflicts as well, coming into contact with disturbing feelings of jealousy, envy, anger, hatred, or fear. The goal of the treatment team in this process must be for the patient to gain insight into the deeper nature of these conflicts and not act them out. Ideally, a patient will learn to understand why they experience a fellow patient as fearful or dominant and what this has to do with their own relational patterns (object-relations dyads). Typically, in the communication with the patient, one uses the terminology of roles or actors to illuminate these sides of the patient ("powerless child" and "critical parent;" "defiant but lonely child" and "humiliated parent," etc.).

The transference-focused work manifests itself on different levels. Ideally, the dominant object relationship theme is pointed out to the patient directly in the transference relationship, clarified and interpreted in its intrapsychic functionality. In addition, transference-focused work can also mean that the object relationships themes are revealed by the interpersonal relationships and conflicts with fellow patients or relevant staff assigned to work with the patient.

TFP-Based Group Psychotherapy In group psychotherapy, the topics of self-perception and perception of others are of particular importance; in addition, the modes of communication as well as the experience of not being an "individual case"—and thus not an "outstanding" patient—will have salience. In this way, patients gain the experience of being "in the same boat" with fellow patients who also appear to be different. Of particular importance is the idea of the therapeutic community, the notion that patients can assume an important therapeutic function for each other, something especially true for borderline patients. Their confrontations can be more precise, sharper and at the same time patients are more likely to accept confrontations from other patients than they do from staff.

The techniques of clarification and confrontation are applied by the whole treatment team. The interpretation and thus the integration of the material is the task of the individual and group therapists. In the work of the nursing caregiver and the social worker, the real world is more strongly emphasized, but also associated with the dominant object-relations dyads.

The inpatient team works as a group in their collective treatment of the patients on the unit using TFP principles. Group dynamics and psychodynamic group therapy are therefore of particular importance. The frequency of group therapy should be coordinated with the frequency of individual therapy. Depending on whether the focus of therapeutic work is group or individual therapy, group therapy sessions generally occur from one to three times a week for 60–90 minutes. The group size should be approximately six to eight patients.

Given the variety of settings in different hospitals, the framework conditions vary, depending on personnel resources on the one hand, but also on the hospital's traditions, on the other. Borderline patients, especially those with paranoid symptomatology should be able to retain a sense of some control. The larger the group, the more difficult this becomes; the anxiety in the patient increases and the ability to communicate decreases accordingly. As a result, larger groups may be more ineffective. In addition, there is a danger that some patients will become disengaged; these are often those patients with social anxiety who would particularly benefit from positive group experiences.

Group therapy should always be led by two therapists—ideally one male and one female. This is not only helpful with regard to transference situations but also convenient in times of vacation and illness so that the group can then continue with only one of the two therapists present. While in some inpatient units' patients have to join the group immediately after admission, in other clinics assignment to the group may take some time, especially when there is an incentive to get to know the patients better beforehand.

In psychodynamic group therapy, the interactions and relationship patterns that occur in the patient group can also be made accessible for reflection and symbolization outside the actual therapy sessions. This is also important because patients with personality disorders in the hierarchically oriented structure of an inpatient unit tend to reenact internalized relationship patterns with treatment team members differently than they do with fellow patients.

As in individual therapy, the treatment technique in group therapy follows the principles of TFP. In inpatient individual therapy, the most affectively significant relationship dyads that are reenacted in the here-and-now are worked on first. The internalized relationship patterns from the past can be updated in the relationship with the individual therapist, but also with another treatment team member, or with a fellow patient. Through clarification, careful confrontation, and interpretation, the patient gradually becomes aware of the relationship patterns and thus is able to experience and understand them in a new way. The procedure in psychodynamic group therapy corresponds to this. The group leader's first task is to create an atmosphere in which free communication about the current mutual experience can be examined.

Clarification and confrontation—the intervention techniques that prepare interpretations—are often carried out by the group members among themselves. The group therapist supports this process through his or her attitude and intervenes, especially when destructive processes take hold or when the working group regresses to a "basic assumption" group and remains stuck in regression [38]. By using the term "basic assumption" group, we refer to Bion's observations of how the recurrent emotional states of groups inform group behavior. Interpretations by the group therapist refer primarily to regressive group processes, as well as to the dominant object-relations dyads [39].

In group therapy—especially in the inpatient setting—it is primarily the transferences that occur between group members or between individuals and the group as a whole that are the subject of reflection and interpretation. The task of the group leader is to provide a space in which reenacting relationship dyads can be recognized and reflected upon together. This is a very complex process with a multitude of constellating aspects of past relationship experiences.

Transference-focused group therapy is experienced by patients as very demanding and often frightening at the beginning. At the end of the treatment, however, it is usually described as a challenging, but also very valuable, experience. In order for the patients to be able to cope with the group sessions, especially at the beginning, the treatment team has to recognize the patients' insecurities and fears and then stabilize them. The team still has to be convinced of this central element of therapy, in much the same way as a parent empathically understands the child's fears of kindergarten but nevertheless helps to confront this challenge and takes the child to kindergarten.

Termination Phase

At least four weeks before the patient is discharged, the final phase of treatment should be initiated by the individual therapist and the primary caregiver. This phase is about separation and the farewell process, about mourning, sometimes also about envy for those who can still stay, and about hope for those who must leave or are allowed to leave. In addition, this phase focuses on planning and preparing the first steps after discharge. Separation and farewell are sometimes a topic even at the beginning of therapy due to the inherent time limit of the inpatient stay.

In connection with the impending discharge and the anticipated loss of support and security, and given the patient's particular sensitivity to separation, it is not uncommon for the original symptoms to manifest themselves again so that a patient can appear at the end of the hospitalization much as he did at the beginning. However, this is usually not a sign of an unsuccessful hospitalization but can, on the contrary, mean that the patient has been able to develop a number of sustainable relationships. In the work with the primary nurse, concrete preparations are made with the patient to facilitate the transition to everyday life (e.g., working out a daily structure). In the context of termination in an individual TFP treatment during the hospitalization, the recurrence of original symptomatology can sometimes be interpreted against the background of the activated object-relations dyad, e.g., the therapist as rejecting parent. To support a disengagement from the ward, it is particularly important to grant the patient more freedom, and opportunities for contact with everyday life during these last days of hospitalization, for example in the form of prolonged therapy exposure trials.

At the end of the treatment, the patient should no longer have pathological anxiety, but also should not display euphoria. He should approach the future challenges with appropriate seriousness. The farewell phase is not easy for the patients. The arrival of new patients underscores to the patient preparing for discharge that the hospitalization is a transitional phase of treatment. The changes caused by new admissions, often met with rejection and fear by those patients facing imminent discharge, occasionally make it easier for those patients to say goodbye.

The team members also have to say goodbye and it is important that they, for their part, name their feelings in this regard in team meetings. An art of experienced teams is the capacity to calibrate the closeness to the patient in such a way that the patient realizes that the inpatient stay should not, and will not, result in a long-term therapeutic relationship. The patient with prominent separation anxiety may react in a way that calls into question the advisability of discharge after that date has been determined. It is optimal if the team can adhere to the discharge date and if the patient can be engaged in a process that allows disposition planning to proceed smoothly. Treatment should not be prolonged if it seems little has been achieved; doing so will usually have no effect. Occasionally, an extension of inpatient treatment may be useful if what has already been positively achieved is to be consolidated. In the final phase of treatment, the patient's further treatment must be planned by the team together with the patient. In some places, further treatment of the patient is possible through the outpatient department of the psychiatric-psychotherapeutic institution until outpatient psychotherapy can concretely begin.

Many inpatient site patients will refer patients to the regular outpatient treatment system. There are usually not enough colleagues among practicing psychiatrists and psychologists who: (1) have experience with borderline patients, (2) are willing to take these patients into outpatient treatment, and (3) can provide treatment that is consistent with prevailing psychotherapy guidelines. Because of this frequently observed problem, it is advantageous for hospital-based clinicians to establish a network of skilled outpatient clinicians and offer basic training in TFP to those who are motivated. In any case, communication between inpatient individual therapists and the outpatient aftercare provider is recommended according to the TFP principles.

As an alternative to transferring to the outpatient treatment system, further treatment in a specialized day-care setting may be indicated as a supportive transition to outpatient psychotherapy.

Dealing with Crisis Situations: Inpatient Crisis Intervention and Acute Psychiatric Treatment

If inpatient crisis intervention appears necessary for BPD patients, it should be carried out for as short a time as possible outside of special inpatient settings, usually only a few days [3]. There are different types of crisis intervention units. Some units accept patients on a voluntary basis, and other units that are locked and secure, accept acutely and severely ill patients on both a voluntary basis and an involuntary basis (against the will of the patient). In the following, we refer to acute wards, where both voluntary and involuntary admissions can be made. Crisis interventions often take place in a unit with a heterogeneous patient population; this setting is distinctly different from the psychotherapy inpatient unit designed specifically for patients with personality disorder pathology, which accommodates patients with lower acuity and less pronounced safety concerns. Treatment for BPD patients very rarely needs to be in a locked setting, something required only when suicidality that can no longer be controlled. Treatments of longer duration on a locked unit often say more about the treatment providers than about the risk posed by patients.

Typically, patients with BPD can stabilize again very quickly in a higher acuity setting. During an inpatient crisis intervention, the expectations for therapy offered should not be excessive; most important are stabilizing conversations with an individual therapist or primary nurse. Given the expectations for the patient's return to a less restrictive setting, an attempt should be made by the unit clinicians to form an alliance with the patient and to be flexible. As a rule, borderline patients are capable of collaboration if an agreement has been negotiated and reached with them jointly and they themselves stand by it. It is not uncommon for a patient to be admitted to a locked unit with suicidality and to be able to be discharged the following day. Admittedly, the assessment of a threat requires a great deal of experience, especially regarding the calculation of whether the patient is genuinely highly suicidal or rather communicating suicidality as a way of expressing distress. Ideally, a locked setting should be avoided.

In addition to psychopathological stabilization through a calming setting and medication [3, 40], the aim of an admission to a higher acuity setting is to identify unclear or destabilizing external conditions (for example, whether a patient can continue her outpatient therapy or keep her housing). Therefore, the relevant parties in the patient's environment should be contacted quickly by the treatment provider.

Despite the recommendation to carry out inpatient crisis interventions for only a few days, long-lasting treatments in acute psychiatric departments, sometimes lasting weeks, or months, occur time and again. Due to serious, repeated suicidal behavior or severe self-injurious acts, forced prolonged admissions take place. In these cases, the patients often find themselves in ward environments with limited structure in which a persistent emergency mood prevails with psychotic, severely depressed, delirious, or agitated fellow patients. If the patient with significant PD pathology also encounters a treatment team that is not well trained and experienced regarding the dynamics of patients with a borderline personality organization level, then profound patient regression, increases in agitation, and divisions within the treatment team often occur in a short period of time. Patients in this context experience the efficacy of their destructive behaviors (such as self-injury, affect storms, or suicidal acts). These behaviors mobilize the treatment team, can lead to increased security, and attempts at control out of fear and concern for the patients, which in turn leads the patients to become even more unstable, further delaying discharge. The divisions in the team, when some team members identify with the projected ideal object representations and others with the devalued or hateful ones, may lead the staff to act out their countertransference feelings. This splitting among staff can become greatly destructive.

Such an environment can also lead to malignant regressions because, through processes of projective identification, patients manage to transform parts of their intrapsychic conflict dynamics into interpersonal, psychosocial conflicts. Typically, the treatment team then attempts to identify with the patient's self-parts that are self- and life-sustaining, while the patient identifies more strongly with the self-destructive, hateful, and object-damaging parts. For the patient, this is a relief as their conflict tension and anxiety can be reduced while at the same time responsibility can be delegated to the treatment team. The "struggle" then no longer takes place intra-psychically, but interpersonally "on the stage" of the acute psychiatric ward. If the treatment team fails in overcoming this split, in digesting and understanding the dynamics, and in returning self-responsibility to the patient, individual cases may even result in years of inpatient psychiatric treatment, in which attempted discharges then lead to new admissions after a very short time due to suicidal behavior. Ultimately, here too there is a conflict between maximum safety on the one hand and effective therapy on the other, which always involves a (calculable) risk. Especially in the case of acutely and severely ill patients, the staff is often (unconsciously) forced to identify with the life-sustaining part of the patients.

The training of acute psychiatric treatment teams in essential TFP principles can help to make these dynamics understandable. This training can help to overcome divisions in the treatment team, to facilitate the separation processes, and to limit the opportunity of the patient to stay connected with the staff through expressions of suicidality, as when the team is taken "hostage" due to the concern about the patient's suicide and the confusion about the patient's personal responsibility and the team's legal responsibility. Supervision by a colleague experienced in TFP can be containing here, strengthening the integrating and "affect-digesting" function of the treatment team, and helping to recognize the enacting dynamics.

What Are Possible Targets for Measurement to Gauge the Effectiveness of Instruction About Applications of TFP Principles?

In the German-speaking countries and the Netherlands, inpatient psychodynamic treatment continues to be an important and successful component of care. The effectiveness of inpatient TFP-oriented psychodynamic treatment is well documented empirically. This is now true not only for symptomatic improvements, but also for structural changes and psychological functioning levels [41]. Sollberger et al. [42] examined the efficacy of disorder-specific inpatient TFP treatment combined with elements of DBT skills training compared to general psychiatric inpatient treatment as part of a prospective group comparison. The results of the study indicate a statistically significant superiority of inpatient TFP treatment over treatment as usual (TAU) and confirm an improvement in the outcome measures of identity diffusion and affective psychopathology in relation to the reduction of anger and depression.

Another prospective, naturalistic longitudinal study with a waiting list control group examined the efficacy of inpatient TFP treatment [43]. Final study results are pending, however initial results suggest improvement in personality organization of participating patients.

What Are the Didactic Materials Required to Impart TFP Principles to this Target Group of Clinicians?

The psychotherapeutic staff of the PD units should at least be in advanced training as psychodynamic, psychoanalytic, or behavioral psychotherapists and should also be trained in TFP. A completed advanced training in TFP for the unit staff is desirable.

At present, there are three TFP-oriented psychodynamic institutes in Germany that are conducting training in TFP. The goal of these institutes is to provide experienced therapists working in a wide variety of clinical settings with a disorder-specific therapy method for the treatment of borderline and other personality disorders. The curriculum is based on the TFP manual by Yeomans et al. [2] and is aimed at physicians, psychologists, and social workers. It also provides a well-founded additional qualification for inpatient and therapeutic teams in psychosomatic and psychiatric clinics.

As previously described, the team of a ward with a TFP orientation can include psychiatrists, psychologists, social workers, nurses as well as specialized therapists. Thus, it is important for the unit to provide a specific therapeutic intervention that all team members feel involved in, and that distinct areas of responsibility are clearly defined and distributed. Efforts should also be made to ensure that all members of the team are aware of the possible effects and consequences of TFP interventions. Therefore, in addition to initial training in TFP, regular, ongoing internal training for all the staff members on the basics, techniques, and strategies of TFP is necessary.

Clinical Case Illustration

Conflicts quickly arose between an inpatient, Ms. A, and her roommates, in which the patient's problems with boundaries, her difficulties in saying no and putting her own interests first, became clear. Ms. A felt helpless, at the mercy of others, unappreciated and exploited. She consciously saw herself only as a "helpless victim." Within a short time, she experienced and felt herself on the ward as she had in previous relationships.

Against the background of an obviously "chronically low self-esteem" (reflected in the diagnosis offered by the nursing staff and self-description in SCID), she placed herself as if automatically in the shadow of others. For example, she worked diligently in the studio, but avoided contact with the art therapist. Motivated by her primary nurse, Ms. A succeeded in the group therapy in addressing an emerging conflict with a fellow patient, Mrs. C, who, from Ms. A's point of view, was constantly putting herself in the center of attention in a very calm and composed manner in a way that deprived Ms. A of attention from others in the group. When this fellow patient, Mrs. C, conveyed her dismay about this observation in the follow-up group, this led to great uncertainty in Ms. A and to the feeling that she had been betrayed by her motivating caregiver. In this situation of mistrust—also toward other team members—her thoughts of leaving the inpatient treatment unit intensified.

During the course of her inpatient treatment, Ms. A was able to explore with her individual therapist, and with the members of her therapy group, the ways she reflexively saw herself as inferior, and how she experienced others, including her therapist and others in the treatment milieu, as superior and devaluing. Through repeated exploration of the dominant emerging object relations dyads experienced in the here-and-now of the inpatient unit, Ms. A became increasingly reflective about certain central aspects of her past.

In her individual sessions, Ms. A described her life history, particularly her experience as a twin who had always been outshone by her brother and exposed to his aggressions without the intervention of their mother. It became understandable why the challenge of asserting herself was so prominent for the patient. The totality of the inpatient therapy facilitated for Ms. A increased contact with previously avoided feelings and split-off parts of the self, including envy of the fellow patient, Mrs. C, envy of the brother, fear of aggression. (Modified according to Rösch and Grimmer) [18].

Conclusion

Inpatient treatment of severely disturbed borderline patients is, on the one hand, a professional and personal challenge for all clinicians involved. On the other hand, work in this setting enables these patients to take developmental steps that would not be possible in an outpatient setting. We described how inpatient treatment settings for patients with severe PD pathology can be organized within a TFP-oriented framework. We also described how the multiple therapeutic elements of these settings (i.e., individual, group, and milieu treatments) can be usefully implemented with TFP principles. Increasing empirical evidence [41, 42] shows that such a TFP-informed inpatient approach is effective in improving symptoms and functional outcomes for hospitalized patients for whom standard individual outpatient treatment would have not been indicated.

References

1. Dulz B, Lohmer M, Kernberg O, Wlodarczyk O, Dammann G. Borderline-Persönlichkeitsstörung. Stationäre Übertragungsfokussierte Psychotherapie. Göttingen: Hogrefe; 2022.
2. Yeomans F, Clarkin J, Kernberg O. Transference-focused psychotherapy for borderline personality disorder: a clinical guide. Washington, DC: American Psychiatric Publishing; 2015.
3. Arbeitsgemeinschaft der Wissenschaftlichen Medizinischen Fachgesellschaften e.V. (AWMF). S3-Leitlinien Borderline-Persönlichkeitsstörungen; 2022.
4. Euler S, Dammann G, Endtner K, Leihener F, Perroud N, Reisch T, et al. Borderline personality disorder: treatment recommendations of the Swiss Society for Psychiatry and Psychotherapy. Swiss Arch Neurol Psychiatr Psychother. 2018;169(05):135–43.
5. DGPPN. Psychosoziale Therapien bei schweren psychischen Erkrankungen. S3-Praxisleitlinien in Psychiatrie und Psychotherapie 2ed. Berlin: Springer; 2009.
6. Häfner S, Lieberz K, Hözer M, Wöller W. Indications for inpatient psychotherapy. When does your patient belong in a clinic? MMW Fortschr Med. 2001;25(143):28–31.
7. Linehan M. Cognitive behavioral treatment of Borderline personality disorder. New York: Guilford; 1993.
8. Bateman A, Fonagy P. Psychotherapie der Borderline-Persönlichkeitsstörung. Ein mentalisierungsgestütztes Behandlungskonzept 2ed. Gießen: Psychosozial; 2014.
9. Young J, Klosko J, Weishaar M. Schema therapy: a practitioner's guide. New York: Guilford; 2003.
10. Puschner B, Haug S, Häfner S, Kordy H. Einfluss des Behandlungssettings auf den Gesundungsverlauf. Stationäre versus ambulante Psychotherapie. Psychotherapeut. 2004;49:182–92.
11. Clarkin J, Caligor E, Stern B, Kernberg O. Structured interview for personality organization (STIPO). 2007.
12. Levy K, Meehan K, Kelly K, Reynoso J, Weber M, Clarkin J, et al. Change in attachment patterns and reflective function in a randomized control trial of transference-focused psychotherapy for borderline personality disorder. J Consult Clin Psychol. 2006;74:1027–40.
13. Hörz S, Rentrop M, Fischer-Kern M, Schuster P, Kapusta N, Buchheim P, et al. Personality structure and clinical severity of borderline personality disorder. Z Psychosom Med Psychother. 2010;56:136–49.
14. Doering S. Transference-focused psychotherapy. Göttingen: Vandenhoeck & Rupprecht; 2016.
15. Walter M, Euler S, Sollberger D. Persönlichkeitsstörungen und Sucht. Stuttgart: Kohlhammer; 2016.
16. Dammann G. Grundprinzipien der psychoanalytisch-orientierten stationären Behandlung von Patienten mit schweren Persönlichkeitsstörungen. Psychoanalyse Texte zur Sozialforschung. 2012;16:514–29.
17. Mattke D, Dammann G, Martius P. Der Transfer von einzeltherapeutischen Behandlungskonzepten auf Gruppenformate: Das Beispiel der Übertragungsfokussierten Psychotherapie (TFP). Gruppenpsychother Gruppendynamik. 2007;43:161–80.
18. Rösch C, Grimmer B. Störungsspezifische stationäre Behandlung von Persönlichkeitsstörungen: Integration von TFP und DBT. Persönlichkeitsstörungen. 2017;21:83–95.

19. Dulz B, Ramb C. Beziehungszentrierte Psychodynamische Psychotherapie: von haltender Funktion, technischer Neutralität und persönlicher Sympathie. In: Dulz B, Herpertz S, Kernberg O, Sachsse S, editors. Handbuch der Borderline-Störungen. Stuttgart/New York: Schattauer; 2011. p. 584–609.
20. Lohmer M. Der Umgang mit Krisen in Institutionen und Teams bei der Behandlung von Borderline-Störungen. In: Lohmer M, editor. Borderline-Therapie Psychodynamik, Behandlungstechnik und therapeutische Settings. Stuttgart: Schattauer; 2013. p. 178–92.
21. Portwich P. The doctor-patient relationship in focus: what Michael Balint has to say to us today. Swiss Arch Neurol Psychiatr Psychother. 2014;165(1):4–9.
22. Seiler D. Balints theme: relationship. Balint J. 2011;12(3):85–9.
23. Yeomans F, Clarkin J, Kernberg O. Übertragungsfokussierte Psychotherapie für Borderline-Patienten: Das TFP-Praxismanual. Stuttgart: Schattauer; 2017.
24. Spitzer R, First M, Shedler J, Westen D, Skodol A. Clinical utility of five dimensional systems for personality diagnosis: a "consumer preference" study. J Nerv Ment Dis. 2008;196:356–74.
25. Watzke B, Rueddel H, Koch U, Rudolph M, Schulz H. Comparison of therapeutic action, style and content in cognitive—behavioural and psychodynamic group therapy under clinically representative conditions. Clin Psychol Psychother. 2008;15:404–17.
26. Beesdo-Baum K, Zaudig M, Wittchen H. SCID-5-PD Strukturiertes Klinisches interview für DSM-5-Persönlichkeitsstörungen [German version of the structured clinical interview for DSM-5—personality disorders MB First, JBW Williams, LS Benjamin, RL Spitzer]. 1st ed. Göttingen: Hogrefe; 2019.
27. Working group OPD. Operationalisierte Psychodynamische Diagnostik OPD-2. Das Manual für Diagnostik und Therapieplanung. 3rd ed. Bern: Huber; 2014.
28. Kernberg O. Structural interviewing. Psychiatr Clinics North Am. 1981;4:169–95.
29. Clarkin J, Caligor E, Stern B, Kernberg O. Manual for the structured interview of personality organization-revised. 2017.
30. Dammann G, Gerisch B. Narcissistic personality disorders and suicidal behaviour. A psychodynamic perspective on treatment difficulties. Swiss Arch Neurol Psychiatr Psychother. 2005;156:299–309.
31. Dammann G. Suizidalität bei Borderline-Persönlichkeitsstörungen. Dynamik und Behandlung. In: Wurst F, Vogel R, Wolfersdorf M, editors. Theorie und Praxis der Suizidprävention. Roderer; 2007. p. 24–36.
32. Dulz B. Lügen in der Therapie. PTT Persönlichkeitsstörungen Theorie Therapie. 2013;3:209–18.
33. Sachsse U. Selbstverletzendes Verhalten als somatopsychische Schnittstelle der Borderline-Persönlichkeitsstörung. In: Dulz B, Herpertz S, Kernberg O, Sachsse U, editors. Handbuch der Borderline-Störungen Stuttgart. New York: Schattauer; 2011. p. 390–405.
34. Ermann M. Die stationäre Langzeitpsychotherapie als Psychoanalytischer Prozess. In: Schepank H, Tress W, editors. Die stationäre Psychotherapie und ihr Rahmen. Berlin, Tokyo, New York; 1988. p. 51–60.
35. Dulz B, Benecke C, Richter-Appelt H. Borderline-Störungen und Sexualität. Ätiologie, Störungsbild und Therapie. Stuttgart, New York: Schattauer; 2009.
36. Kernberg O, Yeomans F, Clarkin J, Levy K. Transference focused psychotherapy: overview and update. Int J Psychoanal. 2008;89:601–20.
37. Dammann G. Chancen und Probleme des recovery ansatzes aus psychiatrischer Sicht. Nervenarzt. 2014;85:1156–65.
38. Bion W. Experiences in groups. New York: Basic Books; 1961.
39. Rösch C. Besonderheiten analytischer Gruppentherapie mit narzisstischen Patienten. In: Dammann G, Sammet I, Grimmer B, editors. Narzissmus. Stuttgart: Kohlhammer; 2012. p. 81–93.
40. Dulz B, Sachsse U. Pharmakotherapie: Freund oder Feind? Oder beides?. PTT Persönlichkeitsstörungen: Theorie und Therapie. in preparation; 26.
41. Kraus B, Dammann G, Rudaz M, Sammet I, Jeggle D, Grimmer B. Changes in the level of personality functioning in inpatient psychotherapy. Psychother Res. 2021;31:117–31.

42. Sollberger D, Benecke C, Schwald O, Walter M, Dammann G. Change in self functioning and psychopathology in patients with borderline personality disorder during TFP-based disorder-specific inpatient treatment: a prospective, controlled study over 12-weeks. Clin Psychol Psychother. 2014;22:559–69.
43. Abel T, Happel M, Daerr F. Borderline personality organization: Changes in psychic structure during an inpatient transference focused psychotherapy (TFP) and follow-up in preparation.

Transference-Focused Psychotherapy (TFP) Principles for Mental Health Professionals in Higher-Acuity Settings

8

Miguel Angel Gonzalez Torres and Luis Valenciano

Who Are the Clinicians?

The public mental health system is Spain is inherently complex, given the decentralization of services, which are directed by the 17 different regional jurisdictions. That said, these 17 different systems share a number of core features, allowing for some generalization about the provision of services nationwide [1]. The public health system in Spain is universal (it covers everyone) and free (paid by taxes). Every person is assigned to a general practitioner and local medical center. The general practitioner will serve as the first-line clinician treating emerging mental health symptoms. If this clinician feels the patient needs specialized attention, a referral is then made to a psychiatrist who works as part of the public system. Patients are assigned to these clinicians in the public system; they are not free to choose a specific individual. The authors work in these public mental health settings, specifically the Psychiatry Department in a general hospital (MAGT) and the personality disorder (PD) unit of the day hospital (LV). The continuum of services offered includes the ambulatory intensive program and day hospital, as well as the psychiatric emergency departments located in general hospitals and the inpatient psychiatric facility.

M. A. G. Torres
Department of Neuroscience, University of the Basque Country Psychiatry Department, Basurto University Hospital, Bilbao, Spain
e-mail: miguelangel.gonzaleztorres@osakidetza.edu

L. Valenciano (✉)
Community Mental Health Centre Molina de Segura, Murcia, Spain

R. G. Hersh, C. De Panfilis (eds.), *Implementing Transference-Focused Psychotherapy Principles*, https://doi.org/10.1007/978-3-031-68062-5_8

Who Are the Patients?

Patients we designate as having severe personality disorder (SPD) pathology often live with elevated levels of emotional intensity and exhibit difficulty in recognizing and controlling their affects, finding themselves overwhelmed by changing and contradictory emotions that consume them. That emotional intensity inevitably taints their interpersonal relationships, which become scenarios marked by distinct behavioral patterns leading to certain conflicts. A common situation would be the patient with SPD expressing distress through actions, rather than being able to express these sentiments through words. Moreover, the patients described may have a diminished ability to "walk in other people's shoes" or sense the other person's mental state; they may also have a limited ability to self-observe and examine their own emotional reactions and behaviors from a distance. This summary captures the familiar prototype of the patient with BPD who uses significant mental health services of all kinds; this description may also fit patients with types of narcissistic and antisocial disorders, and those patients with prominent somatization.

What Is the Contemporary Standard of Care for Clinicians Treating These Patients?

The late John Gunderson, a pioneer in the assessment and treatment of patients with borderline personality disorder (BPD), outlined four levels of care [2] for these patients. He described Level I, what would be called Mental Health Centers in Spain, which provides a general, low-frequency outpatient treatment. Level II would correspond to the Unit of Rehabilitation, offering a more intensive ambulatory intervention; in Spain, such services are in early development and thus far offered only at a few sites. Level III corresponds to the Day Hospital, with intensive programs designed specifically for PD patients. Finally, Level IV would be the inpatient hospital, with either acute, short-term, or long-term options. While the focus of this chapter is on the care of the PD patient in higher-acuity settings, it is useful to first put into a broader context the place of those services in the Spanish system.

Generally speaking, the assistance offered to patients with PD diagnoses in Spain, as in most locales, is highly fragmented [3]. The care offered often stresses pharmacotherapy, even though there is scant data supporting the benefits of medications for PD symptoms. For the patient, the system is often highly frustrating, marked by a lack of coordination, unpredictability, and indifference. Secondary gain, meaning the benefits indirectly derived, consciously, or unconsciously, from a patient's symptomatology, is rife. Disability payments can be a disincentive for improvement, and insufficient attention to the goal of employment is also common. The system described results in many PD patients engaged in treatment focused on symptoms and medications and not on the patient's functioning in life. It is common for psychiatrists in the Spanish ambulatory care setting to see between 18 and 20 patients per day. The syndrome of so-called "compassion fatigue" [4] is common among them. Usually, the psychiatrist in this system will also have 24-hour hospital or emergency room (ER) obligations on top of their outpatient responsibilities. The psychiatrists in the Spanish system have heterogeneous backgrounds, education, and interests [5]. Most of them have a good, solid education in psychopathology and pharmacology. A minority, nowadays a decreasing percentage, will have some sort of psychoanalytic training. Most psychologists in the public system have a cognitive-behavioral therapy (CBT) orientation.

The treatment difficulties for patients with SPD within the Spanish system of care extend to the inpatient level as well. The role of psychiatric hospitalization for the SPD case can be critically helpful, albeit limited. At this time in Spain, psychiatric hospitalization is reserved for specific purposes related to heightened clinical acuity, as both short and extended psychotherapy interventions, when available, generally are conducted in the outpatient clinic or day hospital setting, as is judicious, symptom-focused pharmacotherapy. Inpatient admission serves solely to facilitate the resolution of a crisis or to address a comorbid pathology (affective disorders, anxiety disorders, substance abuse disorders, eating disorders, etc.). In addition, there are important differences among the counties' inpatient psychiatric facilities, some offering both short-term and long-term stays, which can be up to 6–12 months. In these long-term psychiatric facilities without a specific program for patients with PD diagnoses, the general patient population will customarily include patients with primary psychotic disorders. The PD patients treated in these long-term facilities tend to be those exhibiting more clinical severity, often with lower IQ, more prominent functional deterioration, what were called in the past "Cluster A" PD diagnoses, or possibly without easily determined diagnostic presentations.

A subgroup of patients with more financial resources can receive care through the private system. These patients often receive either pharmacologic treatment only or non-specific psychotherapies; only a very limited number of these patients access psychotherapy designed specifically for patients with PD pathology. Of note, in some counties, the patients have organized themselves and formed groups designed for mutual support that may meet on a weekly basis [6].

While there may be a variety of nationwide services offered, what we have reviewed here reflects the typical situation in Spain. Therefore, as described in other parts of the world, the majority of those patients in Spain who suffer from SPD pathology do not receive a specifically designed or empirically validated treatment. Basically, in most cases, they receive pharmacologic treatment almost exclusively, which is combined during periods of crisis with some hospitalization in short-term psychiatric wards. Unfortunately, this patchwork system outlined has historically led clinicians to adopt negative attitudes about the course of treatment for many PD patients, concluding that this population; (1) cannot respond to treatment, (2) by definition, will have a poor prognosis, and (3) are apt to exploit the system, including overusing hospital services without evident benefit.

What Are the Goals for Imparting to these Clinicians the Principles of TFP for Working with These Patients?

The earlier-described specific features of patients suffering from SPD obviously affect the patient-therapist dyad, which is a special form of interpersonal relationship. Two characteristics of this therapeutic relationship make it likely for SPD-specific psychopathology to unfold within this context, with great ease and intensity.

1. Crisis and/or vulnerability. Therapist-patient contact generally comes about in moments of crisis. At this time, the emotions of the patient are particularly intense and overwhelming, which means there is a greater possibility of difficulties in the therapeutic relationship. Simultaneously, because the patient is accessing treatment in a situation of vulnerability and presumably because the patient does not feel able to completely control circumstances without assistance, there can be emerging feelings for the patient of anxiety, mistrust, and fear of abuse.
2. Asymmetry. The therapeutic relationship, as opposed to a normal social relationship, involves an enormous asymmetry. One person, the patient, seeks help, and another person, the therapist, gives it; one reveals his or her life story, and the other explores it; and, above all, one person suffers or causes suffering, and the other does not. This peculiar condition of the professional mental health worker-patient relationship, which can be difficult to endure for many, can have a heightened intensity for those patients described with significant PD pathology, making it more likely in these cases for intense feelings to emerge.

All of the above multiplies whenever there is a situation that is especially critical, such as would be expected in the ER, or a patient's admission to, and stay in, an inpatient psychiatric unit. These tend to be situations of maximum crisis; the mistrust upon entry, the fear of staff and the fear displayed toward the other patients, and the loss or limitations of liberties, together produce the ideal conditions bringing to the fore the relational difficulties that these patients endure.

Furthermore, there is one interpersonal characteristic that is worth highlighting, as it is key in understanding the behavior of subjects with SPD in the healthcare environment. The emotional intensity that they undergo, and their difficulty in simultaneously perceiving the positive and negative aspects of others (splitting), will likely have an impact on the clinician. This aspect of the patient's response can lead the clinician involved to sometimes identify strongly with the patient's point of view, or alternatively, to react with great intensity toward the patient and the position in which the patient has put him or her. The result tends to be hastily made, rash decisions, which may reflect the turmoil of the professional, as well as defensive attitudes on his or her part. Such reactions would not favor the optimal management of the case and might bring about premature conclusions to treatment, and the subsequent difficulties of starting the process over again. What happens frequently is that after the therapeutic relationship is ruptured, the professional is left with a sense of failure and regret. At times, the clinician will feel both ambivalence and relief in finding him or herself freed of this troublesome patient, often upset in recognizing the countertransference aggression that was displayed during the encounter with the patient, aggression that is often difficult to avoid but which ideally should never come up in clinical decision-making.

In light of these unique difficulties in working with SPD patients, the goal for imparting to the clinicians operating in the Spanish health systems transference-focused psychotherapy (TFP) principles is to enable them to provide a structured, coherent treatment rather than impulsively, automatically react to the challenging and often chaotic interpersonal behaviors exhibited by patients suffering from SPD.

In this regard, four TFP-based principles should govern the relationship of the professional with a patient who has SPD.

1. Security. The clinician should feel secure when interviewing the patient and therefore he or she should not proceed whenever those security conditions have not been met. If necessary, we would wait until health personnel or security are available to ensure safety and we would postpone the interview until this condition is met. An intimidated clinician *cannot* properly evaluate a case and thus cannot give the patient the treatment he or she needs and deserves.
2. Training. The clinician should know the pathology he or she is treating, especially in situations of high complexity and demand such as this one. Continuing education in this area is key.
3. Time. The attention given to these patients requires sufficient time for all of its phases. There is no such thing as "brief attention" when it comes to patients with SPD, and the clinician should not allow him or herself to be influenced by pressures coming from either the patient, the surroundings, or the very institution where he or she works.
4. Reasonable conditions. All clinicians need certain minimum conditions to be met in order for an encounter with a patient to be effective. These conditions should be implemented by the institution, or by the clinician himself or herself; in addition, the patient involved should demonstrate sufficient compliance with the conditions outlined in advance. Whenever these minimal conditions are not met, the clinician should humbly acknowledge an inability to treat the patient and redirect the patient or postpone the session until these conditions can be met. When the patient shows a particularly low level of collaboration, making progress impossible, through lack of attendance, compliance, respect, or self-control, it is necessary to halt the treatment taking place until these conditions are remedied.

Finally, mental health systems could benefit from a TFP-informed approach toward structuring the treatment framework. Patients with SPDs, due to what has been mentioned above, tend to challenge and transgress the normal limits of interpersonal relationships, especially in therapeutic situations. For this reason, both outpatient and inpatient treatment should be preceded by a detailed review of the structure of the treatments offered, as well as the obligations of all parties involved. In order to manage these challenges to limits, it is necessary to establish clearly in advance to the patient what those limits are, as well as the consequences expected for breaching those limits. Without those conditions in place, the treatment may not be possible, and therefore the clinician should occasionally acknowledge his inability to work under such circumstances and halt the treatment in progress.

What TFP Principles Might Be of Utility for the Clinicians Working with These Patients?

The theoretical principles of TFP and many of the practical elements outlined in the TFP treatment manual (Yeomans et al. 2015) can be useful even outside of the traditional context of work in individual psychotherapy sessions for patients [7]. We are going to point out, briefly, some areas in which TFP principles can be of help to clinicians on a daily basis in their routine work:

1. Completing and refining the diagnostic assessment process.
2. Making a thorough differential diagnosis.
3. Sharing the diagnosis with the patient and his or her family.
4. Exploring and setting therapeutic goals.
5. Helping in differential therapeutic selection.
6. Establishing the therapeutic contract with the patient.
7. Managing medication in a rational and efficient manner.
8. Helping to develop a working relationship with the patient's family.
9. Controlling acting out impulses, both institutional and individual.

Now, we will review the possible contributions of TFP in the different levels of care, following this schema.

I. Using TFP principles in the ER.

Often for the patient with a PD diagnosis, the ER constitutes the first encounter of the patient with the mental health system. The variables involved in this encounter will include the specific pathology and background of the patient, as well as the personalities of the doctors, nurses, and other staff on duty at that time. In Spain, the typical situation includes trainee physicians working as residents on call together with a more senior psychiatrist for a 24-hour shift. The pressures on those clinicians involved are intense and highly unpredictable, which understandably affects the mental state of psychiatrists on duty, depriving them of more ideal circumstances needed to be able to interview patients in depth. Patients usually present to the ER due to suicidal ideation or gestures, after an outburst of rage following an interpersonal disappointment, or with symptoms of common comorbid conditions, including alcohol or other substance intoxication, or eating disorder-related complications, such as arrhythmias after severe and continued vomiting. Most patients in Spain do not have a therapeutic contract or agreement in place with the assigned outpatient psychiatrist. Very often, psychiatrists on call not only attend the ER but the psychiatric ward too when required, where they will see patients whom they do not know.

They will also see patients at the bedside in a consultative role who are managed on other medical services.

The patient coming to the ER after a suicide attempt will usually be under medical observation by our colleagues in general medicine for hours before clearance for an initial psychiatric interview. If the patient comes for suicidal ideation, perhaps the most common reason for a PD patient to present to an ER, there is sometimes a wait for a number of hours; this may be negatively reinforcing, leading to reluctance to present to the ER under such circumstances going forward. More broadly, the psychiatrist on call in the hospital will not be able to predict in advance the assistance required by patients and other clinicians across a range of services. It is important that the on call psychiatrists keep in mind that, when a patient presents to the ER with suicidal ideation, there is always a good likelihood that he or she will have primary or co-occurring PD pathology.

Our recommendations for training ER personnel using TFP principles would integrate these principles into standard algorithms as follows:

Objectives:

Evaluate the case in order to decide if we will proceed to:

- Discharge with outpatient follow-up
- Admission, voluntary or involuntary

a) Evaluation:

The clinician should be guided equally by a timely interview in the ER and an active exploration of longitudinal information that can be gathered in real time. Information collected from family members and close relations could be of importance. Specifically, we teach ER clinicians to inquire about interpersonal relationships with significant figures (e.g., family, intimate friends, partners), which could reflect with greater clarity the patients' basic patterns of behavior. Additionally, it is key that information is collected regarding dangerous behaviors that may then influence decisions regarding the need for psychiatric admission. These behaviors include self-harm or harm of others, substance abuse, or transient psychosis. Of importance also would be any information about the patient's engagement in critical self-destructive behaviors. Learning about past treatments and details about prior therapies such as modality offered, frequency of meetings, and details of treatment termination, would be expected. To that end, the clinician should have a clear vision of the following key elements at the conclusion of the assessment process:

- The current clinical situation with primary symptoms, provisional diagnosis/diagnoses.
- Prior history and patterns of behavior.
- History of prior treatments received and the patient's response to those interventions.
- Risks that determine the need for hospital admission.

For this evaluation phase, a TFP-informed approach to diagnosis may be particularly helpful to guide clinicians working in the Spanish psychiatric ER. TFP uses as its main diagnostic tool the structural interview, developed by Kernberg [8]. The structural interview as conceptualized by Kernberg might be useful, but likely not practical, for use in the ER. Therefore, we have considered those elements that could be used by clinicians under time pressures.

The attitude of the interviewer should be containing, firm but kind, never apathetic, routinized, or mechanical. The interviewer should demonstrate interest and attention. The psychiatrist must be aware that the attitude displayed, and vitality imparted, will have an important effect on the patient, even in this brief encounter. The purpose of the interview in the ER is three-fold: (1) to gather information to get to an accurate diagnosis, both descriptive (meaning based on DSM-5 nosology), and structural; (2) to estimate risk, and (3) to develop a treatment alliance with the patient and others involved. It may be difficult to obtain a precise diagnosis in the brief time allowed in the ER, thereby dictating for the clinician an emphasis on clarity and prioritization.

As outlined in the structural interview, the first consideration is to rule out a possible organic, or medical, etiology for the presenting condition. If the sensorium is preserved, then a more detailed psychiatric inquiry will consider psychotic symptoms. This would include a focus on the presence or absence of delusions, hallucinations, or any severely bizarre or disorganized behaviors, as well as any evidence in the patient's speaking, behavior, or affect that might seem somehow at odds with social norms. In TFP terms, this questioning about deviations from standard social expectations would be understood as "fine adjustment of reality testing." After having ruled out psychotic illness, the ER clinician would then assess possible bipolar conditions. It is not uncommon to observe confusion among clinicians regarding these diagnoses, requiring both attention to a careful differential diagnosis and the possibility of rare comorbidity.

The ER interview aims to combine goals for diagnosis with therapeutic alliance building. TFP principles stress the focus on four channels of communication; not just verbal communication, but how the patient behaves, how the clinician feels (the countertransference), and the observation of the interaction between both parties.

When exploring the patient's chief complaints, the interviewer should attempt to clarify any stereotyped language and technical jargon the patient might use, inviting the patient to speak as naturally as possible. Symptoms including self-harm, suicidal thoughts or gestures, and disordered eating, are understandably all important in the process of making a diagnosis and decisions about admission. A TFP-informed approach would also stress the necessity to explore other areas of the patient's life, such as work and studies, love and sex, social life, and creativity, given the interviewer's goal of coming to know the patient in more depth.

A TFP approach to the diagnosis also stresses the need to carefully evaluate aspects of antisocial behavior or tendencies, often a salient subject in the ER. Interviewing family or those people closest to the patient in an effort to gauge the patient's truthfulness would be necessary when there is a history of outbursts of rage and violence, putting others at risk, reckless driving, or unprotected sexual activity. In reality, there are always those presentations that are difficult to diagnose. Part of our supervision with psychiatry residents will reinforce that symptoms of impulsivity do not always reflect BPD, and may result from psychosis; conversely, the absence of impulsivity will not necessarily rule out some other kind of SPD pathology.

b) Discharge from the ER with therapeutic advice:

The clinician will consider, if the patient does not present with a critical situation that would require admission, offering the following:

- Pertinent psychoeducation, including a review of current symptoms, related history, past treatments, and current risks and protections. This is imparted to the patient and to his or her relatives, explaining the reasons behind the decision to discharge.
- Pharmacologic treatment, with the goal of alleviating certain symptoms, if required at that moment. It is advisable that pharmacologic treatment is kept to a minimum, given the frequent tendency to misuse medication in these cases.
- Advice, specifically an explanation for the patient about what treatment the ER staff thinks is necessary. At this time, it is feasible to outline different treatment modalities that might be available, the requirement for the patient's efforts in seeking and then committing to treatment as fundamental, and the expected problems in this process. In addition, the staff would review with the patient the details for accessing any follow-up treatment, including a likely timetable for that process. All practical details are included in a report given to the patient upon discharge from the ER.

c) Admission, voluntary or involuntary:

If the ER clinician deems the patient's situation to be critical, concluding that outpatient treatment is insufficient to safely address the issues at hand, the decision is made to admit the patient to the unit. To that end, we have instructed the ER staff the following:

- Outline of the conditions of admission: The patient will be told of the conditions of admission that include: (1) the objectives of an admission are to alleviate the crisis situation. A hospital admission is not expected to "cure" the patient with an SPD, but will instead have more modest, concrete goals; and (2) the hospitalization is framed as one phase of a longer set of treatment interventions. This message is directed both to the patient and to others in his or her orbit.
- Conditions of admission: The admitting clinicians will underscore a requirement for the patient's collaboration with the treatment team. This collaboration is deemed required and essential.

- Commitment for the patient: The patient is expected to accept the conditions and objectives as delineated, and this commitment is expected in writing for the record. The staff stresses that the patient's cooperation is necessary for the inpatient hospitalization to be of benefit. When providing the conditions of admission, the staff avoids any suggestion of punishment should the patient be unwilling or unable to comply with expectations. The attitude of the treaters reflects an understanding that certain conditions are required to be in place if a specific intervention is to be safe and effective.
- Decisions regarding involuntary care: If the patient accepts conditions after they have been explained in detail, admission to the inpatient service will then proceed. If the patient does not accept the conditions and therefore does not sign the record, the admitting clinician would then consider the need for an inpatient level of care and determine the advisability of discharging the patient from the ER with outpatient follow-up or moving forward with involuntary inpatient care. Obviously, if admission is involuntary, the expectations for the inpatient stay may be tempered, as long as the absence of collaboration persists. The objective would then be to lessen the symptoms related to more immediate risks and later move onto discharge and outpatient referrals.

II. Using TFP principles in inpatient psychiatric hospitalization.

Within the hospital system, there may be a prejudice against the admission of patients with PD diagnoses harbored by some senior clinicians in the staff. There is an unacknowledged pattern of approval for the admission of those patients with bipolar or psychotic disorders, but a tacit disapproval of admitting PD patients with comparable acuity. It is paramount that all unrealistic "fantasies" associated with the hospital admission of the PD patient are avoided; on the other hand, it is important to acknowledge that a brief hospitalization, even as short as 1–2 days, can be useful and efficient, while avoiding excessive expense or the risk of fostering passivity. Some short-term goals are clearly reasonable: providing safety for the suicidal patient with intent and plan; stemming a spiral of dangerous impulsive behavior; revisiting the outpatient treatment plan; and addressing problematic polypharmacy, among them. Conversely, it is imperative that the staff directly address the fantasies of patients, family members, and clinicians in the community who may have unrealistic hopes about the benefits of an inpatient stay.

It is vital that the clinician involved share with the patient and family the deliberately made diagnosis in an understandable language and manner, using layman's words, and then clarify ambulatory resources available in the community. This sharing of the diagnosis can have a major impact, often experienced as a coherent explanation, thereby providing reassurance for the patient and family. When sharing the diagnosis, offering expert information about the primacy of psychotherapy in PD treatment, as well as the relative limits of pharmacotherapy, can proactively address unrealistic expectations for medication at the outset.

The following steps highlight the key aspects of a TFP-oriented inpatient psychiatric hospitalization for patients with SPD:

a) Treatment contract
b) Staff organization
c) Treatment objectives
d) Treatment conditions
e) Pharmacotherapy

a) Treatment contact

Voluntary inpatient treatment is based on a therapeutic contract examined in detail and then accepted by the patient. The patient is made aware of the contract at the earliest moment possible, ideally in the ER or during the first hours of the hospital stay. This contract, or agreement, will describe the objectives and conditions for the hospital stay, with tasks and obligations for both the patient and the professionals involved, as well as consequences described in advance for any breach of this agreement.

b) Staff organization.

Ideally, the staff involved should be as consistent as possible, with the goal of fortifying alliances and limiting conflicts. The unit's physician-in-charge (PIC), when feasible, should be consistent throughout the patient's hospitalization. Whenever possible, there should be a member of the nursing team who assumes responsibility for the patient's care, serving as the patient's chief advocate throughout the stay. In the rare situation when any member of the staff, including the PIC or nurse, does not feel able to manage unusual countertransference reactions to a particular patient, the unit supervisor would then work on reassigning the patient to another staff member. The complexity of these cases suggests that, whenever possible, the equitable distribution of patients assigned with this level of acuity is assured.

Working with these patients can be unduly challenging and the creation of a group for staff dedicated to discussion of the details of diagnosis, hospitalization, and treatment options, is highly advisable. A working group formed to meet on a weekly basis to review the SPD cases can have important benefits. In our model in the Spanish system, this group is made up of the PICs involved, the section head of the unit, staff nurses, and clinical psychologists. Along with this group, any member of the staff motivated to do so is encouraged to attend with the goal of addressing concerns and questions related to the care of this specific group of patients. The objective of this group is to examine and resolve the inevitable difficulties associated with caring for these patients in this context. The overarching aim is to improve therapeutic interventions and minimize adverse events for the milieu and the unit professionals.

c) Treatment objectives.

Objectives for the hospitalization should be specified within the first hours following admission. In general terms, they will target alleviating the crisis and/or treating and comorbid pathology. It is important that these objectives are explicitly reviewed with the patient, his or her family, and the entire treatment team. It is advisable to take advantage of the hospitalization to educate the patient regarding his or her illness, his or her therapeutic options, the personnel resources that he or she can utilize, and the steps that are to be taken upon discharge.

d) Inpatient treatment conditions
- Respect: The patient should be treated with respect by staff throughout the hospitalization. Likewise, he or she should also show respect for the rest of the patients, the visitors, and families, and, of course, for the professionals involved. Failure to comply with these conditions could put treatment at risk to the point that it becomes impossible.
- Violence: No form of physical violence is permitted in the unit, nor is any relevant form of verbal violence.
- Activity schedule: The schedule will be communicated to the patient in the emergency department or in a timely manner immediately following admission. The schedule is the same for all the patients in the unit.
- Participation in activities: Expectations for participation in unit activities will be communicated along with the schedule, and, again, these are expectations communicated to all patients.
- Visits: This will be decided as in the other cases.
- Interviews: It is particularly important that the nursing staff know, in detail, the therapeutic objectives established as well as the eventual progress and evolution. The participation of a nurse in these interviews, together with the PIC, can be of help to that end.
- Discharge against medical advice (AMA): This is solely decided by the PIC. In all aspects that are problematic, the PIC should be the one to weigh the relevant clinical decisions, avoiding a situation in which professionals who barely know the patient are faced with complex decision-making that could potentially have negative consequences for the treatment. AMA discharge is a breach of the commitment on the part of the patient with the consequence that the patient does not return to the inpatient unit for a set period of time (four months is our recommendation). In this period, only the most extreme conditions should make admission advisable, and should always have very specific objectives. In such a case, whenever possible, it would always be better to opt to extend the stay in an emergency unit (if the patient arrives there) or to authorize the inpatient admission for a short duration only.
- The role of the psychiatrist on call: While the psychiatrist on call may be asked to make administrative decisions during off hours, ideally the PIC should be consulted before any critical clinical decision is made. It is preferable that the treater familiar with a particular case is the one to sign off on

challenging decisions, especially those that concern the continuance of treatment.

- Relations with family: The PIC will interview the family and relatives in order to obtain relevant information as well as to take steps to ensure collaboration in both present and future treatment.
- Relations with the outpatient therapist: It is expected that the inpatient team will make contact with a patient's outpatient treater during the course of a psychiatric hospitalization. This would allow for obtaining pertinent parallel information, ensuring the necessary continuity of care, and imparting of relevant information as part of discharge planning.
- The discharge. This should occur when the objectives initially set forth have been reached and when continuing treatment is no longer likely to advance the patient's goals. It is important that the patient and, if indicated, his or her relatives, are aware of the reasons for the discharge and of the therapeutic steps to follow.

The fundamental consequence of a relevant breach in the therapeutic commitment on the part of the patient should be the termination of the inpatient treatment and its eventual resumption only after an extended period. The structure of our public network complicates the application of this principle; the specific team should design steps that could facilitate its application.

It is important to reiterate that there are certain conditions in which safe and effective treatment of the patient is not possible. These measures we have outlined thus far when in place can allow the team and the therapist to identify those conditions that would make the clinical task possible again. Repeated hospitalizations after a voluntary discharge will likely be of limited use to the patient and may lead to serious deterioration in the team morale and effectiveness. The limitations of a public system are evident in this case; inpatient care is a scant and valuable resource that merits protection. It is possible to structure inpatient care in an effective way that reduces the chances that the patient will destroy his or her therapeutic goals; these destructive impulses are often expressed in serious relational difficulties with the staff and others. It is critical that the unit staff directly address the abusive behavior of the patient; failing to do so will undermine the effectiveness of the treatment for the individual patient and can also contaminate the milieu, thereby impacting other patients as well. There is a risk when inpatient staff are not able to set appropriate limits. A particularly concerning outcome would be staff moved to express punitive sentiments or engage in unprofessional behavior as a result of experiencing a patient's persistent aggression or abusiveness that has gone unchecked. Such an unfortunate outcome will have serious negative repercussions for all involved.

e) Pharmacotherapy

Hospitalization is an excellent moment to simplify the medicine regimen. Too often, the patient arrives at the ward with a complex plan that includes many medicines that in fact are taken irregularly or misused. The TFP model can help to examine the psychological aspects of prescribing and de-prescribing. It is possible to understand pharmacological interventions in light of the object-relations dyads activated in the exchange between the patient and the prescriber. In those moments, the patient will communicate with the prescriber in a complex way that combines: (1) the more concrete information related to identifiable components of prescribing (e.g., target symptoms, side effects, symptom reduction), and (2) the psychological currents in the dyad activated in the situation. The inpatient psychiatrist has the opportunity in the relative calm of that environment to address iatrogenic complications. One frequently observed scenario might be the following: a patient on the ward is asking assertively to be prescribed a new antidepressant and possibly an adjunctive stimulant, but the staff does not see him as depressed. The patient may rationalize his confrontational behavior, genuinely believing that his distress reflects a diagnosis of major depressive disorder. The patient's behavior may cause the prescribing physician to feel some mix of impotence, oppression, and confusion polypharmacy. If the clinician does not stop and examine the configurations in place, he could enact any of these two countertransference urges: he might submit and prescribe despite his misgiving about doing so, or he could refuse to do so in a way that leaves the patient feeling unheard or mistreated. If the clinician has the frame of mind that allows him to avoid acting in ways dictated solely by his negative countertransference, he or she will then have the chance not to answer in an automatic, unreflective way, and choose instead a more calm, strategic, and potentially useful way. An intervention along those lines might be: "I understand that your suffering is genuine, but I firmly think that adding more medications would only make things worse. In addition to this, what about looking together what seems to be happening between the two of us now? Perhaps we could learn something from doing that."

The clinician unfamiliar with the phenomenon of projective identification can have in their practice, whether they communicate it aloud or not, a more "paranoid" view of patients with PD pathology. They may view this population as not truly mentally ill, motivated to undermine their therapeutic efforts, and bent on purposefully challenging their skills and value. Projective identification, a psychoanalytic concept introduced by Melanie Klein [9], is the means by which the patient matches his internal experience with his external world. For example, if the patient has had an abusive father, he may adopt mocking or provoking behavior expecting that the physician act aggressively in return, doing so without an awareness of having of his contribution to this exchange. If the clinician understands that the behavior of the patient is not "personal" and he can name what is happening between them, it is less likely that the treater will attack or withdraw and more likely that he can be of help to the patient.

III. Using TFP principles in managing the transition between different levels of care:

It is always advisable that the clinicians in the psychiatric ward and the ambulatory psychiatrist work in a coordinated way and share information regarding the patient, with his permission, of course. For example, the information conveyed by the outpatient clinician to the inpatient staff would include many aspects of the patient's history including prior treatments, therapeutic modalities employed, medication trials, and the patient's response to specific drugs. Conversely, the inpatient team would alert the receiving outpatient clinicians about how the patient was perceived while on the unit and those target symptoms to be addressed in future work as an outpatient. A range of variables will inform recommendations from the inpatient team for future care. These variables include the working diagnosis or diagnoses, comorbid conditions, intellectual capacities, as well as the patient's level of motivation. Together these factors will determine a referral either to treatment as usual or a more specific psychotherapy.

It is important that clinicians in the psychiatric ward appreciate different intensities of treatment that the patient with PD may need. The point would be to match the intensity of treatment with the patient's openness to engagement and level of motivation. It is not possible to determine in advance the ideal treatment for any particular patient presenting with PD pathology. Even if we faced the unlikely scenario of being able to choose among TFP, mentalization based therapy (MBT) [10], dialectical behavioral therapy (DBT) [11], schema focused therapy (ST) [12], or any other evidence-based treatment for BPD, the clinician would be required to guide himself by his past experience or intuition rather than solid data. However, we can reflect here on the possibility of offering the patient TFP, supportive therapy, or standard case management. If the patient shows enough ability in terms of intelligence, introspection, and verbal capacity, in addition to a clear motivation reflected by a pattern of attending to tasks, schedule and limiting acting out behavior, clinicians in our system might recommend TFP, if available. Those patients with less ability (with a low IQ, for example), but good motivation could be candidates for psychodynamically oriented supportive psychotherapy. Patients with a very chronic condition, who have a demonstrated pattern of obtaining secondary gain through monetary benefits or more generally with limited motivation for change, could be transferred to standard case management in the community with the frequency of visits customarily managed by the mental health public center. Of course, a change in the type of intervention is possible if circumstances change; for some patients the access to a more intensive treatment may serve as a positive reinforcement for improved functioning and treatment adherence.

What Is the Source of Institutional or Government Support for this Initiative?

In general, support comes after the initiative has been set up. These are teams that already have professionals trained in TFP and whose leader is familiar with the model and supports its extension beyond the traditional framework of individual psychotherapy. Local authorities view these advances positively as long as they lead to measurable and relevant outcomes: days of admission, relapses or reduction of conflict situations in the units where the new model is applied.

What Are the Didactic Materials Required to Impart TFP Principles to this Target Group of Clinicians?

The materials are varied, depending on the interest of the different professionals in deepening their understanding of the model. Slide presentations are used and readings from both articles and books are recommended. The Spanish translations of the texts by Clarkin et al. (2016) and Caligor et al. (2018) play a key role [13, 14]. It should be noted that what we have proposed requires the participation of the whole team, including orderlies, nurse aids, nurses, clinical psychologists, and psychiatrists. The basic principles should be known to all of them, the further elaboration of more detailed aspects depends on the interest of each professional and the responsibility of each one in the care of the patient.

What Is the Format for Instruction of TFP Principles to this Audience?

As we have pointed out, it is not just a matter of teaching a series of concepts to team members. A new way of working and dealing with the relationship problems that these patients generate should be built. There are several ways, and the choice may depend on the idiosyncrasies of each team. We believe that an approach based on the real problems that professionals have to face is especially useful. Through successive team meetings, interventions can be discussed that are based on the TFP model and its fundamental elements. In our opinion, a purely didactic top-down model in which the TFP expert "enlightens" the rest of the team is not very useful. If we are talking about an inpatient ward the genuine involvement of the nursing staff, starting with the supervisors, is absolutely key. It is important to keep in mind that in an inpatient ward, it is the nursing staff who live 24 hours a day with the patients. If they do not believe in the model, the initiative will not prosper.

What Are Possible Targets for Measurement to Gauge the Effectiveness of Instruction about Applications of TFP Principles?

In the case of initiatives such as the ones we propose, effectiveness should be measured through variables that reflect changes in the atmosphere of the ward and a clear reduction in problems. We have achieved for example drastic reductions in mechanical restraints in the ward [15].

Clinical Illustration

Dr. P. is a psychiatrist attending working in the Emergency Room (ER) of a general hospital in a mid-sized Spanish city. She is the only psychiatrist working late on a Friday evening; she has two nurses and a social worker who are also present, and a senior attending psychiatrist who is available for phone guidance when needed.

This particular Friday evening has been unusually busy as Dr. P. is called upon to provide consultation for a number of patients on the medical units with co-occurring psychiatric conditions. Just as the ER is quieting down at midnight, the local police bring in a new patient, Mrs. M., who was seen by her neighbors to be distressed and agitated, pacing on the roof of her apartment building.

Dr. P. has a particular interest in treating patients with schizophrenia and she is planning to do research on this topic as her career advances. Her orientation has been primarily on pharmacotherapy; she does not plan to do additional training in psychotherapy and envisions a career where her work as a psychotherapist will be limited. She was therefore surprised to find that the course and supervision provided to her during her residency on the uses of TFP in the multiple acute-care settings where she works is of significant, practical use. Because she had seen Mrs. M., the patient brought in by the police, once before the past year when Mrs. M. was in the ER following an altercation with her teenage daughter and the team had speculated about the contribution of personality disorder symptoms at that time, Dr. P. now begins to review the basic TFP principles familiar to her of use in guiding ER clinicians when assessing and managing a patient with a possible primary or co-occurring personality disorder diagnosis.

Dr. P. has uppermost in her mind her goals of first assessing the active diagnoses contributing to Mrs. M.'s current presentation, and then determining whether she requires an inpatient admission or can be safely discharged for possible outpatient treatment. The police had reported that Mrs. M.'s neighbors had heard her repeating "I can't go on like this!" as she paced the building's rooftop, at times going to the edge and peering over the six stories. Dr. P. systematically addresses possible contributing factors of organic processes (intoxication, medication side effects) and active psychiatric conditions (mania or mixed state, panic), before initiating a series of questions aimed to clarify whether Mrs. M.'s current symptoms reflect some aspect of personality pathology. Dr. P. reviews with Mrs. M. some important interpersonal contributions to her current distress (another altercation with her daughter, a recent break-up with a new boyfriend), and evidence of impaired coping strategies (combining small doses of benzodiazepines with alcohol, making multiple urgent calls to her estranged boyfriend threatening to disrupt his workplace). Dr. P. approaches this line of questioning with active interest and her full attention; she is careful not to let her countertransference (annoyance, disapproval) impact her ability to collect sufficient data so that she can make a thoughtful decision about hospitalization. Dr. P. learns that Mrs. M. is not currently in treatment and has likely been misusing alcohol and taking medications without sufficient supervision for many months. Dr. P. is also able to learn from the record of Mrs. M.'s hospitalization the past year that the team had documented a diagnosis of borderline personality disorder traits, as well as an alcohol use disorder, noting that Mrs. M. had an extended history of difficulties staying in outpatient treatment, often stopping treatment when she found a new boyfriend.

Because Mrs. M. is not able to convincingly contract for safety, Dr. P. recommends admission for a focused inpatient stay. Dr. P. outlinesthe conditions of this admission and works with Mrs. M. to consider some modest, achievable goals. Mrs.

M. can work with Dr. P. to formulate some practical objectives for the hospitalization: safely taper her use of benzodiazepines; identify an outpatient program for alcohol use treatment; arrange a meeting with her daughter to begin to plan for longer-term family support, given their frequent, disruptive arguments; consider restarting individual treatment. Dr. P. is clear in framing this hospitalization as a single, first step in a likely extended path of treatment. She draws up an agreement to review with Mrs. M. as part of the process of admission. This agreement details the steps required for Mrs. M.'s participation and the conditions necessary to move forward. Mrs. M. supports some of these conditions (a meeting with her daughter, obtaining information from her prior treaters), and balks at others (contact with her present prescriber, contact with her daughter's father to assess the wellbeing of Mrs. M.'s daughter). Dr. P. is clear with Mrs. M. that admission to the hospital would not proceed until they had obtained some kind of agreement, which was then documented in a contract signed by both parties.

Dr. P. reflects that the use of TFP-informed principles has allowed her to assess Mrs. M. in a deliberate and systematic way, and to establish certain expectations that should improve the likelihood that the hospitalization would be of some genuine benefit to Mrs. M. By conveying a set of expectations for Mrs. M.'s participation and adherence from the start, the hospitalization is framed as a collaboration between two parties, and not an intervention by clinicians on a passive participant. Dr. P. had in the past often felt demoralized by the repeated, rote admissions of patients with BPD that often seemed counterproductive or even damaging. She felt that using TFP principles allowed her to frame this hospitalization in a more productive and realistic way.

Conclusion

We have outlined our approach to introducing the valuable tools derived from TFP to clinicians in the Spanish mental health system. The use of psychoanalytically informed interventions in General Hospital Psychiatric Units is not currently a common practice; however, based on our observations of the high prevalence of patients with primary or co-occurring PD pathology in settings such as the emergency room and inpatient units, we believe that the use of TFP principles can provide significant advances for those responsible for the care of this population. Incorporating TFP principles into the standard of care currently provided can help limit the harm a patient can do to themselves or others, ensure the safety of the clinicians involved, and help foster a treatment alliance even in difficult circumstances. The key to an appropriate inpatient approach is not necessarily the implementation of sophisticated psychotherapeutic models, which are often difficult to apply outside of specialized academic and research settings. Rather, the presence of an informed, trained, and cohesive team will provide real support in these difficult situations. The team can provide a safe and therapeutic atmosphere that minimizes iatrogenic risks. The use of TFP principles to support hospital-based clinicians is a project in its early stages that holds promise for both our Spanish system and beyond.

References

1. Sistema Nacional de Salud de España 2010 [monografia en Internet]. Madrid. Ministerio de Sanidad y Política Social, Instituto de Información Sanitaria. Disponible en: http://www.msps.es/organizacion/sns/librosSNS.htm
2. Gunderson JG, Gratz KL, Neuhaus EG, Smith GW. Levels of Care in Treatment. In: Oldham, JM, Skodol, AE, Bender, DS, editor. The American Psychiatric Publishing textbook of personality disorders. American Psychiatric Publishing, Inc; 2005. p. 239–255.
3. Gonzalez Torres MA. Las psicoterapias en los equipos públicos. De la preferencia personal a la respuesta terapéutica necesaria. Revista de la Asociación Española de Neuropsiquiatría, ISSN 0211–5735, Vol. 39, N°. 136, 2019, págs. 189–203.
4. Rothschild B. Help for the helper: the psychophysiology of compassion fatigue and vicarious trauma. W Norton & Co.; 2006.
5. Chouza Perez JM. Actitudes y práctica de la psicoterapia en España. Implicaciones en la formación de residentes. Tesis Doctoral. Universidad del País Vasco—Euskal Herriko Unibertsitatea; 2011.
6. Asociaciones de Trastorno Límite de España. https://www.amaitlp.org/asociaciones-trastorno-limite-espana/. Accessed 10 Oct 2021.
7. Yeomans FE, Clarkin JF, Kernberg OF. Transference-focused psychotherapy for borderline personality disorder: a clinical guide. Arlington: American Psychiatric Publishing, Inc.; 2015.
8. Kernberg OF. Trastornos Graves de La Personalidad. Manuel Moderno. Mexico; 1995.
9. Klein M. Notes on some schizoid mechanisms. In: Spillius E, O'Shaughnessy E, editors. Projective identification: the fate of a concept. New library of psychoanalysis. New York: Routledge/Taylor & Francis Group; 2012. p. 19–46.
10. Bateman A, Fonagy P. Mentalization-based treatment. Psychoanal Inq. 2013;33(6):595–613.
11. Linehan MM. Cognitive-behavioral treatment of borderline personality disorder. New York: Guilford Press; 1993.
12. Young JE, Klosko JS, Weishaar ME. Schema therapy: a practitioner's guide. New York: Guilford Press; 2003.
13. Clarkin JF, Kernberg OF, Yeomans FE. Psicoterapia centrada en la transferencia: su aplicacion al trastorno limite de la personalidad. Bilbao: Desclee De Brouwer; 2016.
14. Caligor E, Kernberg OF, Clarkin JF, Yeomans FE. Psychodynamic therapy for personality pathology: treating self and interpersonal functioning. American Psychiatric Publishing, Inc.; 2018.
15. Miguel Angel Gonzalez-Torres MD, Aranzazu Fernandez-Rivas MD, Sonia Bustamante MD, Fernando Rico-Villademoros MD, Esther Vivanco RN, Karmele Martinez RN, Miguel Angel Vecino RN, Melba Martín RN, Sonia Herrera RN, Jorge Rodriguez NA, Carlos Saenz NA. Impact of the creation and implementation of a clinical management guideline for personality disorders in reducing use of mechanical restraints in a psychiatric inpatient unit. Prim Care Companion CNS Disord. 2014;16(6) https://doi.org/10.4088/PCC.14m01675.

Using Transference-Focused Psychotherapy (TFP) Principles in an Integrated Care Continuum

9

Maria Jesus Rufat and Joan Vegué Grilló

Abbreviations

BPO	Borderline personality organization
CPB-SSM	Centre Psicoterapia Barcelona—Serveis Salut Mental (CPB-SSM), a public psychiatric treatment network located in Barcelona (Catalonia, Spain), composed of eighteen different treatment facilities treating patients in a variety of settings
BPOTP	The Borderline Personality Organization Integrated Care Continuum Treatment Program (BPOTP), is a program within the CPM-SSM network, providing services specifically for patients with personality disorder pathology, across a range of treatment options
CLINICA LLURIA	An inpatient subacute unit organized as a therapeutic community that includes, but is not limited to, patients with personality disorder diagnoses
RSBPO	The Specialized Rehabilitation Service for BPO Patients (RSBPO) developed to address employment difficulties that patients with BPO may exhibit

M. J. Rufat (✉) · J. V. Grilló
Centre Psicoteràpia Barcelona – Serveis Salut Mental (CPB-SSM). Grup TLP Barcelona, Barcelona, Spain
e-mail: mjrufat@gruptlpbarcelona.org; mjrufat@cpbssm.org; jvegue@gruptlpbarcelona.org; jvegue@cpbssm.org

R. G. Hersh, C. De Panfilis (eds.), *Implementing Transference-Focused Psychotherapy Principles*, https://doi.org/10.1007/978-3-031-68062-5_9

Introduction

The goal of this chapter is to outline the development of a specialized service for the treatment of patients with personality disorder (PD) diagnoses within a network of public mental health settings in Barcelona (Spain), with a specific focus on this service's use of transference-focused psychotherapy (TFP) as a treatment intervention and as a set of overarching principles. This program, an integrated care continuum, uses TFP in multiple ways, as both individual and group treatments, and as a tool for staff supervision. This innovative program and its employment of TFP elements evolved as follows:

- The creation of a public treatment network called the Centre Psicoterapia Barcelona—Serveis Salut Mental (CPB-SSM) composed of 18 different facilities.
- The implementation of a program within the CPB-SSM, called the Borderline Personality Organization Integrated Care Continuum Treatment Program (BPOTP), designed to serve patients with PD diagnoses across a continuum of services within the public mental health network.
- The introduction of the use of TFP as an individual and group modality within the BPOTP.
- The utilization of TFP principles in clinician supervision throughout the BPOTP.

The design and implementation of these specialized services using TFP in treatment and supervision is a novel, innovative program. The support of the government, and the commitment to interventions tailored to meet the needs of patients with PD diagnoses and the clinicians who treat them, represent a unique model.

Who Are the Clinicians?

Centre Psicoterapia Barcelona – Serveis Salut Mental (CPB-SSM) is a public institution located in Barcelona (Catalonia, Spain). It was created in 1980 following the deinstitutionalization of a significant number of patients from large psychiatric institutions; in this context, the first day hospital for adults in Barcelona was started by the late Dr. Josep Fabregas. Since its founding, CPB–SSM has implemented a public network of 18 community services to treat different pathologies, among others, borderline personality organization (BPO). These services are informed by the concept of institutional psychotherapy, or an emphasis on the patient's transference to the institution as a whole. This concept was innovative, even revolutionary, in 1980, since it was at odds with the traditional treatment model that dominated at the time. Dr. Fábregas explained his rationale for this approach to the mental health teams in his own words: "The best psychiatric treatment begins with a caring relationship with the patient". This sentence contains an explicit reference to the instrument that he considered a first-order therapeutic tool: the clinician's relationship with the patient. This relationship is now the main tool in the 18 mental community public health services created then; thus, institutional psychotherapy is conceptualized as a multiple transferential field or "institutional transference" [1, 2].

To this end, a systematic review of scientific evidence about the efficacy of public specialized treatment programs for BPO patients developed in other mental health networks worldwide was performed almost 20 years ago and periodically actualized. Clinical guidelines were also consulted to reach expert agreement [3]. The BPOTP was designed to include those characteristics and components that are deemed necessary to provide a specialized attention to these patients in optimal conditions.

The professionals in each sub-team of the BPOTP are psychiatrists and clinical psychologists trained and accredited in various therapy modalities, as well as nurses, social workers, social educators, and psychiatric caretakers (assistants to the treatment team providing supportive services).

Who Are the Patients?

The BPOTP of the CPB-SSM treats adult patients (from 18 years old) who meet criteria for BPO, following Kernberg's classification of personality pathology [4], which includes some PD according to the Diagnostic and Statistical Manual of Mental Disorders, Fifth Edition (DSM-5), including borderline PD (BPD) [5]. Kernberg [6, 7] proposed the concept of BPO as a way of assessing the personality structure that underlies PD symptoms. Using the structural interview, this approach evaluates multiple spheres including reality testing, aggression, and defenses (particularly the existence of primitive, splitting-based, defenses), identity diffusion versus identity consolidation, object relations, and moral values. Patients showing prominent impairments in functioning and varying degrees of identity diffusion are hence described as BPO, as opposed to those patients organized at a neurotic level, who exhibit relatively circumscribed areas of conflict and dysfunction.

Many BPO patients show extensive comorbidity with other mental disorders, such as affective disorders, anxiety disorders, eating disorders, and substance use disorders. BPO patients typically have different levels of clinical and functional severity, which is reflected in highly variable levels of vocational achievement. Patients with antisocial personality disorder as a main diagnosis, mental retardation, and psychotic disorders are excluded from the patient population treated at BPOTP; those patients with active substance use disorders will require treatment for those symptoms before participating in the BPOTP.

The multiple services comprised in the BPOTP are considered an integrated care continuum, with a focus on transference elements, as noted, as a core tool in the treatment. This model started from the clinical observations of seriously ill institutionalized patients employing predominantly primitive defense mechanisms and of their relational patterns with other patients and with clinicians [1, 3, 8, 9] reflecting the particular nature of transferences noted in their interactions.

The patients referred to the BPOTP by other public health services within the CPM-SSM, complete the following assessing protocol (structured interviews, scales, and self-reports validated in Spanish):

- Informed consent documentation
- Structural Interview [4]
- Structured interview of personality organization revised Spanish version (STIPO-R) [10]
- Structured diagnostic interview for personality disorders (SCID–II) [11]
- Diagnostic interview for borderline patients revised, DIB-R [12]
- Personality inventory for the DSM-5 (PID-5) [13]
- The childhood trauma questionnaire (CTQ) [14]
- The borderline personality disorder checklist (BPD-CL) [15]

If the patients are accepted into the program, they are also administered the following measures of change one week before treatment begins, every 6 months during the course of treatment and one week after treatment completion.

- Structured interview of personality organization revised Spanish version (STIPO-R) [10]
- Clinical global impression for patients with borderline personality disorder [16]
- Symptom checklist – 90 – revised; (SCL-90) [17]
- Barratt Impulsiveness Scale; BIS-11 [18]
- World Health Organization Quality of Life Questionnaire; WHOQOL-brief Group [19]
- Reflective functioning questionnaire [20]

Thus, this assessment process aims: (1) to accurately assess the patient's diagnosis at intake, in order to establish that the patient meets the criteria for BPO on entrance to the program; and (2) to reliably assess the patient's progress over time, thereby enabling the team to adjust treatment interventions accordingly.

Furthermore, the assessment helps the team to determine the appropriate level of care for the individual patients, based on the specific features of their clinical picture and functional impairment. The results of the assessment phase are shared with the patient and in the most severe cases with the family too, in a preliminary visit arranged before the treatment begins.

What Is the Contemporary Standard of Care for Clinicians Treating these Patients?

Within the CPB-SSM, the BPOTP was created in 2006 in response to the specific needs of a subset of the patients in the CPB-SSM services, that is, BPO patients, including those with BPD, who did not respond to the usual treatments offered by the public mental health network. Up to that time, patients with a diagnosis of BPO were treated together with other patients with different psychiatric diagnoses.

Clinical experience and trial and error showed that if patients with BPO were offered specifically designed therapeutic options, the results of their treatment experience were more positive. Therefore, CPB-SSM staff started to think about a differentiated, and specialized, treatment program for BPO patients across all the local public services in the Barcelona area. Because most of the existing treatment research for patients with PD focused specifically on BPD, the BPOTP professionals used those research findings as a foundation for their clinical work, which addressed not only BPD patients but also other patients meeting criteria for different PD.

This treatment approach was informed by Gunderson's [21] work with BPD patients and included: (1) providing specialized services for BPD patients across all the levels of care; (2) recruiting professionals with extensive and proven experience, who are then specifically dedicated to treating the BPO patient population; (3) providing services with all of the available evidence-based therapy modalities; (4) developing research teams on BPD; and (5) implementing services with specialized learning programs to help and advise BPO patients' families. These components were deemed necessary to solve the enormous problems concerning health costs in this clinical population and the high economic consequences of labor disability of BPD patients. The program's goals included both symptom reduction and an emphasis on functional rehabilitation over time. Following Gunderson's recommendations [21], the BPOTP was organized to offer different levels of treatment that are sequenced and developed in different public mental health services: an outpatient service, two day hospitals, and one subacute inpatient unit organized as a therapeutic community (Clinica Llúria). All of these services included patients with different psychiatric diagnoses, among others, BPO. More recently, a specialized rehabilitation service for BPO (RSBPO) was created, dedicated to BPO patients only. The BPOTP may also collaborate with community-based mental health teams which can offer domiciliary treatment interventions if necessary.

Thus, the BPOTP included multiple, specialized components that employ different evidence-based BPD treatments; as a public service, it was deemed necessary to have a wide range of treatments adaptable to the heterogeneous profiles of patients with BPO pathology, their individual needs, and the variable course of their illness. Day-to-day experience showed that the multiple treatments offered were effective, as patients improved in all the outcome measures studied. However, difficulties in continuity of care between services were observed, and treatment outcomes regarding the resolution of the core aspects of BPO pathology (i.e., identity diffusion and psychosocial functioning), were noted to be limited.

The BPOTP has five axes of treatment: (1) psychotherapy; (2) affiliation (meaning artistic expression or leisure time activities); (3) psychotherapeutic general strategies (emotional regulation, mindfulness, relaxation); (4) body-centered activities (a "health workshop," body awareness, scenotherapy [22], which use dramatization for educational or therapeutic purposes, or dance therapy) [23]; and (5) social adjustment or work-promoting activities (workshops on orientation and motivation, vocational objectives, or general planning). The extent and specific ways in which elements of these five interventions are articulated in the individual patient's specific treatment plan is determined by an ongoing assessment of the patient's needs and the severity of illness.

Importantly, the history of the BPOTP as an organization was marked by logistical and practical problems at its inception. Some of the different services were attached to a more traditional, "sole-service" model that resisted integration, which prevented the team from optimizing both treatment and continuity of care. Conversely, the creation of an integrated system of care necessitated: (1) a single assessment process for all patients; (2) a therapeutic contract used consistently throughout a patient's pathway of care; (3) a care coordinator working with the teams across multiple settings/services offered; and (4) a standard protocol used to measure change over time.

Furthermore, other conditions emerged as useful ways to optimize therapeutic benefits. Because the patients can rotate between the different levels of the BPOTP, special attention is paid to transitions among levels of care (i.e., residential, day hospital, and outpatient). Some rigid, idiosyncratic, and traditional organizational aspects had to be eliminated in the transition from one level of treatment to another to ensure the continuity of care. When the patient begins treatment in a new level of care within the BPOTP, such as an admission to the day hospital following an inpatient stay, the treatment team will review with the patient the specific details of the therapeutic contract and the treatment goals. This is done during a coordinated meeting that is held at admission with the patient, the referring therapist from the former service (i.e., the inpatient unit), and the new therapist working at the patient's new level of care (i.e., the day hospital). In this meeting the therapeutic contract is revised, as well as the treatment goals of the patient, with the formulation of new goals to be worked on in the next level of treatment. This continuum of care has to be outlined from the beginning of the treatment, with continued monitoring at different treatment stages to facilitate improvement over time with attention to especially fragile moments.

What Are the Goals for Imparting to These Clinicians the Principles of TFP for Working with These Patients?

While results of the systematic assessments of the BPOTP showed its efficacy, the goals of further improving core aspects of the psychopathology of BPO patients remained less fully developed. Aspects such as identity diffusion and psychosocial functioning, as reflected, for instance, in the inability to sustain employment, did not improve substantially, leading the BPOTP clinicians to consider how to increase the effectiveness of the program, in line with longitudinal follow-up studies on BPD, showing that treatments were clinically useful in promoting symptomatic remission, but functional impairment remained more severe as compared with many other major psychiatric disorders. These studies pointed out the necessity to develop more effective therapies by improving functional outcomes. They also highlight the imposing public health issue these patients represent and the embarrassingly disproportionate lack of attention the disorder has received [24]).

The implementation of TFP in the BPOTP explicitly aimed to pursue this goal.

The introduction of TFP principles followed the progression below:

- The structural diagnostic interview [4] was included in the 2006.
- Teams were trained in TFP individual and group psychotherapy, which were included in BPOTP in 2013.
- TFP individual and group psychotherapy (TFP-G) model tools were incorporated in the institutional work model [25] in 2013, as a way to help with the identification and management of transference patterns that take place in institutional relationship spaces between the patients within their groups, and between the patients' group and the staff members.
- The structured interview for personality organization revised (STIPO- R) was included in 2016 [10].

Thus, beginning in 2006, TFP was progressively included as a core component of BPOTP along with the other therapies with scientific evidence offered including mentalization based therapy (MBT) [26], dialectical behavioral therapy (DBT) [27], eye movement desensitization and reprocessing (EMDR) [28] and systems training for emotional predictability and problem solving (STEPPS) [29]. The main reason was TFP's unique focus on the resolution of identity diffusion and improved functionality. Identity diffusion is a core component of BPO [6, 30] and a well-described clinical domain in BPO patients [10, 31] with severe consequences in relationships areas (e.g., intimate relationships with significant others) and in work and leisure time areas, thus in psychosocial functioning generally [30]. Identity diffusion engenders in BPO patients the experience of intense instability and splitting in patients' relationships with the members of the treatment team (transferential patterns). These are based on primitive defensive dynamics so that patients often saw staff as either ideally good or totally bad. These patterns of primitive defenses provoke in the treatment team members intense countertransference reactions; if the team is not helped in their containment, treatment team members can act out in unproductive ways. The main consequence of this division of the team into good and bad figures, a common scenario observed with BPO patients, is the undermining of therapeutic work. The recurrence of such patterns was clearly one of the main goals in the utilization of TFP as a therapeutic model, as its principles helped the treatment team to have tools to systematically analyze such transferential patterns. Two concurrent general objectives throughout the entire integrated care continuum emerged influenced by TFP principles were: (1) to take care of the team in its capacity to think clearly and contain countertransference feelings, and (2) to help the patients in resolving identity diffusion and in improving psychosocial functionality.

Benefiting from familiarity with TFP principles, the team endeavored to incorporate aspects of the TFP treatment model in work in all services of BPOTP. TFP as an individual psychotherapy was made available in 2013 directly addressing identity diffusion and relationships with others undermined by splitting. It had been observed over the years that these two elements, (1) lack of consolidated identify for the individual, and (2) relationships with others, marked by lack of integration of positive and negative qualities, could have severe consequences in vocational, interpersonal, and social functioning. To this end, the creation of the aforementioned RSBPO directly targeting vocational impairment, well-documented in this population, was a landmark initiative. To summarize, the goal of the treatment at this point in a patient's trajectory within the BPOTP, informed by TFP principles, included further consolidation of the patient's identity with associated improvement in socialization and meaningful participation in the community facilitated by participation in the RSBPO.

TFP principles were also introduced as guidance for the treatment team in their roles more broadly [32, 33]. These TFP principles informed the clinicians' understanding of the transference constellations taking place within various treatment programs. The clinical teams were trained to monitor the multiple therapeutic relationships occurring across the continuum of services. They were oriented to TFP principles including the clinicians encouraging patients to speak freely, maintaining technical neutrality, and considering the dominant object relations dyads in play, and monitoring for associated role reversals.

What TFP Principles Might Be of Utility for the Clinicians Working with These Patients?

Patient Assessment in the BPOTP

A comprehensive and detailed diagnostic assessment is done with all patients that present to our services asking for diagnosis and treatment, as was explained earlier. The STIPO-R [10, 34] assists the clinical staff: (1) to employ a comprehensive and flexible assessment process that explores all of the core clinical domains that define BPO, thus facilitating BPO diagnosis when appropriate; (2) to measure the patient's severity of illness in terms of the impact of each clinical domain on the patient's functionality; (3) to identify preliminary treatment goals in all of assessed areas; and (4) to plan treatment assigning patients to levels of treatment (services of BPOTP) depending on severity of illness.

The patients are assigned to one of two general levels of treatment depending on their diagnosis and requirements. One of these levels of treatment corresponds to a profile of affective instability, impulsivity, and emotional dysregulation as central symptoms, with specific alterations in the control of emotions and in decision-making [35, 36]. Most patients with this profile have impulsive self-harming tendencies and dysfunctional behavior marked by externalization of aggressive impulses. Thus, these patients receive more intensive treatment (18–25 hours per week) during three months in the day hospital, or two months in the subacute service (Clinical Lluria), or up to two years in the RSBPO. These patients receive DBT or MBT in the first phases as individual and group psychotherapy modalities, or STEPPS as a group psychotherapy intervention.

The other level of treatment is offered to those patients who present with defining disturbed relationships, which are characteristic of, and central to, their clinical and functioning problems [36]. Patients with this profile, who show more passive destructive and dysfunctional behavior, with more dissociative symptomatology and core problems in interpersonal relationships, receive less intensive treatment: between 8 and 12 hours per week, for six months in the day hospital, or to two years in the RSBPO depending on their requirements. This group responds more robustly to dynamic [37, 38] and cognitive [39, 40] therapies. Therefore, this group receives either individual TFP or TFP for groups (TFP-G) as a group intervention.

Involving Family in Treatment Including Negotiation of the Treatment Contract

The BPOTP fosters the treatment alliance with family members. At the time of the first meeting with program staff, a therapeutic contract is developed, to be signed by all parties involved. The alliance with family members rests on consistent, good-quality communication [41]. This is reinforced by clarifying at the start with the patient and family the expectations for the treatment. The main objective during the first contact with patients and families is to ensure the viability of the treatment by developing a consensus about the basics of the treatment frame. These negotiations are done to minimize the risk of patient dropout. Patients who are well-prepared are significantly more likely to participate meaningfully and comply with treatment and are much less likely to stop therapy prematurely [42]. The patient's objectives will be addressed then, as part of the treatment setting.

The team will address confidentiality concerns at the outset; the therapist will outline stipulations for communication about privileged information among team members. The team will also review confidentiality issues that relate to contact with family members, including those crisis situations that might involve communication without direct patient authorization because of the emergence of risky situations for the patient or others. In addition, patients are educated about the need to protect the privacy of other participants in the program, specifically the obligation to avoid sharing information about patients with those outside of the program. Many of the patients enrolled in the program with more severe PD pathology will be at risk for secondary gain of illness or gratification related in some way to their symptoms, which could compromise the treatment intervention. These benefits could be primarily psychological, or they could be financial. Psychological benefits could include special treatment or indulgences by family members. Economic benefits could mean family support or government stipends for disability. Such secondary gain of illness can reinforce self-destructive attitudes causing patients to destroy opportunities for improved functioning. Improved functioning is central to the mission of the BPOTP and is expected as an outcome of TFP as an individual treatment. The risk of secondary gain of illness is identified in the first interviews, with an explicit communication that the treatment is designed to help the patients improve their lives. The patients are asked specifically for a commitment to finding and initiating a productive activity during the BPOTP, as is done usually in TFP. It is explained that work for pay, volunteer work, or meaningful studies will help the patient bring to the treatment those most pertinent issues in their lives, thereby facilitating the deep work involved and its effective resolution.

Another important objective communicated at the start of treatment is the expectation for a continuous informed consent process. This process stresses the importance that the patient and family members understand the details of the treatments available and the evidence for their use. The informed consent process at the BPOTP is concerned with all the components of the program, and changes in those components over time, and the duration of treatment and the roles and functions of the various team members.

Identifying Patient Goals

Following a TFP approach, the BPOTP now emphasizes the need to identify specific goals that serve as a basic guide to be followed by the teams from the beginning of the treatment and continuously throughout it. These goals reinforce the essential tasks to be carried out by the team and constitute part of the therapeutic setting.

The first specific goal is promoting patients' motivation. As is known, BPO patients show, as a core characteristic, extensive difficulties in maintaining stable views of self and significant others. This inevitably affects their changing and unstable attitudes toward treatment. The patient's motivation for treatment fluctuates, often reflecting conflicts with the therapist or other members of the group. The emergence of prominent negative affects in certain BPO patients will be associated with attacks on others, including the treatment team members, sometimes leading to ruptures in treatment.

Elucidation of the patient's goals is also a fundamental step. The patient is asked to elaborate a list of goals, and at the same time, the therapist considers his or her goals for the patient. These two lists are shared to try to find some common treatment goals. The patients' goals will continue to be monitored and revised periodically.

It is widely recognized that a prerequisite to achieving an effective treatment consists of three interdependent components of the therapeutic alliance: the patient's and therapist's agreement on goals, the patient's and therapist's agreement on tasks, and the quality of the bond between patient and therapist [41]. Therefore, establishing personal goals with the BPO patient is a fundamental task, which can directly address common challenges faced by these patients including passivity or inhibition [43, 44]. Formulating personal goals and treatment goals starts during the assessment and anchors the treatment as it begins. When the agreement is settled, the goals are sequenced according to the treatment phase, taking into account the hierarchy of priorities described in standard TFP, and the length of stay in each service. These goals are also periodically monitored and modified if necessary, during treatment. Before initiating treatment, an informed consent process is carried out, defining the details about the therapy methods and the management of the confidentiality commitment. In addition, the patient is aware from the beginning that all of the team will be informed about their identified goals and that the therapist will share the minimum information necessary for clinical coordination. The primary therapist and the other members of the treatment team will keep in mind the patient's goals as a way to shape and define the interventions over time.

The patients' goals depend on their clinical situation and functioning. There are common general goals and more personal individual patient goals. For instance, a significant proportion of the patients treated endorse numerous comorbid pathologies. Most of them have co-occurring affective disorders, anxiety disorders, eating disorders, substance use disorders, and/or complex trauma. The destabilizing effect of these co-occurring pathologies risks undermining the treatment; thus, a key initial goal is addressing comorbid conditions.

Therefore, the patient may be asked to add some other goals to the list they generate, such as maintaining abstinence from psychoactive substances, or maintaining an adequate body mass index, for example. The patient's goals will correlate with specific personal factors. There may be goals shared by other participants in the program, but some goals may be narrower as suggested earlier; for example, the patient with a substance use disorder requiring ongoing support, or the patient with obesity referred to adjunctive treatment for that concern.

Establishing a Treatment Contract

The therapeutic contract symbolizes the commitment of the two parties that are involved in the therapeutic relationship and structures the treatment process between the patient (and eventually their family) and the team. Within the contract, the tasks and responsibilities of the patient and family in the treatment and the tasks and responsibilities of the team are made explicit and follow the TFP individual contract principles [45] adapted to an institutional framework. These points are discussed in detail with the parties involved in order to define a consensual agreement (e.g., if the patient cannot come to treatment, the patient, not the family, is responsible for notifying the team).

As outlined by Yeomans et al. [45], the contract tries to: (1) establish a mutual understanding of the problems to address in treatment; (2) define the responsibilities of the parties involved (the team, the patient and, in some cases, the family), and (3) ensure the protection and safety of all parties. It is important to clarify the details of the patient's responsibilities; for example, if we agree with the patient and family that the patient is responsible for supporting himself financially, then the family would know to refrain from intervening and stay committed to the expectation that patient must work and pay for his expenses.

The BPOTP combines individual and group treatment in all of its services. However, the BPOTP is essentially a group treatment experience. Because treatment groups are the main components of the program, the therapeutic contract must include some points related to group therapy. A contract that describes in detail the expectations for the patient as a participant in the program's groups will be of benefit both to the patient and to the other group members, and the treatment process generally [46–48]. For all of the above, the therapeutic contract is accurately worked out in detail before starting treatment.

The contract is always both a written and verbal agreement, in contrast to standard individual TFP, which customarily includes a verbal agreement only. Possible threats to the treatment customarily addressed in TFP are detailed in the contract. The contract includes: psychoeducation about the different interventions that are part of the BPOTP, as well as the weekly group activities schedule, the frequency and duration of psychotherapeutic sessions (individual and family), the program's cancelation policy, vacation schedule, expectations for attendance and policies for absences, and measures of treatment required during the course of participation.

The contract also includes some specific aspects that must be taken into consideration throughout treatment and especially during the group sessions. These aspects combine more practical questions (such as punctuality, the prohibition of drinking, eating, or using mobile telephone during the sessions, among others), with other questions typically considered in a TFP contract. These include an effort to limit patients' aggressive behavior toward themselves or others (members of the team or fellow patients), the commitment of the patients to speak to the entire group, not to only one member, and the maintenance of confidentiality regarding anything they have heard during the group sessions required for trust within the group. Also included in the contract are the commitment to bring to the treatment the inevitable conflicts arising between the members of the group, and the expectation that patients refrain from interpersonal relationships with other group members outside of the treatment sessions (including sexual relationships). The contract details will guide the material explored in both individual and group therapeutic sessions; as with the standard TFP agreement for individual psychotherapy, the hierarchy of priorities is determined in advance and thereby informs the areas of focus of exploration.

Of note, the COVID-19 pandemic required adjustments in both individual and group treatment interventions at the BPOTP. At the start of the pandemic, treatment was offered remotely only, using virtual or on-line tools. This transition from in-person to virtual settings for treatment required review and adjustment of the therapeutic contract. Because of the pandemic and its sequelae, it was noted that those patients with more severe conditions, even if superficially motived to participate in on-line groups, deteriorated in their functioning with worsening of social capabilities and, at times, more passive or resistant attitudes toward engagement in treatment.

The same dynamics that were observed previously during in-person groups, such as paranoid transferences, were observed in on-line groups too. During the first weeks of the pandemic, some technical problems added difficulties for the groups, such as failures in connections, doubts about the security and confidentiality of the on-line spaces, and those times when instability in the computer network underscored the instability in the group itself. Some patients described problems in maintaining a sense of security because they did not have their own private space. This concern required patients and families to make appropriate accommodations. The team observed an increase in "acting in" in the sense of inappropriate or exhibitionistic behaviors and a blurring of the public versus private sphere in on-line contacts. The patients therefore were asked to conduct themselves in on-line sessions in an appropriate way, similar to expectations conveyed for behavior in when seen previously in-person.

Using TFP Principles to Structure the Work of the Team

The BPOTP employs a wide range of different evidence—based treatments for BPD, as described earlier, such as: TFP [45, 46], MBT [26], DBT [27] and more recently EMDR [28] and STEPPS [29]. The professionals in each sub-team are psychiatrists and clinical psychologists trained and accredited in these therapies. The teams also include nurses, social workers, social educators, and psychiatric caretakers. While clinicians in the BPOTP may offer any one of these specialized treatments, all these clinicians are also engaged in the ongoing application of certain TFP principles including reflection about emerging dyads between patients, between patients and clinicians, and among clinicians. They have specific instructions to keep in mind the hierarchy of priorities of treatment and the personal goals of the patients. They also work with a commitment to maintain technical neutrality in interactions with patients individually and in group settings.

One of the most difficult tasks to manage when working in an integrated care continuum like the BPOTP is the integration of the multiple component parts, or sub-teams, which are part of the larger organization. There are several explanations for this difficulty. One commonly observed phenomenon is the tension between different parts of the organization. There is a chronic risk that the different services will "speak different languages" and therefore present to the patient in fragmented, sometimes contradictory, ways. There can be highly problematic situations when there is a more pronounced conflict between the services, marked by devaluation or invalidation, creating a negligent and aversive experience that many of the BPO patients have already lived in their personal history. These situations also increase the tendency within the team to somehow repeat aspects of the patients' underlying pathology, expressed mainly in splitting dynamics. The impact of splitting within treatment teams in many different psychiatric settings has been well-documented. In general, we have observed that smaller services within more expansive networks such as the BPOTP will tend to focus primarily on dynamics within their own treatment sub-team, with limited attention to broader trends within the larger organization. Familiarity with TFP principles facilitates appreciation of team dynamics as a whole. It may be useful to monitor how the sub-teams operate, as each particular service provides care in what they consider to be the best way possible. In doing so, there may be activation of more primitive defensive operations between teams. There may be a subtle devaluation of the contribution of other teams and questioning of their competence. This lack of trust displayed may reflect the projection of negative elements, seeing other treatment providers as incompetent or defective. These primitive dynamics can be understood as transferential patterns between sub-teams, such as narcissistic or paranoid transferences, undermining the mutual trust between groups of clinicians. It is useful if these dynamics between sub-teams can be explored in an unthreatening and constructive dialogue.

In summary, the BPOTP follows TFP principles in its organization of teamwork. Patient care is carried out by a large team specializing in the treatment of patients with severe personality disorder pathology, which is composed of multiple small sub-teams located in each service or level of treatment. They work together as a single, large team, within a unified treatment program, with a common therapeutic contract and consistent coordinator.

Using TFP Principles to Coordinate the Teams' Work

The importance of the role of the treatment coordinator in the clinical setting that is essentially a group treatment and where a variety of psychotherapy groups are available, has been widely studied. The coordinator serves as a crucial, ongoing communication link between patients and clinicians on the team, between different teams of clinicians, and between the clinical staff and institution management. Ideally, the treatment coordinator should be both an effective therapist and an effective resource manager (e.g., human, technical, or organizational resources) [49]. This professional figure has been regarded as essential by therapists who have had considerable experience in such settings [49, 50].

In the TFP-oriented approach described here, the first major coordinator's role includes analyzing, both within the large team and the various sub-teams, the splitting processes that occur routinely when treating BPO patient populations. To do so, the coordinator pursues active monitoring of transference currents between patients and between patients and clinicians that emerge in the milieu and explores them in a way that reinforces stability and safety for the program and supports increased reflective functioning and integration for the patients.

This process enables the team to achieve interrelated core goals: (1) helping the team of clinicians acquire a deeper and richer understanding of the patients, (2) assisting the team of clinicians as they manage familiar patterns of projection and splitting, as would be anticipated with work with these patients; and (3) increasing integration of self and object splitting processes characteristically altered in BPO patients and observed by the team. The program coordinator serves a supervisory role, assisting the team members as the collective projections of the patients can impair the team members' ability to think clearly. Because the team is immersed in a maelstrom of massive projections and transference constellations, there is inevitably a deep impact on their capacity to stay focused without undue reactivity. If the patterns of projection and splitting have not been elaborated, the therapeutic work is impossible in this model.

After this elaborative process related to the entire patient group has been shared with the team, a second important task is necessary: to supervise the team members in their efforts with each individual patient in the BPOTP, again informed by the proposed model. It is useful to help the team to monitor the short, medium and long-term goals of each patient (including broader life goals), as well as the treatment plan crafted for the patient throughout participation in the program. This last phase is a kind of "navigation notebook" shared by all parties in the treatment that guides the step-by-step progression of the treatment process and also helps collectively to avoid getting lost within the impact of borderline pathology.

Using TFP Principles to Focus on Identity Diffusion

The process of addressing the patient's observed patterns of splitting follows TFP principles. All team members use TFP principles to interpret and respond to patients' behavior in the treatment milieu, and what emerges in this context is then used by the TFP therapists during individual and group sessions. Specifically, the various team members employ clarification and confrontation, but not interpretation, during their interactions with the patients in the milieu, and then report on the transference patterns they have identified in the team meetings. The coordinator uses TFP principles to clarify with the team the emerging dominant object relations observed, so that this understanding can eventually be conveyed to the patient in an individual or group psychotherapy. Multiple transferential constellations are analyzed in detail, looking for dyadic patterns. This process helps the team to gain a deep understanding regarding what the patients and the group are feeling and to return to the individual patient, in both individual and group therapy, a more integrated image of self and others, using these elements of the interpretation cycle of TFP.

Then, in individual sessions, the therapist aims to identify the dominant affect, considering the material that the patient brings to the session, with a goal of identifying the emerging transference patterns and fostering the interpretive cycle. Ordinarily, the patients can spontaneously talk about their relationships with the team or the rest of the group members in individual and group psychotherapeutic spaces, expressing the conflicts that they are experiencing within the treatment process. This is facilitated by the previous work of the team outside of the sessions, using clarification and confrontation interventions in exploration of transference patterns and evidence of splitting.

What Are Possible Targets for Measurement to Gauge the Effectiveness of Instruction about Applications of TFP Principles?

Data collected since 2006 has confirmed that patients have benefitted greatly from the BPOTP services. The majority of the patients treated in the day hospital (72% of a sample of 350 patients participating in the treatment program from 2006 to 2014) have improved significantly in different clinical and psychosocial variables. These variables are suicide attempts, self-destructive behavior, paranoid symptoms, impaired interpersonal relationships, fear of abandonment, identity diffusion, impulsivity, and feelings of emptiness, with more improvement correlated with the longer the patient participated in the day hospital [43]. However, 28% of the patients in the sample prematurely ended their treatment in DH. These results are similar to those obtained by other treatment programs [44]; this subset of patients leaving treatment in the day hospital prematurely have been identified as those patients with the greatest impairment in functioning [52]. Notably, those patients who do improve are able to maintain these gains 5 years after completing treatment in the day hospital; improvement is most robust in the resolution of impulsivity. However, they continue to endorse impoverished psychosocial functioning [51, 53]. These results indicate that treatment for BPO patients is effective in terms of clinical improvement in all of the core typical areas of BPO and results in greater treatment adherence for the majority of patients. Nevertheless, the follow-up data also indicates the necessity of searching for therapeutic strategies to improve psychosocial functioning.

Because of the well-documented impaired psychosocial functioning that persists even after remission from certain BPO symptoms, the RSBPO was created in 2015. Preliminary results from an initial assessment [52] of the program showed positive results; the chief goals of the program relate directly to the patients' functioning and capacity to sustain meaningful employment. Summarizing the main results, 56.9% of a sample of 68 patients who enrolled consecutively in the service during 13 months from 2015 to 2017 had improved. The admissions to inpatient services in this group enrolled in RSBPO were reduced significantly; 94.9% of the patients in the sample did not need any hospital admission. The patients consolidated improvement in clinical variables such as unstable relationships, suicide attempts, feelings of emptiness, paranoid ideation, aggressive behavior, use of substances disorder, psychotic symptoms and affective disorders. The same proportion of patients (94.9%) who did not require rehospitalization also improved in psychosocial and functional variables such as family relationships, global activity, community activities, daily life activities, general functioning, social adjustment and quality of life, as well as in symptom variables such as impulsivity and feelings of emptiness.

What Is the Source of Institutional or Government Support for this Initiative?

Results of evidence of efficacy of the BPOTP were reported annually to the government, which made it possible to include TFP in the BPOTP developed by CPB-SSM in public network mental health services.

What Are the Didactic Materials Required to Impart TFP Principles to this Target Group of Clinicians?

The didactic tools used to impart TFP principles to this target group of clinicians are the following:

- Training sessions included in the current annual institutional training program.
- Weekly supervision sessions of all the BPOTP teams.

- Four supervision groups (every other week) on individual TFP therapy led by external TFP teachers and supervisors.
- Two supervision sessions focused on TFP group therapy (every other week) led by Dr. Otto Kernberg and two TFP teachers and supervisors of the institution.
- Annual meetings for all the BPOTP sub-teams, where sub-teams present cases that are analyzed and supervised using the institutional TFP model by a TFP teacher and supervisor.

Clinical Case Illustration

Maria is a 26-year-old single woman who moved with her family to Barcelona when her father's work transferred him from a more rural part of Spain. Beginning at age 18, Maria had three psychiatric hospitalizations, all in the context of threats of suicide during periods of turmoil in her romantic life. Maria was diagnosed with depression and anxiety and started on a series of medication trials, mostly with antidepressants, which did not help address her chronic affective instability and periodic threats to harm herself. On the few occasions when she was able to find and begin a job, she was often overwhelmed and resorted to binge drinking and self-mutilation to manage her feelings of despair.

When Maria's prescribing psychiatrist arranged for her follow-up care in Barcelona, he referred her to an outpatient unit of the CPB-SSM, not far from the new home where Maria and her parents lived. This psychiatrist had often considered a primary or co-occurring diagnosis of BPD for Maria but did not feel he had the time or skills to provide her with the necessary specialized treatment. He conveyed his observations to the CPB-SSM staff; therefore, at the time of Maria's first appointment, she was referred to the intake process at the BPOTP. Maria was irritated with the extended assessment period, often becoming demanding and saying, "Why can't you just give me refills of my medication!"

At the time the intake assessment phase was completed, Maria was told of the clinicians' diagnostic impression, which included a personality disorder diagnosis and informed about the BPOTP. The team met with Maria and her parents who strongly supported Maria's participation in this novel program, especially since they had become increasingly concerned about Maria's failure to identify work or school options and her pattern of spending her days meeting friends at a local park and becoming involved in disruptive and tumultuous relationships with young men she tried to date. While Maria no longer displayed the kind of impulsivity and affective instability she had in earlier years, she nevertheless displayed a pattern of recurrent, dysfunctional interpersonal relationships.

Maria and the BPOTP identified and agreed on some preliminary treatment goals, which included a return to school parttime, engagement with an exercise program, and meetings with a nutritionist, given Maria's weight gain associated with prior medication trials and her general level of inactivity. Maria was referred to an individual TFP therapist and 10 hours per week in the day hospital, for six months. Maria's family was actively involved at the outset of treatment; furthermore, the treatment frame included periodic family meetings with the treatment team throughout the day hospital program. Based on Maria's personal history of self-injuring behavior, the treatment contract also included an agreement to move to the inpatient level of care in case of severe suicidal ideation and uncontrolled self-harming behavior. The treatment goals and frame, which were agreed upon in the contract phase, were shared and addressed both by the day hospital treatment team and the individual TFP therapist.

Maria's participation was rocky at the beginning, as she often became embroiled in conflicts with other members of the patient group, whom at times she would consider "the best friends I could ever find in my life," but at other times she would find disappointing and uncaring, ultimately accusing others of being rude and insensitive to her profound inner pain. The team members used clarification and confrontation in their interactions with Maria in the day hospital milieu, with the aim to identify and illuminate the various object relations dyads activated between her and her peers. These observations were then reported and discussed in team meetings, and consistently addressed during group and individual therapy. Gradually Maria became more reflective and gained increased understanding of the ways her overinvolvement with friends and rapid move to distrust in stressful situations undermined her functioning generally. She was able to understand that her rapidly shifting opposite views of others, occurring within the day hospital but also in her real life outside the treatment, corresponded to her profound inner conflict between wanting desperately to be loved and cared for, and fearing that this cannot ever happen, thus resulting in feeling mistreated and attacked in actuality. Maria took one accounting course at the beginning and managed to lose a significant amount of weight, which generally brightened her mood. The treatment team continued to focus on the agreement made with Maria at the outset that included her participation in the program, her family's involvement, and her commitment to her class in accounting.

At one point, Maria met a man in her accounting class and began a romantic relationship that ended abruptly, leading Maria to drink in a binge pattern and threaten her parents that she would take an overdose of her medications. Maria and her alarmed parents met with the BPOTP team. Mindful of the treatment frame and the contract, the clinicians introduced the possibility of an inpatient admission to the Clinica Lluria for stabilization. This possibility was received with great relief by Maria's parents, who were seriously concerned by her escalating dangerous behaviors. The team members used their supervision work with TFP principles and explored their countertransference reactions: they felt overwhelmed by an urge to "act" and to immediately hospitalize Maria to control her suicidal risk. Instead of acting this urgency, the team members tactfully told Maria that, based on her apparent suicidal risk, she could indeed require full-time hospitalization, as they previously agreed on during the contract phase, and that they would surely admit her to Clinica Luria if this was the only way to save her life. However, at the same time, they reminded Maria of their shared understanding of her object relation patterns repeatedly identified over the course of the day hospital program, both in the treatment milieu and in the individual and group therapy settings. Thus, they also empathically communicated to Maria that she was likely struggling with an inner conflict between two parts of self, one destructive, and the other with the motivation to live. It looked like Maria was desperately trying to solve this conflict by denying that part of self that wanted to survive and acting "as if" only the others in her life wanted her to survive. For this reason, she was forced to attribute to her parents and to the team that part of self in favor of life, in such a way that she could then more fully identify with the part of self that was trying to destroy her. Because this situation could indeed be life-threatening, hospital admission could actually be indicated. However, this would prevent further exploration, by the day hospital treatment team, of Maria's devastating inner conflict – therapeutic work that, they reminded Maria, had helped her so often in the past to develop and maintain a greater sense of self-efficacy and more gratifying interpersonal relationships. At the same time, the clinicians also pointed out that the day hospital program would not be suitable if Maria remained actively suicidal and asked her opinion about this. Maria looked surprised by the direct, though empathic, communication modality of the clinicians. While maintaining the point that for her it was not easy at all to be fully committed to survive in this difficult moment, she acknowledged that the team had helped her in the past to overcome her difficulties by focusing on what was happening inside her. She said that she was willing to "start again," and agreed to continue the day hospital program, confident that she would be able to immediately inform the clinicians if she would lose control over her suicidal ideations in such a way that would require hospitalization to preserve her safety.

Maria was soon able to regain stability and complete her six-month participation in the day program. She was then referred to the RSBPO to focus on her engagement in looking for paid work. This transition required additional attention by Maria's team, given their concerns that she would have had challenges with the transition from the day hospital to the new program. For this aim, the team coordinator arranged a meeting between the day hospital and the RSBPO sub-teams. Previous treatment goals were reviewed together with the patient and her parents and based on Maria's progress during the day hospital program, the new goal of finding a full-time job was identified. The mutual agreement on this treatment contract by all the parties involved was re-emphasized, thus ensuring integrated continuity of care between the day hospital and the outpatient levels. During this time, Maria continued in individual treatment, but her improved stability allowed her to shift her focus to the challenges of developing a resume, going on interviews, and eventually finding a job as an assistant in an accounting company.

Conclusion

Working in a comprehensive, multi-faceted program for patients with personality disorder pathology using TFP principles as a guiding influence can be highly rewarding for clinicians and beneficial to patients. This chapter illustrated the experience of the Barcelona borderline personality organization integrated care continuum treatment program (BPOTP). Here, using TFP principles has proven particularly effective for structuring treatment across multiple levels of care (i.e., outpatient, day hospital, inpatient) and treatment modalities (i.e., group therapy, individual therapy, treatment milieu interventions). The significant support given to the BPOTP from institutional leaders and the strong commitment to the TFP approach of the various professionals allowed the implementation of this novel, integrated, and particularly promising treatment model.

References

1. Tosquelles F. Que faut-il entendre par psycho-thérapie institutionelle ? Informations psychiatriques;1969:45(4).
2. De Vicente F. La palabra en psiquiatría: ¿Todavía eficaz? Barcelona: Xoroi; 2016.
3. Oury J. Psychiatrie et psychothérapie institutionnelle. Paris: Payot; 1976.
4. Kernberg OF. Structural interviewing. Psychiatr Clin North Am. 1981;4(1):169–95.
5. American Psychiatric Association (APA). Diagnostic and statistical manual (Fifth edition). DSM-5. Washington, DC: American Psychiatric Publishing; 2013.
6. Kernberg OF. Psicoterapia focalizada en la transferencia para trastornos límite de la personalidad. Bilbao: Desclée; 2016a.
7. Klein M. Envy and gratitude, a study of unconscious sources. New York: Basic Books; 1957.
8. Diamond M, Allcorn S. The cornerstone of psychoanalytic organizational analysis: psychological reality, transference and countertransference in the workplace. Hum Relat. 2003;56(4):491–514.
9. Clarkin JF, Caligor E, Stern B, Kernberg OF. Manual for the structured interview of personality organization—revised (STIPOR). 2019. https://www.borderlinedisorders.com/assets/STIPORmanual.July2019FINALMod.pdf Rufat MJ. Validación al castellano de la Structured Interview of Personality Organization Revised (STIPO-R) como instrumento diagnóstico de los Trastornos de la Personalidad. Tesis Doctoral. Psicología Clínica y de la Salud. Barcelona: Universidad de Barcelona. (España). 2024.
10. First MB, Spitzer RL, Gibbon M, Williams J. The structured clinical interview for DSM-III-R personality disorders (SCID-II). Part I: description. J Personal Disord. 1995;9(2):83–91.
11. Barrachina J, Soler J, Campins M, Tejero A, Pascual JC, Álvarez E, Zanarini M, Perez V. Validation of a Spanish version of the diagnostic interview for Bordelines- revised (DIB-R). Actas Esp Psiquiatr. 2004;32:293–8.
12. Gutiérrez F, Aluja A, Peri JM, Calvo N, Ferrer M, Baillés E, Krueger RF. Psychometric properties of the Spanish PID-5 in a clinical and a community sample. Assessment. 2016;24(3):326–36.
13. Hernandez A, Gallardo-Pujol D, Pereda N, Arntz A, Bernstein D, Labad A, Valero J, Gutierrez-Zotes A. Initial validation of the Spanish childhood trauma questionnaire-short form: factor structure, reliability and association with parenting. Journal of interpersonal violence. J Interp Viol 2012. 2012;28(7):1498–518.
14. Calvo N, Valero S, Arntz A, Andión O, Matalí JL, Navascues V, Ramos-Quiroga JA, Casas M, Ferrer M. Validation of the Spanish version of the borderline personality disorder checklist (BPD checklist) in a sample of BPD patients: study of psychometric properties. Eur J Psychiat. 2018;32(1):26–35.
15. Pérez V, Barrachina J, Soler J, Pascual JC, Campins MJ, Puigdemont D, Alvarez E. Global clinical printing for patients with limit personality disorder (ICG-TLP): a scale sensitive to change. Spanish Psychiat Acts. 2007;35(4):229–35.
16. González de Rivera JL, Derogatis LR, De las Cuevas C, Gracia Marco R, Rodríguez Pulido F, Henry Benítez M, Monterrey AL. The Spanish version of the SCL-90-R. Normative data in the general population. Towson: Clinical Psychometric Research; 1989.
17. Oquendo MA, Baca-García E, Graver R, Morales M, Montalban V, Mann JJ. Spanish adaptation of Barratt impulsiveness scale (BIS). Eur J Psychiatry. 2001;15:147–55.
18. Lucas R. Spanish version of WHOQOL. Majadahonda, Madrid: Ergón, d.l.; 1998.
19. Fonagy P, Luyten P, Moulton-Perkins A, Lee YW, Warren F, Howard S, et al.

20. Development and validation of a self-report measure of mentalizing: the reflective functioning questionnaire. PLoS One. 2016;11(7):e0158678. https://doi.org/10.1371/journal.pone.0158678.
21. Gunderson JG. Borderline personality disorder: clinical guide. Barcelona: Ars Medica; 2006.
22. Daurella N. Reseña de la obra de V. Cabre (comp.): "Escenoterapia. Aplicaciones clínicas y educativas". Clínica e Investigación Relacional. 2015;9(1):306–11. [ISSN 1988-2939] [Recuperado de www.ceir.org.es]
23. Levy FJ, Fried JP, Leventhal F. Dance and other expressive art therapies: when words are not enough. New York: Routledge; 1995.
24. Gunderson JG, Stout RL, TH MG, Shea MT, Morey LC, Grilo CM, Zanarini MC, Yen S, Markowitz JC, Sanislow C, Ansell E, Pinto A, Skodol AE. Ten-year course of borderline personality disorder: psychopathology and function from the collaborative longitudinal personality disorders study. Arch Gen Psychiatry. 2011;68(8):827–37. https://doi.org/10.1001/archgenpsychiatry.2011.37.
25. Rufat MJ. 5th International Society of Transference Focused Psychotherapy (TFP) conference. TFP groups in severe BPD patients treated in an institutional psychotherapeutic – TFP setting: BPD an integrated care continuum program (day hospitals, subacute service and rehabilitation service). 2018; 30 Sep. – 2 Oct. Barcelona (Spain).
26. Bateman A, Fonagy P. Psychotherapy for borderline personality disorder: mentalization based treatment. Oxford: Oxford University Press; 2004.
27. Linehan M. Cognitive-behavioral treatment of borderline personality disorder. New York: Guilford Press; 1993.
28. Shapiro F. Eye movement desensitization and reprocessing basis principles, protocols and procedures. New York: The Guilford Press; 2001.
29. Blum N, Pfohl B, Stuart S, McCormick B, Allen J, et al. Systems training for emotional predictability and problem solving (STEPPS) for outpatients with borderline personality disorder: a randomized controlled trial and 1-year follow-up. Am J Psychiatry. 2008;165(4):468–78.
30. Kernberg OF. What is personality? J Personal Disord. 2016b;30(2):145–56.
31. Clarkin JF, Caligor E, Stern B, Kernberg OF. The Structured Interview for Personality Organization (STIPO). 2007. Downloaded from https://www.borderlinedisorders.com/assets/Structured-Interview-of-Personality-Organization.pdf
32. Kernberg OF. Leadership and organizational functioning: organizational regression. Int J Group Psychother. 1978;28:3–25.
33. Kernberg OF. Ideology conflict and leadership in groups and organizations. Barcelona: Paidós; 1999.
34. Clarkin JF, Caligor E, Stern B, Kernberg OF. Structured interview of personality organization (STIPO). New York: Personality Disorders Institute-Weill Medical College of Cornell University; 2003.
35. Salvador R, Vega D, Pascual JC, Marco J, Canales-Rodríguez EJ, Aguilar S, Anguera M, Soto A, Ribas J, Soler J, Maristany T, Rodríguez-Fornells A, Pomarol-Clotet E. Converging medial frontal resting state and diffusion based abnormalities in borderline personality disorder. Biol Psychiatry. 2014;79(2):107–16.
36. Gunderson J. Disturbed relationships as a phenotype for borderline personality disorder. Am J Psychiatry. 2007;164(11):1637–40.
37. Kernberg OF. Borderline personality organization. J Am Psychoanal Assoc. 1967;15:641–85.
38. Bateman A, Fonagy P. Effectiveness of partial hospitalization in the treatment of borderline personality disorder: a randomized controlled trial. Am J Psychiatry. 1999;156:1563–9.
39. Westen D, Klesper J, Ruffins SA, Silvermna M, Lifton N, Boekamp J. Object relations in childhood and adolescence: the development of working representations. J Consult Clin Psychol. 1991;59:400–9.
40. Young JE, Klosko J, Weishaar ME. Schema therapy: a practitioner's guide. New York: Guilford; 2003.
41. Bordin E. The generalizability of the psychoanalytic concept of the working alliance. Psychother Theory Res Pract. 1979;16:252–60.

42. Richetin J, Preti E, Costantini G, De Panfilis C. The centrality of affective instability and identity in borderline personality disorder: evidence from network analysis. PLoS One. 2017;12(10):e0186695. https://doi.org/10.1371/journal.pone.0186695.
43. Rufat MJ, Barrachina J, Verdaguer E, Vegué J. Evaluation of the effectiveness of a TLP Treatment Program in Day Hospital. 2014 (unpublished manuscript).
44. Bateman A, Fonagy P. Treatment of borderline personality disorder with psychoanalytically oriented partial hospitalization: an 18-month follow-up. Am J Psychiatry. 2001;158(1):36–42.
45. Yeomans FE, Carkin JF, Kernberg OF. Transference focused psychotherapy. Application to Borderline Disorders. Bilbao: Desclée; 2016.
46. Kernberg OF. The inseparable nature of love and aggression. Clinical and theoretical perspectives. London: American Psychiatric Association; 2012.
47. Rutan JS, Stone WN. Psychodynamic group psychotherapy. 3rd ed. New York: The Guilford Press; 2001.
48. Yalom I, Leszcz M. The theory and practice of group psychotherapy. 5th ed. New York: Basic Books; 2005.
49. Lonergan EC. Discussion of group therapy program development. Int J Group Psychother. 2000;50(1):43–5.
50. Roller B. The promise of group therapy: how to build a vigorous training and organizational base for group therapy in managed behavioral healthcare. San Francisco: Jossey-Bass; 1997.
51. De Angel I. Study on improving functionality in TLP patients treated in Day Hospital. 2015 (unpublished manuscript).
52. Rufat MJ, Marí C, De Ángel I, López M, Caupena S, Fernández M, Zarauza E, Ureña T, Vegué J. Specialised rehabilitation for patients with borderline personality disorders: does it work? 5th international congress on borderline personality disorders and allied disorders. 2018; Sep. 27 -29 Sitges (Barcelona, Spain).
53. Verdaguer E, Castillo JA, Plaza A. Efectividad del tratamiento y seguimiento longitudinal de pacientes con TLP tratados en Hospital de Día (Tesis Doctoral). Barcelona: Universitat Ramon Llull; 2017.

Transference-Focused Psychotherapy (TFP) Based Group Therapy

10

Bernhard Grimmer, Benjamin Kraus, Maya Krischer, Christiane Rösch, and Sandra Vohl

Introduction

Decades of research on the efficacy of group psychotherapy suggest that this treatment modality demonstrates outcomes comparable to those of individual psychotherapy [1]. Based on its cost-effectiveness and accumulated evidence, group psychotherapy is now widely used in outpatient settings and constitutes a substantial part of psychotherapeutic inpatient and day hospital treatment. Clinicians have implemented a wide range of group therapy interventions modified for various theoretical orientations and patient populations; this process has been akin to the development of different individual psychotherapy approaches over the years. The evolution of group psychotherapy techniques has been significantly influenced by theoretical concepts introduced for individual psychotherapy. However, these concepts could not be transferred directly in the context of the group setting but required modification for that treatment format.

In this chapter, we address the question of to what extent basic principles of Transference-focused psychotherapy (TFP), an established and evidence based psychodynamic psychotherapy derived from object relations theory for patients with personality disorders (PD) [2], can be transferred to the group psychotherapy setting. Similarities and differences between TFP as an individual psychotherapy and TFP-oriented group psychotherapy, as well as specific modifications necessary for

B. Grimmer (✉) · B. Kraus · C. Rösch
Psychiatric Services Thurgau, Münsterlingen, Switzerland

University Hospital for Psychiatry and Psychotherapy, Paracelsus Medical University, Salzburg, Austria
e-mail: bernhard.grimmer@stgag.ch; benjamin.kraus@stgag.ch; christiane.roesch@stgag.ch

M. Krischer · S. Vohl
Department of Child and Adolescent Psychiatry, Psychotherapy and Psychosomatics at the University Clinic of Cologne, Cologne, Germany
e-mail: maya.krischer@uk-koeln.de; sandra.vohl@uk-koeln.de

R. G. Hersh, C. De Panfilis (eds.), *Implementing Transference-Focused Psychotherapy Principles*, https://doi.org/10.1007/978-3-031-68062-5_10

the group setting, will be discussed. In addition, those modifications required for different treatment environments (e.g., inpatient versus day hospital) and different age groups (adults versus adolescents) are detailed. It is beyond the scope of this chapter to review all of the details of group TFP as outlined by Kernberg in work done under his supervision at New York Presbyterian Hospital-Westchester Division in the past. The two examples offered here use Kernberg's work as an inspiration while building on that model with different patient populations and settings [3].

TFP-Based Group Therapy for Adults with Personality Disorders: The Munsterlingen Program

Who Are the Clinicians?

The treatment programs in Munsterlingen, Switzerland are staffed by psychiatrists and psychologists providing direct care to patients across a continuum of services. These clinicians are customarily introduced to group treatment theory and practice in their training. Generally, the clinicians are also trained in TFP as an individual psychotherapy. The clinicians in the Munsterlingen programs work in inpatient, day hospital, and outpatient settings, informed by the overarching goal of providing patients with continuity of care across a continuum of services. TFP-informed groups have been offered since 2008.

Who Are the Patients?

Psychiatric Hospital Munsterlingen (PHM) is a hospital with 210 beds and compulsory admission for psychiatric patients in Canton Thurgau in Switzerland. It is part of a state-supported system that accommodates all local residents. The patients are a heterogeneous group who are offered treatment in a variety of settings based on clinical acuity:

- The system's outpatient program offers TFP-informed groups for those patients with all kinds of diagnoses. These patients are usually sufficiently stable to live at home and work while accessing treatments.
- Patients who are more impaired require the structure and supervision of the day hospital setting. TFP-informed groups are offered as part of a psychoanalytically oriented treatment design [4], which consists of a coordinated integration of individual and group psychotherapy, psychopharmacological treatment, music, movement, art and milieu therapy, social work, and relaxation techniques.
- The inpatient psychotherapy unit at the PHM treats patients who are medically or psychiatrically unstable and therefore require more intensive therapy. These patients suffer from high comorbidity, significant symptom load, and severe interpersonal problems. TFP-informed groups are offered as part of a psychoanalytically oriented treatment design established by Janssen [4], with consists of a

coordinated integration of individual and group psychotherapy, psychopharmacological treatment, music, movement, art and milieu therapy, social work, and relaxation techniques.

What Is the Contemporary Standard of Care for Clinicians Treating these Patients?

As noted, group treatment options have been a key element in mental health services for decades. These groups have been identified as offering a significant additional dimension to treatment, which allows for examination in real time of interactions among patients and the group process that emerges organically in such situations. Psychodynamic or psychoanalytically informed groups grew in popularity in the 1970s with wide dissemination for patients with a variety of diagnoses and different levels of acuity. In more recent years, the empirically validated treatments for patients with borderline personality disorder (BPD) or other moderate to severe PD presentations, have included group elements in their design. For example, dialectical behavioral therapy (DBT) [5], mentalization-based therapy (MBT) [6], and systems training for emotional predictability and problem solving (STEPPS) [7] all include a group component as part of their intervention.

In many mental health services, groups of different kinds are offered, in part because of the cost-effective nature of these options, which allow more patients to be treated as compared to individual modalities only. Group therapies can also be delivered in combination with various individual modalities. TFP-informed groups were developed originally in the inpatient setting, at a time when patients with PD diagnoses were sometimes hospitalized for many weeks or months. Changing healthcare economics in some countries eventually led to a marked reduction in such long-term psychiatric hospitalization opportunities, but group interventions grew in outpatient settings, including those like the day hospital, which were put together to offer some of the support and supervision no longer available with the demise of long-term inpatient PD institutions. As described in Chap. 7 of this volume, extended inpatient hospital units for patients with PD diagnoses do still exist in the Netherlands and the German-speaking countries, Germany, Austria, and Switzerland. The development of TFP-informed groups adds to group interventions of different kinds already firmly part of the inpatient treatment schedule.

The development of TFP-informed group therapy by Kernberg built on landmark observations outlined by Bion. These observations were understandably influenced by the currents of psychoanalytic thinking dominant at the time. It is useful to put into context Kernberg's introduction of a group TFP modality by reflecting on Bion's landmark contribution from an earlier time. On the basis of his studies, Bion [5] described three typical forms of regressive group constellations, what he called "basic assumptions groups." Kernberg [3] summarized them as follows:

1.) Mode dependence

Oral-dependent conflicts predominate. The group leader is initially idealized and fantasized as omnipotent and omniscient, while dependence and experienced incapacity, as well as feelings of impotence, dominate in the group. The group participants strive to receive attention, encouragement, love, and recognition from the group leader, of whom they are at the same time envious. If the group leader fails to satisfy their desires, the group reacts with massive disappointment and devaluation. Under certain circumstances, an attempt is made to remove the leader and look for a new one who will fulfill the expectations. Typical immature defense mechanisms in this constellation are idealization, projected omnipotence, denial of aggression, envy, and greed.

2.) Mode combat escape

The group climate is characterized by anal conflicts over power and control as well as feelings of persecution. The group feels threatened from the outside or a split develops within the group between an inner and an outer group. The leader is supposed to be a powerful protector defending the group against enemies. Alternatively, splitting occurs between those who admire and submit to the group leader and those who want to depose and fight him. The dominant defense mechanisms are splitting and projection of aggression, omnipotent control, idealization, and generally a paranoid climate.

3.) Pair formation mode

There is a tendency from within the group to create an idealized couple that will ensure the continuity of the group as ideal and powerful parents. This is to replace the leadership and make it independent of him. At the same time, aggression and conflicts within the group are avoided through defense in the form of eroticization and sexualization. The level of pair-building groups is clearly more oedipal than the other two modes, where pre-oedipal themes dominate.

Along with those conceptualizations, Bion [5] postulated a more mature mode, i.e., the working group mode. In this mode, the group deals with the internal and external realities and works goal-driven and rationally towards solving tasks and challenges. In this way, the working group mode serves as the ego function of groups. The group culture is driven by a cooperative basic attitude, in which strong conflicts can occur in order to be mastered. Thus, the level of the defense mechanisms in this group mode is higher than in the basic assumptions groups. Depending on the internal and external threats that the group is exposed to, the level of personality functioning of the individual group members, and the group constellation, there are oscillations between basic assumption and working group modes.

For Kernberg's conception of TFP-oriented group therapy [3], the further development of Bion's model of regressive work groups by Ezriel is of importance [6]. In psychotherapeutic groups where the focus is on the treatment of individual patients, the exclusive analysis of the current group mode, and the conflicts affecting the group as a whole, is not sufficient. Ezriel combines the analysis of the current dominant group themes with the question of how the individual members of the group position themselves in relation to the current central conflict theme of the group [6]. The starting point is the question of which conflicts preoccupy the group, which conflict resolution strategies emerge in terms of group pressure, and which conflict components (the central fear and threat in the group) are thereby averted. In other words, the aim is to decipher the psychosocial, interpersonal conflict constellations and defense mechanisms. At the same time, the group process explores how its members position themselves as these conflicts emerge and what side an individual may take on a particular subject. The behavior of the individual group members is understood as reflecting both the prevailing group pressures, as well as the dyads activated for the individual in this moment.

The initiative to use TFP principles in group treatment was therefore launched building on the foundation of work by Bion and others who were not necessarily focused on groups comprised of individuals with confirmed PD diagnoses. TFP-informed groups were developed specifically for patients with PD diagnoses, with particular attention to those pitfalls associated with offering a group intervention better suited to higher functioning patients to those patients with prominent PD pathology, thereby requiring the adjustments to standard group offerings referenced earlier.

What Are the Goals for Imparting to these Clinicians the Principles of TFP for Working with These Patients?

TFP was developed as an individual psychotherapy for patients with personality disorders functioning at a borderline level of organization. This group, described as meeting criteria for a borderline personality organization (BPO), encompasses patients with BPD and other personality disorder presentations. The therapeutic relationship is designed so that the multiple aspects of the patient's sense of self (termed self-representation), the patient's experience of another (sometimes someone in the patient's life, sometimes the therapist), and an associated affect, can be named and explored in the here-and-now. These experiences of self and others are described as object relations dyads; the emergence of these dyads in the context of the treatment relationship, or transference, are described and then systematically explored in TFP. The TFP therapist maintains an attitude of technical neutrality (meaning making an effort not to identify with a particular side of a patient's conflict), and uses clarification, confrontation, and eventually interpretation, to bring into the patient's awareness what might be denied or split off. The overarching goal of the treatment is to help address the patient's identity diffusion and reflexive use of defenses that reinforce a rigidity in their experiences of themselves and of others. This change is also described as the evolution from the paranoid-schizoid position to the depressive position [7–9]. This process is supported by a stable long-term setting and the limitation of destructive acting out [10].

In the group therapy setting, patients encounter each other and the group leader, bringing to the interactions their specific, individual patterns of experiencing self and others (what in TFP would be called object relations dyads). Along with those object relations dyads in evidence, there are also those dyads that are split off and not necessarily in evidence on the surface. In the group process, conflicts emerge between group members and between the group and the leader.

As in individual therapy, the group leader can name the emerging object relations dyads in evidence, informed by transference and countertransference currents, and bring this into the awareness of the patients involved. This approach can be described as individual therapy in the group. The group leader's interventions address the patient or patients interacting and describe role assignment and role assumption.

Along with a focus on the individual in the group, the group leader attends to the dynamics of the group as a whole. The group therapy situation cannot be understood only as the sum of individual dyadic interactions and relationship patterns. Regardless of the size of the group, the presence of other patients creates a triadic situation for everyone, which brings certain psychological challenges: shared attention; being the center of attention or being overlooked; belonging or being excluded; admiration or shaming; or envy and competition.

Groups develop their own dynamics, peer pressure, specific group tensions, and issues. These phenomena reflect the central conflicts that are dominant in a particular group at a certain time. The behavior of any group member can only be partly explained by the individual's psychology; this behavior of an individual is also an expression of current group dynamics and conflicts within the group at a particular moment in time.

In unstructured and poorly controlled group situations, strong pressures toward regression usually arise. In all psychoanalytically informed group therapies, including a TFP-oriented group, the group leader can sometimes initially act mostly observant and restrained, refraining from introducing topics; this can both motivate the group members to associate and interact as freely as possible but also can engender regression and anxiety among group members. When a TFP-oriented group therapy involves patients with moderate to lower levels of personality organization with associated impairments in functioning, this dynamic of possible regression is further enhanced.

Outpatient Group Therapy

For an outpatient TFP group therapy, Kernberg recommends five to eight participants and a session duration of 90 minutes with two sessions per week [3]. The group should work together as cohesively as possible over an extended period of time and, if possible, have no contact with each other outside of the group sessions. The group leader reserves the right to discuss confidential information about individual patients when necessary; this information may come to the group leader's attention outside of the group process. This policy serves to limit any individual group member's divisive tendencies or attempts to control the group process. Establishment of this policy requires that it is discussed and agreed upon in advance with all patients involved.

Inpatient Group Therapy

In inpatient TFP group therapy, the setting is influenced by the fact that patients also interact intensively with each other and with the group leader outside the group sessions. Inevitably, the interactions and transferences in the here-and-now in the group session and outside of group therapy become the topic in the sessions. Group therapy thus becomes precisely the place where the interactions, acted partial self-affect-object relations, and conflicts that take place in the everyday life of the ward can be named, made conscious, and integrated. It follows that it is even more important for the group leader to have the freedom to address and interpret what happens inside and outside of group therapy during a patient's inpatient treatment. All patients on a ward should participate in group therapy if possible. This can lead to a group size significantly larger than five to eight participants. If the group becomes larger, the danger of regressive processes and the anxiety of individual members will increase. The possibility that patients will withdraw from the group and not participate for the entire duration of hospitalization also will increase. Therefore, the group leader's even more active role is required to promote communication and interaction addressing individual patients directly. In addition, a higher frequency of at least three weekly sessions is recommended, so that there are not extended periods between groups in which patients interact with each other without an opportunity for reflection on these interactions in the group. In this way, group therapy has the function of not only making patients aware of the themes, group tensions, and transferences currently affectively dominant in the group but also facilitating the exploration of group dynamics with the goal of enhancing the working atmosphere on the ward.

Because inpatient treatment is limited in time, it is important to follow TFP's considerations about the early phase of therapy and Bion's concept of working groups [5]. The group setting is usually unfamiliar and frightening for patients. It creates tension and activates regressive individual and group processes. The attitude of the group leader is oriented toward the anxiety and tension level of the individuals and the entire group. Accordingly, interventions are sometimes more supportive and sometimes more confrontational. Above all, it must be kept in mind that progress and integration are only possible through the patient's recognition and the acknowledgment of destructive patterns, which is often painful.

Sexual and romantic relationships often develop among inpatients; these relationships can be impulsive and secretive and occur despite stated unit policies discouraging such activities. These relationships can be understood as manifestations of expressions of primitive idealization, often serving as protection against the threatening group situation. The revelation of this kind of sexual or romantic relationships among inpatients requires processing within the group therapy. In a similar vein, the group therapy situation is the appropriate venue for exploration of expressions of externalization, as in the "bad" authorities outside, the "stupid" people outside the therapeutic setting, etc.

As described, it is evident that outpatient and inpatient TFP-informed group therapy share several central tenets. These tenets include reflection on group processes as oscillations between basic assumption groups and working groups, thereby regulating anxiety and tension within the group, and limiting the activation of participants' destructive impulses. While in the inpatient setting the function of containing is predominantly performed by the group leader; in an effective outpatient group, the containing can be done by the group itself.

What Is the Source of Institutional or Government Support for this Initiative?

The programs in Munsterlingen are supported by the Swiss government and initiatives like TFP-informed group therapy are vetted by administrative bodies overseeing use of government funding.

What TFP Principles Might Be of Utility for the Clinicians Working with These Patients?

Free Association in the Group

The role of the leader in TFP-oriented group therapy is much more active than in a traditional analytic group therapy. Nevertheless, sufficient attention must be paid to free association, to the group members' ideas, and their significance in the group context must be appreciated.

The group leader limits long periods of silence and encourages the group members to interact among themselves and participate actively. Extended periods of silence are avoided given the risk that they can lead to an even stronger regression of the group; other associated risks include the withdrawal of individual group members and increased anxiety, expressions of more pronounced primitive defense mechanisms, and more intense paranoid transferences for some participants. As in individual TFP therapy, the group leader intervenes from a position of technical neutrality and deviates only temporarily in the case of behaviors that endanger the patient, others, or the therapy itself. These problematic behaviors can include aggressive attacks on other group members or the group leader. It is also advisable to negotiate an individual therapy agreement with each patient for participation in group therapy and to define responsibilities within the group and in crisis situations outside the group.

Employing the Three Channels of Communication

As in individual TFP, in a TFP-informed group treatment attention is paid to the three channels of communication. In addition to what the patients say, special attention is focused on how the patients behave, with an emphasis placed on the discrepancies between verbal and non-verbal communication. As mentioned, the group members' sentiments about each other are often expressed non-verbally. In TFP-oriented group therapy, these reactions expressed non-verbally are actively identified by the group leader, sometimes requiring the group leader to interrupt an interaction, depending on multiple contributing factors. In doing so, the group leader tries to label the non-verbally expressed feeling in a descriptive, non-judgmental, and curious way: "You averted your gaze…" or "You seem to be getting restless…" The group leader also uses his countertransference as a basis for these interventions, less frequently in relation to an individual group member and more often in relation to the group as a whole.

Management of Negative and Positive Transferences

In the situation of group therapy, it is inevitable that both positive and negative transferences are activated simultaneously for group members. The patient's mixed positive and negative reactions will involve all the other group members and the group leader. It is likely that intensely positive transferences (marked by idealization), and intensely negative transferences (marked by devaluation), will be in evidence, and the interplay between these transference reactions will be fluid and meaningful.

As in individual TFP, the exploration of expressions of negative transference is a priority in a TFP-informed group treatment for patients with PDs. In the case of open hostility, this seems self-evident; the group leader is compelled to take up the affectively dominant aggressive affect. When comparable negative affects are expressed non-verbally, the group leader is similarly obligated to make this a priority. Patients with PD pathology frequently have conflicts related to aggression. Aggression may not be integrated, ambivalence cannot be tolerated, and subsequent expression of aggression can be intense. The group leader is challenged to examine negative transferences, label them, and interpret these sentiments for individuals in the group and as they reflect aspects of the group as a whole. The first step toward the integration of purely positive (idealized) or negative (devalued) experiences of self and others requires the therapist or group leader to tolerate and name the dyads as they emerge in treatment.

It is possible to understand certain symptoms of significant PD pathology such as somatization, self-harm, suicidality, or promiscuity as reflecting a patient's challenge in tolerating experiences of self and others imbued with powerful hatefulness. A critical situation in group therapy arises when group members adopt a condemning attitude toward a group member to protect themselves from confronting their own destructiveness. A major task for the group leader is ensuring that the group allows for examination of expressions of destructiveness. If negative transferences do not appear in the context of group therapy, it may be assumed that the group leader is in denial because of fear, or that there are processes of projective identification between the group and the group leader. Motivation for participation in group therapy and the experience of the effectiveness of group therapy depend crucially on whether negative effects can be expressed. It is expected that these negative reactions will be part of *all* effective therapy groups. The new, corrective experience for the patient is that the negative affect can be experienced, regulated, and metabolized through discussion, reflection, and understanding.

As outlined, the processing of negative transferences is imperative in an effective TFP-informed group treatment; similarly, the emergence of idealizing transferences should also be described and discussed. It may be possible to tolerate an initial idealizing transference of the group leader, which is expected to wane. When the idealizing transference of the group leader occurs in tandem with a split-off negative transference, it is of benefit to interpret this circumstance.

The idealization of the group leader can be understood as: (1) a regressive defense of the whole group (the basic assumption group of dependence described by Bion), (2) a regressive defense of the individual group member, or (3) a reflection of a defensive stance ascribable to the group leader. The group leader may assume the role of the "expert" as a reflection of a group process that can be understood as a group "seduction." The group leader may need to actively resist the tendency to respond to the collective idealization of group members and risk becoming a disappointing object; doing so may make the group leader vulnerable to the expression of aggression by the group. The group leader's ability to manage experiences of narcissistic vulnerability, thereby relinquishing the idealized role and fostering a position of being a "good enough" group leader, is critical.

Maintaining Technical Neutrality

When working through the manifestations of negative transference (open devaluation, covert devaluation expressed through contempt, rule violations, and violation of the setting) and interpretation of these negative transferences, the use of technical neutrality is of central importance. The patients´ experiences and negative affects expressed in different ways (acted out non-verbally or expressed verbally) are not immediately sanctioned, morally condemned, or devalued, as long as they are not threatening to the other group members.

The group leader's use of technical neutrality will be challenged when couples are formed; this is the case in both inpatient and outpatient group situations. Often the emerging pair in a group situation will express unalloyed positive affects; in this case, self and object are endowed with ideal qualities, often of "unreal quality" [11] that protect the pair from the threat of the group. The group leader has to maintain technical neutrality and work out the individual and group psychodynamics given the inherent threat to the capacity of the group when pair formation occurs.

Basically, in all analytic groups, one can assume an oscillation between regressive and progressive group processes reflecting respectively an alternating pattern between basic assumption and working group modes. The interventions of the group leaders are not primarily aimed at the re-establishment of a working group, but rather at making conscious the etiologies of the regressive defense processes observed. The technically neutral attitude of the group leader employing TFP principles ensures that the individual group members, and the group as a whole, will benefit from a well-functioning intervention. In situations that threaten to derail the group marked by activated aggressive affects, however, the group leader must immediately abandon technical neutrality and protect the setting, returning to technical neutrality as quickly as possible. Technical neutrality does not mean passivity. Particularly in outpatient groups for patients with PD pathology, it is important especially at the beginning of a group session to identify and "name" emerging disorder-specific interpersonal problems. The members of an outpatient group may hope for progress through harmonious togetherness rather than painstaking exploration. Clinical experience shows that even in groups that have been running for a long time, the group leader is always challenged to maintain a constructive group culture through timely interventions.

The Process of Interpretation in the Group: Clarification, Confrontation, and Interpretation

The goal of TFP-oriented group therapy corresponds to that of TFP in the individual setting. Through an in-depth exploration of the complex cognitive and emotional processes in the interactions of the here-and-now, the aim is to focus and modify the patient's cognitive self-concept in his or her relationship with others [10]. In individual TFP, the interpretive process, which consists of clarification, confrontation, and interpretation, is guided by the therapist. In TFP-oriented group therapy, the interpretive process is directed only in part by the group leader. Clarification, confrontation, and also interpretation will be done by the group members, if the group functions at a working group level. The leader has the task to intervene in such a way that the group members take over especially the first two steps in the interpretative process among themselves: clarifying and confronting.

The group leader might intervene, for example, when one group member responds with guidance or advice to another member who has described an active internal or external conflict. This is more common with new group members who are not yet familiar with the therapeutic stance of a TFP-oriented group. This same pattern also occurs when tensions and anxiety within the group are activated, sometimes for the individual offering advice and guidance, or sometimes for the group as a whole. Depending on the total situation and the group leader's impression, an early intervention may be indicated. The group leader might acknowledge the relief conferred for the individual offering the guidance (thereby conveying validation, as might be appropriate for a new group member), while also naming the defensive aspect of the patient's actions. Although the group leader intervenes very cautiously when the group is functioning on a working group level, when there is a risk for regression to a basic assumption group because of defensiveness, a timely intervention is necessary. Thus, on the one hand, a certain amount of tension is imposed on the group, while on the other hand, the group leader ensures that the working group culture is maintained consistently through active, validating, and confrontational interventions. These interventions consist of mutual exploration, inquiry, and clarification; simultaneously the group leader actively monitors countertransference reactions to the material raised.

Kernberg formulates the TFP interventions in the context of group therapy as follows [3]:

1. Clarification: working out what the affectively dominant group issues are at any given time.
2. Confrontation: naming contradictions, especially between verbal and non-verbal behavior, as well as contradictions between different verbally expressed positions in the group.
3. Interpretation: The dominant group theme is named, based on the exploration by the group leader of conscious and preconscious experiences in the group. After naming the theme observed, the group leader describes how it is introduced and speculates about the pertinent motivation of group members. The group leader formulates hypotheses about what themes may be avoided and how this might

reflect a dominant fear in the group; in this way, the group leader interprets the unconsciously averted parts of the group conflict.

What Are Possible Targets for Measurement to Gauge the Effectiveness of Instruction About Applications of TFP Principles?

TFP is intended not only to achieve symptom reduction and patient satisfaction, but also has the goal of bringing about change in personality structure. This change in personality structure results from a joint examination of the transference relationship between patient and therapist as well as the exploration of the patient's pattern of object relations. Kernberg and his colleagues have described their sophisticated treatment intervention focusing on the here-and-now of the patient's experience, transference currents, and the exploration of defensive operations [10]. The same goals for symptom reduction, patient satisfaction, and change in personality structure would be expectable targets for measurement in TFP-informed group therapy interventions.

What Are the Didactic Materials Required to Impart TFP Principles to this Target Group of Clinicians?

This involves the application of video material and discussion of the dynamics of the group processes in the supervision.

What Is the Format for Instruction of TFP Principles to this Audience?

Clinicians learn the principles of TFP in ongoing training and supervision.

Clinical Illustration

Ms. E., a confectioner of about 30 years of age, was approached in her third inpatient group therapy session by Ms. W., who was in her mid-twenties. Ms. W. said that she had heard that Ms. E. was taking care of her because she considered her weaker than herself. Ms. E. confirmed that she had said this, but that she had not meant it in a malicious or degrading way. Ms. W. actually triggered pity and the need to mother her. The 30-year-old Ms. R., a very well-groomed, attractive, caring mother with long black hair, who shared a room with her, then intervened. She stated, that she did not understand Mrs. E. and she was afraid of her. She said that Mrs. E. had been very affectionate and friendly in the conversations in the shared room, but seemed aggressive and hostile outside the room when they were interacting with the fellow patients. She added that she had become afraid since Ms. E. had told her about her dream in which she, Ms. R., no longer had long hair. She had felt the need to change her room and wondered why she had not been threatened.

In a very short time, the self-object dyads dominating the inner world of Mrs. E. and defending against each other were revealed during the group therapy session. Toward Mrs. W., who was experienced as weaker and needy, Mrs. E. felt and behaved as a caring and superior ideal object in relation to a needy self, which was projected onto Mrs. W. In the relation with Mrs. R., on the other hand, a role reversal of this self-object-dyad seemed to be activated at first. Mrs. E. was identified with her needy self, longing for a gratifying provider, whose role was now projected onto Mrs. R. However, this dyad was defending against an opposite one, where Mrs. E. was identified with a needy but rejected and uncared for child in relation to a superior but neglecting object. The intense negative affect linking these split-off selves and other representations could not be overtly expressed at the same time toward Mrs. R. but could only emerge in Mrs. E.'s awareness at different times or expressed toward other fellow patients. Intuitively, Mrs. E.'s dream was interpreted coherently by Mrs. R. perceiving Mrs. E.'s split-off aggression.

These dyads, split between two group members and dominating Mrs. E.'s inner world, could be worked out in this group session with the help of the group leader. The group leader paid special attention to the tolerance of the occurrence of the negative, hostile affect expressed in the dream, which was activated in the context of a disappointment during Mrs. E's relationship with Mrs. R. He then named the various dyads as they emerged during the session, and tactfully pointed out that Mr. E. was facing an inner conflict between the desperate wish to be perfectly cared for and the belief that the others would be rejecting her. Thus, negative affect, anger, and aggression toward others would emerge when Mr. E. was more fully identified with a representation of self as neglected by cold, distant others—while the corresponding idealized representations of self and others were split-off and denied. By tolerating the negative affects that emerged in the session and by verbalizing them openly together with the other group members, the group leader fostered the process of integration, within Mrs. E's internal world, of purely negative (devalued) and positive (idealized, but equally unrealistic) experiences of self and others.

Conclusion

We have presented a novel program where principles of TFP have been integrated with the analytic group therapy of adult patients with BPO. This has been accomplished by introducing unique TFP elements into the practice of group therapy, both at the inpatient and outpatient levels of care. Such unique elements include the active monitoring of the three channels of communication within the group dynamics, the examination of both positive and negative transferences among group members and between them and the group leader, and an emphasis on the process of interpretation and on maintaining technical neutrality. This application of TFP principles to the group modality of therapy is rooted in previous work by Kernberg [2,

11–17] and may represent a useful and cost-effective treatment option for patients with personality disorders.

TFP-Based Group Therapy for Adolescents with Personality Disorders: A Day Hospital Program

Who Are the Clinicians?

In January 2014, the Department of Child and Adolescent Psychiatry, Psychotherapy and Psychosomatic Medicine at the University Clinic of Cologne University opened a new specialized psychotherapeutic unit–a day hospital for adolescents with borderline pathology. Two of the authors of this chapter (MK, SV) were in charge of the implementation of group therapy in this ward. There was no previously developed concept of group therapy for adolescents with personality development disorders using techniques of TFP. Therefore, the methodology was developed along with the therapeutic work and was continuously improved under supervision. The concept of applied TFP for borderline adolescents in a day clinic program is further explained in Chap. 6 of this handbook [18].

We consider group psychotherapy as an especially essential treatment element for adolescents. Taking the developmental tasks for juveniles in general into account, adolescence is a transition phase from childhood to adulthood in which separation and individuation are essential, the dependence on parents needs to be reduced, and, finally, in which aggressive and sexual drives can lead to severe anxiety [19]. In borderline adolescents, these tasks can lead to severe episodes of crises and breakdowns. Based on these general developmental difficulties, their ability to reflect is not as pronounced as in adults [20, 21]. During treatment, the adolescent patient can be helped in the consolidation of identity by peers who can function as a transitional object and as a mirror of split-off self-representations. These interactions with peers thereby support the adolescent patient in developing capacities for reflection and for separation-individuation.

The group is led by a therapist specialized and certified in treatment of children and adolescents and in individual TFP for Adolescents (TFP-A) (Sandra Vohl) with a further qualification in group-based psychodynamic therapy as well as a co-therapist who is part of the care and education service of the day hospital unit and is trained in TFP-A theory [22].

Who Are the Patients?

The group therapy in the day hospital for adolescents is embedded in a multimodal treatment concept and takes place twice a week. Every session lasts 75 minutes. After being admitted to the hospital, the adolescents will have a one-on-one conversation with the therapist who is in charge of the group therapy (SV). The therapist informs the patients about the setting, rules, and possible contents of the group sessions. Furthermore, another purpose of this conversation is to find out about fears, worries, and expectations of the patients. Due to new admittances and discharges from the day hospital, the group is half-open, meaning new patients may join a pre-existing group while the other group members may be discharged early.

What Is the Contemporary Standard of Care for Clinicians Treating These Patients?

Prior to the development of the TFP-A day hospital program described in Chap. 6, these patients were treated in regular inpatient and outpatient units designed for a heterogeneous patient population.

What Is the Source of Institutional or Government Support for this Initiative?

This TFP-informed group intervention is part of the TFP-A day hospital program described in Chap. 6. This program was newly developed for adolescent patients with BPO, and the treatment is paid for by the German healthcare system.

What Are the Goals for Imparting to These Clinicians the Principles of TFP for Working with These Patients?

The clinicians at the Department of Child and Adolescent Psychiatry, Psychotherapy, and Psychosomatic Medicine at the University Clinic of Cologne University were versed in both TFP-A, the treatment modality developed for adolescents adapting TFP for this age group, and in various group therapy interventions. Integrating TFP principles into a group format, used in pilot programs as detailed earlier by Kernberg, had not been tried before in therapeutic work with adolescent patients. The innovative clinicians involved used their familiarity and experience in conducting group treatments with adolescent patients in this new way informed by the ambitious goals of individual TFP. Thus, implementing the day hospital treatment with the TFP-oriented group intervention aimed at further fostering the effectiveness of the program in promoting identity integration, symptom reduction, and good psychosocial functioning among borderline adolescents.

What TFP Principles Might Be of Utility for the Clinicians Working with These Patients?

Establishing Goals

Among other tasks, the patients need to learn to talk about their goals for the treatment. This TFP element—defining a treatment goal—was implemented into the treatment frame for borderline adolescents admitted to the day hospital program. This implementation aimed to address the predominantly regressive attitude of borderline adolescent patients who identify very often with the split-off self-representation of a helpless child who has no sense of responsibility. By agreeing to name a treatment goal during their day hospital treatment (of 12 weeks) the goal is to bring a split-off, or dissociated, responsible self-experience into their awareness and thereby reduce the tendency for self-destructive behavior, which is often based upon this passive-aggressive attitude.

The treatment goals are usually defined before attending the group session for the first time and are put on record in a conversation with the patient's counselor at the start of hospital treatment. The aim is to make the goals transparent and open for discussion with the whole group. This means the adolescents who are admitted into treatment have agreed upon an obligation to mention what they are working on and what they would like to change. The patient's agreement, or contract, for group participation, includes the following:

- Accepting help and support in order to limit those behaviors linked to self-harm and harm to others
- Aiming to be approachable and therefore tolerating confrontation
- Agreeing to confront others about their destructive behaviors when evident

When formulating these objectives, it is important to keep them realistic. This means it must be possible for the treatment team and other patients to monitor adherence to the elements of this agreement. Moreover, the patients are asked to formulate their objectives in explicitly constructive ways. Instead of saying: "I don't want to cut myself anymore," they would be asked to be more concrete, with an objective outlined as thus, "If I feel pressured to harm myself, I will look for alternatives, such as contacting another person seeking connection, rather than cutting myself."

A newly added group member may disclose her objectives, or a more senior group member may talk about changes in their objectives or the state of her treatment. The idea is to make the developments visible to everyone and to make resistance against the process, and the possible reasons for it, understandable.

The group helps to substantiate the individual patient's goals:

When an adolescent patient describes treatment goals, for instance: "When I am in a fight with my mother or a friend and want to harm myself, I would like to find an alternative way to deal with my anger." Then the group therapists might ask a number of specific clarifying questions:

- How do you usually harm yourself?
- In what kind of situations?
- What would you like to achieve in these kinds of situations?

The group will then be included in reflecting on the transference aspect (or interactional aspect) in these situations, thus avoiding an "individual therapy session within the group." Sometimes the group will ask more questions because some things may not be clear enough to understand what is going on. As a result, the group members often refer to themselves and describe that they have similar feelings in these situations, or that they feel differently but that they can at least partially understand what has been described. Alternatively, they may have experienced similar problems but learned how to deal with them in a different way. Whatever the feedback may look like, it usually provides great relief for the patient who just talked about their treatment objectives and thus revealed her/ his inner difficulties. This relief often provides the basis for dealing with their own difficulties in the group and reduces feelings of shame when the group acts tactfully. Also, it encourages the other patients to open up about their inner difficulties and the feelings of shame that come with them. They realize that there are peers with similar difficulties. Shortly after being admitted to the clinic a 15-year-old patient said in her first group therapy: "Finally, I do not feel like the weirdest person in the world anymore!"

When working on these specific objectives, the patients should connect with their healthy ego-parts. These are dissociated parts of the ego that represent progression instead of regression. Focusing on the therapeutic objectives means putting the progressive part into the spotlight.

Establishing a Treatment Frame

In the TFP-based group therapy the customary rules for other group modalities will apply, such as respecting the conditions of treatment (i.e., being on time, not leaving the room during the session if possible, and so forth), keeping personal information of other group members confidential, and being respectful toward the other members.

The group therapists usually do not suggest any topics. At times, there are situations that are considered relevant for the group and the therapeutic process. When this is the case then the group therapists may address this in the group. In general, the therapists are only as active as necessary. Their level of activity depends on the composition of the group: sometimes they help to keep the central theme in mind, and at other times they moderate the process. Occasionally, they will need to be more active, for instance when they summarize the content, or when they want to activate a passive group by structuring the meeting and addressing the group members. Additionally, they keep the time. Sometimes, patients who may dominate will be instructed to refrain from doing so, so that everyone has a chance to speak.

Monitoring Various Channels of Communication

Systematically paying attention to the various channels of communication has been proven useful in group therapy. This can help to clarify and reveal contradictions in messages:

Channel 1: Verbal messages of the patient
Channel 2: Nonverbal messages of the patient
Channel 3: Countertransference
Channel 4 The therapeutic alliance

Whenever the messages of the patients do not match their mimicry, tone of voice, or whatever is transmitted by countertransference, the TFP-A group therapist will address it.

Adding a Novel Intervention to Add a Dimension to a TFP-Specific Group

Using Photograph Cards Newly admitted members of the group, in particular, tend to address only the therapists during their first group meetings when they talk about themselves. The therapists pick up on that quickly and redirect the patient in order to establish a conversation between the new patient and the other adolescents instead.

Most group sessions in the unit begin with a roundtable. For this part, 10–12 photograph cards are placed in the middle of the room. Every adolescent picks a card and uses the image to describe how they are feeling or what could be a possible topic for group discussion. This is not a TFP-specific approach but from our experience, it is helpful to reflect on possible topics and to acquire a more active role for the adolescent. Additionally, it facilitates access to the therapeutic process. In particular, new members perceive this exercise as lowering their fear levels.

After finishing this task, current topics can be discussed. The patients use this opportunity often, but there are situations or group constellations in which the group members passively wait for someone else to take the lead. For instance, there also may be an unexpressed theme, perhaps a conflict between some members, which is on everyone's mind or unsettles the group. When a contradictory and fragmented mindset becomes obvious in a patient, we sometimes ask them to present this by using a technique from Gestalt therapy [23]. It is a possibility for deepened clarification, which is especially helpful when we think the patient can explain different points of view but is not in touch with the underlying emotions.

Role Play From our experience, it can be effective to use two different chairs for two oppositional representations of self and object dyads in order to address the affect. The patient in question first sits on one of the chairs, which represents one of these perspectives. The patient then describes what goes through their mind regarding that particular perspective. After that, the patient moves on to the second chair and repeats the procedure but with a different point of view. The second chair represents the other perspective, which mostly conveys a position contrary to the one of the first chair. A patient who had ambivalent feelings about the process in the clinic named the first chair "getting healthy" which meant staying in the day hospital. The second chair was called "staying ill" which symbolized a premature end of the treatment.

When such work with chairs is done, there is a lot of resonance from the group members who proceed to give feedback at the end of the session. In regard to the aforementioned patient, it became clear that she had considerable secondary gain in being sick, which led to an open discussion about which "advantages" of being ill the patients observed.

What Is the Contemporary Standard of Care for Clinicians Treating These Patients?

Before the creation of the TFP-A day hospital, juvenile patients with PD diagnoses were in treatment in regular inpatient and outpatient units.

What Is the Source of Institutional or Government Support for this Initiative?

The TFP-informed group treatment for adolescent patients with PD diagnoses is part of the TFP-A day hospital supported by the German health care system as outlined in Chap. 6.

What Are Possible Targets for Measurement to Gauge the Effectiveness of Instruction About Applications of TFP Principles?

Results of a study examining changes after treatment [24, 25] at the aforementioned University of Cologne adolescent day clinic suggested that group therapy plays an important role for any change. Group therapy increases the patient's ability for self-reflection, especially because adolescents are not only challenged to deal with their own difficulties and perspectives but also provide the group with an entire spectrum of perspectives, which represent different fractions of their self. Patients usually accept comments, feedback, or objections from peers more easily than by therapists, which enables them to change perspectives and thereby loosen their defensive rigidity. As is known from the literature, based on common developmental anxieties and feelings of shame, peers are of great importance in reducing anxiousness [19, 21]. At the same time, building a therapeutic alliance with adult therapists is often accompanied by resistance in juveniles. Adolescents tend to react in a tense and defensive fashion against adults' tactful remarks or confrontations due to their reflexive mistrust of certain adult figures.

Clinical Illustration

In the following excerpt from a group session the therapists aim to gain insight into what could have led a patient to have a violent and impulsive outburst in the day hospital unit. In the course of the session, it becomes obvious which affect was dominant, how she expressed it, and which part was separated and was directed at another person as part of a process not in the patient's awareness [26]. *The previous day, the patient, Carolin, hurt herself by banging her head against a wall. It was difficult to prevent her from doing this. This was probably triggered by anger about a staff member.*

Co-therapist	*"So, I was worried in that situation and felt somewhat helpless. How will you manage going forward? What will you do when you feel bad again? And I was wondering whether you know this feeling from other situations, that the other person feels helpless? Or how it is at home when things get difficult and how … how that plays out. That is what I've been thinking about."*
Carolin (laughs uncomfortably)	*"Ehm…shall I answer that question?"*
Co-therapist	*"Maybe you can start by telling me whether you can relate to this observation: Your peer feels helpless and doesn't know how to continue. So, do you know that this can happen? I feel like this is also a really bad situation for you."*
Carolin	*"Yes."*
Therapist (to the co-therapist)	*"You mean when the peer feels powerless, what does that mean to Carolin? That there is someone there who does not know what to do?"*
Co-therapist	*"Yes."*
Carolin	*"Yes, I am always worried that people are helpless in that case. So, that I think I caused this … and that I get even worse because I keep thinking: Yes, you caused this … now you have to keep throwing something at them (laughs). I don't know, somehow this is funny but … when someone would tell me 'I am helpless' when I am acting out … then I would probably get even more mad … I mean, I could also sit there and start crying like some … but that is out of the question for me. Then I would feel helpless myself!"*

In this case, the co-therapist starts the session by confronting the patient in the beginning with a current situation in front of the group, which is uncomfortable for the patient at first. At the same time, the co-therapist describes the role of feeling helpless, which was projected onto her and possibly represents a split-off part of Carolin's self, which she possibly denies in this situation. Following this exchange, the therapist invites the other group members to share their impressions about the reasons that could have caused Carolin's acting out the day before in the unit. One participant says he can possibly understand, at least in part, what Carolin was expressing. At times in the past, he also had angry outbursts at home, which were even more intense when he felt that his parents did not know how to help him to feel better or how to calm him down. This caused him to become more and more enraged, both at them and at himself. The therapist encourages the group members to clarify what strategies, in their experience, could be applied to interrupt this kind of "vicious circle". It turns out that some of them had learned to consider that when they are angry with others who don't seem to be of any help, in that circumstance, these friends or family members likely want to help but find it difficult to do so, as they are intimidated by the patient's angry and impulsive behavior. Another group member adds that, even in the unit, it helped her a lot to consider that, although at times she had felt irritated or frustrated by some staff members, they were actually doing their best to help her—in the same way she was doing her best to get better, although it required a lot of effort. "This is not anyone's fault," she commented quietly, "but it will take a lot of work and time to overcome my difficulties." Carolin was particularly relieved by the fact that other fellow patients experienced similar difficulties in regulating their levels of anger, especially when they perceived their carers as helpless. This reduced her shame about being responsible for others' painful feelings, as well as her fear of feeling weak and helpless. At the same time, the feedback from the group instilled hope in her that she could manage to change her behavior and ways of thinking and encouraged her to consider alternatives in managing challenging periods of anger without acting them out in counterproductive ways.

Overall, this is an example of using TFP techniques derived from individual therapy within the group setting while at the same time avoiding individual therapy within the group.

Conclusion

Adolescents are "in a transitional period of their physical and psychological development, in which (…) the relationship to peers is of great importance." [27]. The importance of the peer group becomes evident in the day clinic treatment of adolescents with BPD in a group setting. As already described in the first part of the chapter by Roesch and Grimmer, this leads to a triadic situation and due to this, several challenges (envy, competition, fear of humiliation, being included or excluded, being at the focus of attention or being overlooked) are in place that play an important role in the life of adolescent borderline patients. Tactful clarification and confrontation by other juveniles can help to loosen split-off and rigid defense mechanisms and support reflective capacities in borderline juveniles. The psychotherapy group based on TFP-A seems to be a unique place for juvenile borderline patients where they can learn from each other by taking in alternative perspectives in a safe and innovative opportunity.

Summary

TFP was originally conceived as an outpatient individual therapy. In this chapter, we have discussed the extent to which TFP principles can also be applied to TFP-oriented group therapy in both adult and adolescent populations with personality disorders. The similarities between individual TFP and TFP-oriented group therapy are: (1) the therapist assumes an active role, maintaining technical neutrality, when possible, (2) the focus of the intervention is on the "here-and-now" and not exclusive review of the past, (3) techniques included clarification, confrontation, and interpretation are used, and (4) the establishment and maintenance of a treatment contract help to limit acting our behaviors of different kinds.

That said, we have also proposed several modifications of individual TFP techniques to meet the specific characteristics and needs of groups. In groups, unlike in individual therapy, the group members, the group leader, and the group as a whole are confronted with a triadic situation mobilizing fear and consecutive regressive processes. This regression offers a complex matrix of transference-countertransference currents between the individual group members and between them and the group leader. Groups may be characterized by oscillations between modes of a "basic assumption group" and a "working group" as defined by Bion [5]. The major task of the group leader is to make conscious the respective inner tendencies toward regressive defense processes, while also promoting a "working group" atmosphere. In addition, we also have described the specifics of TFP-A-based group psychotherapy with adolescents as conducted in the context of a day clinic. There are special needs of adolescents, that can be addressed in TFP-A-based group psychotherapy.

References

1. Rosendahl J, Alldredge CT, Burlingame GM, Strauss B. Recent developments in group psychotherapy research. Am J Psychother. 2021;74(2):52–9.
2. Kernberg OF, Yeomans FE, Clarkin JF, Levy KN. Transference focused psychotherapy: overview and update. Int J Psychoanal. 2008;89(3):601–20.
3. Kernberg OF. Psychoanalytische Gruppenpsychotherapie. PTT-Persönlichkeitsstörungen: Theorie und Therapie. 2009;13(2):79–93.
4. Janssen PL. Zur Theorie und Praxis psychoanalytisch begründeter stationärer Psychotherapie. Forum Psychoanal. 2012;28(4):337–58.
5. Bion WR. Experiences in groups and other papers. London: Tavistock Publications; 1961.
6. Ezriel H. A psycho-analytic approach to group treatment. Br J Med Psychol. 1950;23:59–74.
7. Klein M. Notes on some schizoid mechanisms. Int J Psychoanal. 1946;27:99–110.
8. Klein M. On the development of mental functioning. Int J Psychoanal. 1958;39:84–90.
9. Klein M. Some theoretical conclusions regarding the emotional life of the infant. In: M. Klein PH, Isaacs S, Riviere J, editors. Developments in psychoanalysis. London: Hogarth Press; 1952. p. 198–236.
10. Yeomans FE, Clarkin JF, Kernberg OF. Transference-focused psychotherapy for borderline personality disorder: a clinical guide. Washington, DC: American Psychiatric Publishing; 2015.
11. Kernberg OF. Innere Welt und äussere Realität: Anwendungen der Objektbeziehungstheorie. 1988:237–267.
12. Clarkin JF, Kernberg OF. Transference-focused psychotherapy for borderline personality disorder: a clinical guide. Washington, DC: American Psychiatric Publishing; 2015.
13. Clarkin JF, Yeomans FE, Kernberg OF. Psychotherapy for borderline personality. Wiley; 1999.
14. Kernberg OF. Borderline personality organization. J Am Psychoanal Assoc. 1967;15(3):641–85.
15. Kernberg OF. Schwere Persönlichkeitsstörungen: Theorie, Diagnose. Behandlungsstrategien: Klett-Cotta; 1992.

16. Kernberg OF. Object relations theory and clinical psychoanalysis. New York: Jason Aronson; 1995.
17. Kernberg OF, Caligor E. A psychoanalytic theory of personality disorders. In: Lenzenweger MF, Clarkin JF, editors. Major theories of personality disorder. New York: Guilford Press; 2005. p. 114–56.
18. Krischer M. Transference Focused Psychotherapy for Adolescents with borderline personality pathology in the outpatient and day hospital treatment. In: Kinderanalyse, 2, p. 147–166. Peer Review, R. 2020.
19. Tschuschke V. Gruppenentwicklung—unverzichtbar für gruppentherapeutische Effekte? In: Langwalter W, Schiepek G, editors. Selbstorganisation und Dynamik in Gruppen. Münster: LIT-Verlag; 1995.
20. Krischer M, Drust M. Transference focused psychotherapy for adolescents—case example from the treatment of a 15 year–old patient with borderline personality organization. Persönlichkeitsstörungen, Theorie und Therapie. 2018;77:235–42. Peer Review
21. Krischer M, Drust M. Shame and guilt in treating adolescents with Borderline Personality Organization. In: Persönlichkeitsstörungen Theorie und Therapie, 25. Peer Review. 2021.
22. Normandin L, Ensink K, Weiner A, Kernberg OF. Transference-focused psychotherapy for adolescents with severe personality disorders. American Psychiatric Publishing; 2021.
23. Perls FS, Hefferline RF, Goodman P. Gestalttherapy. Stuttgart: Klett-Cotta; 2019.
24. Krischer M, Ponton-Rodriguez T, Gooran GR, Bender S. Übertragungsfokussierte Psychotherapie von Borderline-Jugendlichen im tagesklinischen Setting. Praxis der Kinderpsychologie und Kinderpsychiatrie. 2017;66:445–63.
25. Jahn C, Wieacker E, Bender S, Krischer M. Reduction of self-mutilative behavior in juveniles with Borderline Personality Organization treated with Transference-focused Psychotherapy for Adolescents (TFP-A) in a day clinic setting.Praxis der Kinderpsychologie und -psychiatrie. 2021.
26. Kehr G, Köpp W. Superego pathology in narcissistic personality disorder (NPS): the importance of sensing guilt and shame. Persönlichkeitsstörungen, Theorie und Therapie. 2021;25:47–63.
27. Tschuschke V. Research results in regard to therapeutic factors and outcome in group therapies with adolescents. Prax Kinderpsychol Kinderpsychiatr. 1996;1:38–45.

Part III

Transference-Focused Psychotherapy (TFP) Principles with Specific Patient Populations

11 Using Transference-Focused Psychotherapy (TFP) Principles in the Treatment of Forensic Patients

Fritz Lackinger

Introduction to the History of Transference-Focused Offender Treatment

The Psychoanalytic Tradition in the Treatment of Delinquents

This chapter deals with new initiatives informed by psychoanalytic concepts in a small number of forensic therapy facilities in German-speaking countries. In these facilities, the large-scale reorientation of forensic psychotherapy toward cognitive-behavioral methods that has taken place in this field since the 1990s has been responded to not by abandoning but by further developing traditional psychodynamic/psychoanalytic therapy approaches.

Forensic psychotherapy traces its earliest beginnings to psychoanalysis. Donald Winnicott once said, "*More than anyone else, Freud pioneered the understanding of antisocial behavior and crime as the result of unconscious criminal intent and as a symptom of failure in the care and upbringing of the child.*" ([1], p. 28). Indeed, as a young physician at the Vienna General Hospital, Freud had the opportunity to see many violent patients. He also treated at least one pedophile, which was quite unusual in the early part of the previous century, and although forensic patients were not a focus for him, he supervised the therapy of a pedophile by Theodor Reik [2].

Freud's work "*Some Character-Types Met with in Psychoanalytic Work*" [3] has achieved particular fame because it contains that section on "*Criminals from a Sense of Guilt,*" which was to become the starting point of forensic psychotherapy. Freud formulated for the first time the idea that criminality begins in the delinquent's

---

Dedicated in friendship with Gerhard Dammann.

F. Lackinger (✉)
Vienna, Austria
e-mail: fritz.lackinger@gmail.com

R. G. Hersh, C. De Panfilis (eds.), *Implementing Transference-Focused Psychotherapy Principles*, https://doi.org/10.1007/978-3-031-68062-5_11

fantasy world and that unconscious ideas underlie deviant behavior. By emphasizing that delinquency has understandable motivational causes, Freud provided the foundation of most, later theories of forensic psychotherapy. The first pioneer inspired by Freud was August Aichhorn [4], but the psychodynamic tradition of forensic psychotherapy that emerged is also reflected by the following contributors: Alexander & Healy 1935, Bowlby 1944, Glover 1944, 1960, Friedländer 1947, Eissler & Federn 1949, Schmideberg 1949, Johnson & Szurek 1952, Winnicott 1956, 1985, Joseph 1960, Goudsmit 1964, 1974, Menninger 1968, Klüwer 1976, Schorsch et al. 1985, Berner 1985, 1986, 2001, 2011, Glasser 1988, Meloy 1988, Cordess & Cox 1995, Morgan & Ruszczynski 2007, Lackinger et al. 2008, Meloy & Yakeley 2014, Lackinger 2016, 2017 [5–32].

Behavioral Therapeutic Turn and Its Limits

In the 1990s, the debate in forensic psychotherapy was very much under the influence of empirical recidivism studies that seemed to show a superiority of cognitive-behavioral treatment (CBT) approaches over psychodynamic ones [33–36]. Against the background of publicized recidivism of released or treated sex offenders, and a change in the general socio-political climate, these studies accompanied a turn in offender treatment that was partly anti-psychodynamic, partly generally anti-therapeutic in character. However, a methodological critique of this type of research was soon advanced, maintaining that the effectiveness of psychotherapeutic offender treatment according to strict criteria had not been empirically demonstrated in general, including for cognitive-behavioral programs [37–40].

Doubts about the effectiveness of cognitive-behavioral programs (particularly for sex offenders) led to the development of so-called relapse-prevention (RP) programs [41, 42]. Pfäfflin questioned whether these programs could, in fact, decisively reduce sex offender recidivism [43]. He showed that new methods can always demonstrate impressive success as long as they are in a kind of pioneering stage. In everyday practice, when confronted with the complex disorders of unselected patients, the RP programs did not demonstrate robust effectiveness in real-world conditions. Nevertheless, today classical psychodynamic psychotherapy is often no longer considered appropriate for offender treatment (see, for example, Fiedler [44]). Since 1999, the American Psychiatric Association (APA) has recommended exclusively multimodal CBT broad-spectrum programs in this context [45 , p. 146].

Justified Criticism and a Psychodynamic New Beginning

The psychodynamic tradition was criticized for placing too much emphasis on the offender's personality, his interpersonal relationships, and especially the transference to the analytic psychotherapist, while ignoring the criminal offense as a meaningful behavioral phenomenon [46]. This emphasis on elements other than the criminal offense was problematic, as the offense was understood (analogously to the psychological symptom) only as a surface manifestation of a deeper psychological conflict constellation, which would almost disappear by itself if the unconscious or split-off parts of the personality were made conscious or integrated. In addition, the approach of depth psychological forensic therapists was said to be too much process- and too little result-oriented, with the consequence that such therapies often lasted several years without leading to a relapse-preventive change in behavior.

Despite all the problems inherent in empirical efficacy research in real life, these criticisms were likely justified to some extent. However, it can be argued that this approach "threw the baby out with the bathwater" by ignoring completely certain important observations endorsed by clinicians with a psychodynamic orientation. As a result of this dialectical development, many psychodynamically-oriented forensic psychiatrists and psychotherapists began to actively explore the extent to which the psychodynamic concepts in delinquency treatment could be enriched by the cognitive-behavioral critique.

In this context, two new psychodynamic treatment methods have been developed and disseminated internationally: mentalization-based therapy for antisocial personality disorder (MBT-ASPD) [47, 48] and transference-focused forensic psychotherapy (TFFP). TFFP is the forensic application of transference-focused psychotherapy (TFP) [49, 50], conceived in the 1990s as specific to the treatment of borderline disorders. The TFFP approach developed in an international collaboration between forensic institutions in Austria, Germany, and Switzerland, is reflected in the editorship and contributions to the 2008 book "*Psychodynamische Therapie bei Delinquenz. Praxis der Übertragungsfokussierten Psychotherapie*" [29] (Psychodynamic Therapy of Delinquency. Experiences of Transference- Focused Psychotherapy). The application of this approach specifically to the treatment of the pedosexual offender (defined as an adult who is sexually involved with children, synonymous with pedophile) was first presented at the IATSO[1] conference in Oslo in 2010 ("*TFFP as a sexual offender treatment modality*," 52) and published in German in first approaches [29–31, 51–59].

Forensic Patients and Their Psychopathology

Descriptive Psychopathology and Offense-Analysis

In the psychiatric examination of lawbreakers, offense-relevant psychopathological disorders may be found primarily in three fundamental areas:

- Impulse control disorders.
- Antisocial behavior and attitudes.
- Sexual deviations.

[1] IATSO: International Association for the Treatment of Sex Offenders

These three domains correspond to phenomenologically describable behavioral problems (impulse control disorders with and without personality disorders, conduct disorders, antisocial personality disorder, paraphilic disorders, and others), and also reflect complex psychological disorders related to deeper psychological structures and conflicts. It is essential to note that pathologies from these domains can occur relatively independently from each other but are often combined in offenders. The relative weight of the different factors, when diagnosed not only superficially at the behavioral level but also as manifestations of psycho-structural patterns, allows an initial prototyping that is highly relevant for the practice of forensic diagnostics. Thus, the following types can be distinguished according to the predominant area of pathology, so that they can be further differentiated by combining them with the respective second- and third-rank disorder areas:

- Offenders with overt identity diffusion and poor affect regulation (“*borderline delinquents*”).
- Offenders with pronounced narcissistic and superego pathology (“*psychopathic offenders*”).
- Offenders who act out their pathologically sexualized inner world (“*perverted offenders*”).

The goal of first identifying a predominant area of pathology and then exploring co-occurring areas of disturbance is explained by the following. As an example, a patient evaluated might demonstrate a pedophiliac disorder as a strong and dominant feature. It nevertheless remains important whether a second-rank disorder, e.g., impulsive features is identified, which may or may not be strong enough to diagnose a borderline personality disorder. It may also be relevant to explore whether there are antisocial features as well. While less prominent, these antisocial features may still present as a third-rank diagnosis. If these are present, it is, therefore, quite a different case than one where the antisocial features are dominant (first rank) but pedophiliac and fetishistic tendencies are identified as well as second and third-rank features, meaning still important but not the dominant elements of the clinical presentation.

The characteristic features of these prototypes cannot be described with sufficient depth until the descriptive features of psychopathology are considered together with the descriptive features of the offenses committed. The goal of the assessment process would be an investigation of the deep psychological structure and dynamics expressed in both the subtypes of pathology and the offense in question.

The examination of the actual, specific criminal offense in psychodynamic forensic psychotherapy has long been neglected in comparison to the attention paid to either the treatment relationship or the transference. Psychiatric nosologies have also failed to address numerous forensically relevant features. For example, the diagnosis of pedophilia in ICD-10 is quite irrelevant from a forensic diagnostic point of view, as no differential diagnostic features have been included to distinguish dangerous (those acting on pedophilic impulses) from harmless pedophiles (those with pedophilic fantasies but no history of actual pedophilic behaviors).

In recent decades, attempts have been made to compensate for these deficiencies by establishing numerous so-called forensic offender typologies [60–64]. These offender typologies organize characteristics of the external circumstances of the crime, characteristics of the victims, and information about the sexual orientation of the offenders into statistically relevant clusters.

Such type formations are especially important for recidivism prognosis, but they are also therapeutically relevant, although they do not initially contain any consideration about the inner, psychodynamic situation of the offenders. It is the task of psychodynamic diagnostics to establish such connections.

Psychodynamic Contexts and Prototypes

The contemporary psychodynamic diagnostic assessment process aims at elucidating both descriptive disorders, as reflected in DSM-5 nosologic terms, and exploration of deeper, unconscious causal mechanisms. Traditional psychoanalytic thinking focuses on the conflict between underlying drives and associated defenses. Kernberg [65] is of the opinion that drive conflicts are difficult to elicit in an initial interview; instead, he recommends focusing on psychic structures. These structures reflect the history of the drive conflicts and the extent to which these conflicts were resolved and overcome by the individual under study.

The concept of psychic structure can be illuminated by focusing on five elements of the structural interview with particular relevance for a forensic psychodynamic diagnostic assessment:

- *Reality testing*: Can the patient make a fundamental distinction between internal and external reality (which includes social reality) even in stressful situations? What is the nature of the patient's impairment in reality testing? Is this impairment linked to a specific or non-specific stress condition, a substance-induced psychosis, or a significant thought or mood disorder?
  - Are antisocial acts related to the loss of reality testing? If yes, how destructive are the contents of the delusion?
  - Was the loss of reality testing possibly deliberately produced by drug use?
  - To what extent does impaired reality testing contribute to deficits in superego functioning?
- *Identity and object relations*: How mature and integrated are the basic conceptions of self and object? Can positive and negative aspects be brought together? How stable and with what quality does the differentiation of the self from the main object representations take place? What is the patient's capacity for mentalizing his own affects [66]?
  - To what extent is the perception and mentalization of affects impaired in the context of the offense?

  - Can evidence be found that offense victims were endowed with split-off self-aspects (self-swapping acting out,[2] projective identification)?
  - Does the perpetrator somehow appropriate some psychological aspects of his/her victim in the offense? (This has been termed extractive introjection in the psychoanalytic literature.)
- *Narcissism and superego regulation*: Does self-esteem regulation function on the basis of infantile or mature values? Does a pathological grandiose self mask the lack of integrated self-concepts? If yes, to what extent does the grandiose self absorb the contents of the ego ideal and with what degree of intensity do the projections of unbearable self- and superego-parts take place? (This concept of projection of unbearable self- and superego elements is an essential element of the defense of projective identification. For the patient with prominent narcissism, for example, the feeling of dependency on a partner may be unbearable; in this situation, via projective identification, the dependency is located in and ascribed to the partner. In another vein, the unbearable super-ego element could be a relentlessly harsh self-criticism because of feelings of uncertainty and neediness. Projective identification of this aspect would lead others to be critical of the narcissistic subject who is then relieved from inner pressure and can treat the criticism as proof of envy or hostility emanating from external sources.)
  - Does the offense essentially serve to stabilize a sense of self-worth based on infantile values?
  - Does the offense serve to stabilize a pathological sense of grandiosity? Does it serve the satisfaction of narcissistic claims to power?
  - Are sadistic representations of relationships, which are part of a grandiose self-dramatization, acted out unscrupulously?
- *Affect regulation and aggression*: How integrated are affects and how functional is their regulation? Are there split-off aggressive representations of relationships? To what extent are these acted out and to what extent are they part of the pathological grandiose self? Is destructive aggression tolerated in an ego-syntonic way or even idealized?
  - Do impulsive delinquent acts occur in the context of derailed affect regulation?
  - Is it primarily a matter of situationally triggered, impulsive anger, or are there chronic relationship representations behind it that are dominated by feelings of hate?
  - Are the feelings of anger and hatred conflictual or are they experienced and acted upon from an attitude of entitlement and legitimacy?
- *Sexuality*: To what extent is sexual satisfaction possible within the framework of an intimate relationship that respects the partner? Is the partner used as an inanimate object (fetish) to stabilize one's own identity? Is sexuality used to humiliate or harm others?

[2] *Self-swapping acting out* is a translation of the concept of "*Selbstvertauschungsagieren*", which was developed in German-speaking psychoanalytic literature in the 1970ies and 1980ies [22, 63, 67].

- With property or violent offenses: Are the offenses in a sexual context or could they have an unconscious sexual function?
- In the case of a sexual offense: Does the sexual aggression acted imply a momentary exposure or disturbance of the victim, or a longer term psychological (or even physical) harm?
- Does the offense essentially represent acting out of a paraphilic fantasy, or does it result primarily from affective loss of control or from a narcissistic claim to power?

These sets of questions can provide background considerations for a diagnostic interview. For general interview guidelines, following Kernberg's "*Structural Interview*" [68] is suggested, since Kernberg already takes a central look at all topics related to aggression and antisociality (see also the *Structured Interview on Personality Organization* [STIPO], standardized according to Kernberg's ideas, which contains a separate section on aggression) [69–71]. It is relatively easy to integrate the forensic questions into the structural interview and thus add a dimension to the assessment process.

Prototypes and Their Features

The prototypes of delinquent patients mentioned in Section "Descriptive Psychopathology and Offense-Analysis"— "borderline delinquents," "psychopathic offenders," "perverted offenders"—can now be described in more detail in psychodynamic and offense-focused terms. For each prototype, ten characteristic features are named. The operationalization of the assessment process, already partially contained in various diagnostic instruments, would require additional adaptation and systemization for the purpose of a more comprehensive psychodynamic diagnosis of antisocial disorders.

Overt Borderline Delinquency

The term *overt borderline delinquency* refers to offenders in whom the borderline personality organization [65] is overtly evident, i.e., not masked by narcissistic pseudo-integration, as it is typically found in "psychopathic offenders." In these cases, it is primarily the low capacity for impulse control that leads to delinquent acts (Table 11.1). This has characteristic effects on the course of the crime and the crime pattern. The varying degrees to which these characteristics are expressed lead to a scaling of severity, which is reflected in subaxis 4.1 (see Section "Axis Model", Table 11.7). The combination with narcissistic-psychopathic or perverse aspects in the mental structure is expressed in corresponding values in the other structural sub-axes.

"Psychopathic Offenders"

It is characteristic for "*psychopathic perpetrators*"that the diffusion of identity, especially in the area of self-image, is masked by narcissistic pseudo-integration

Table 11.1 Characteristics of offenders with manifest identity diffusion and poor affect regulation (*"Overt borderline delinquency"*)

1	Identity Diffusion
2	Splitting and projective identification as central defense mechanisms
3	Impulsivity
4	Other signs of ego weakness (especially pronounced anxiety and low sublimation ability)
5	Weaknesses in mentalization (typically a reflective self functioning scale (RSFS)-score of 1.0–3.0)[a]
6	Low degree of planning for offenses
7	Prevalence of anger and fear in the context of the offense
8	Mood swings or subsequent feelings of guilt instead of mature (cautionary) feelings of guilt
9	Pronounced self-damaging tendencies
10	Role of addictive substances in the context of the offense

[a]A study by Levinson & Fonagy [72] compared the mentalizing skills of different groups: Violent prison inmates scored an average of 1.4 points, non-violent prison inmates 2.82, non-delinquent patients with personality disorders 3.77, and a non-clinical control group 5.0

Table 11.2 Characteristics of offenders with narcissistic pseudo-integration and superego pathology (*"Psychopathic offenders"*)

1	Grandiosity, excessive ambition, excessive dependence on admiration.
2	Shame, and shame defense; envy, and envy defense
3	Avoidance of depressive feelings
4	Emotional flatness, feelings of emptiness and meaninglessness, lack of empathy
5	Lack of warning guilt and of guilt at all
6	Exploitation and parasitism in relationships, pathological lying
7	Aggressive-paranoid world view ("the world as a jungle")
8	Sense of entitlement to aggression and appropriation of other people's property
9	Idealization of violence
10	Inability to show concern for and loyalty to others, complete devaluation and dehumanization of others disobjectification of others [73].

and is therefore often diagnostically overlooked. This pseudo-integration is managed by the existence of a fragile compensatory defensive operation described as a "pathologic grandiose self." A pathological grandiose self has all positive aspects of the self, together with the positive aspects of its partial objects and the most important contents of the ego ideal combined and condensed. The negative aspects of both self and significant others, along with the prohibitive and persecuting layers of the superego, are split-off and typically projected into the external world in some form (Table 11.2). "*Psychopathic offenders*" are often able to deceive others, including treaters. Their offenses are often planned rather than impulsive. The degree of violence tolerated or even intended by the pathological grandiose self varies according to severity (see Section "Axis Model", subaxis 4.2, Table 11.8).

The conceptual distinction between overt borderline structure and narcissistic pseudo-integration has recently found confirmation in neurobiology. According to Christopher Patrick [74], the central factor of psychopathy, the so-called "meaness", results from a primary fearlessness (associated with a hyporeactivity of the amygdala) that interacts with an interpersonal aloofness that can be characteristic of the parent, the child or both in early relationships. Thus, psychopathy is by no means exclusively genetically determined. As always in such cases, there is likely to be a spectrum between more genetic and more experiential forms of psychopathy. In any case, the characteristics described as disinhibition or impulsivity are neurobiologically located elsewhere, namely mainly in the prefrontal cortex. Impulsive and planned aggression thus have distinctly different neurobiological correlates.

"Perverted Offender"

Although the language "perverted offender" might sound potentially stigmatizing, at the structural level of personality organization this term implies a deeper, psychostructural dimension than the purely descriptive terms paraphilia and disorder of sexual preference. The structural dimension addressed here refers to the instrumentalization of sexuality for the purposes of identity stabilization and aggression channeling (Table 11.3). Perversion means, on the one hand, a defense against intimacy (reflecting fear of proximity to an object that is fantasized as absorbing or even devouring) and, on the other hand, simultaneously the binding and bundling of destructive aggression in a perverse pseudo-relationship. In this way, perversion mitigates the acting out of pure aggression. The extent of channeled aggression forms the basis of the severity levels depicted in subaxis 4.3 (see Section "Axis Model", Table 11.9). Since the "aggression binding capacity" of perversion (i.e., its "coping function") is unstable, progressive forms of deviant development may arise. In extreme cases, a complete failure of the aggression binding, "perverse" coping attempt can lead to sexual murder.

Axis Model

In addition to a psychodynamic interview, further information must be collected on the offense, the history of the offense, current attitudes toward the offense, social circumstances, and other treatment prerequisites. In addition, for an overall

Table 11.3 Characteristics of perpetrators who act out their highly sexualized inner world (*"Perverted offenders"*)

1	Inadequate capacity for sexual satisfaction in the context of an intimate relationship
2	Sexualization as a defense against intimacy and against depressive feelings
3	Sexualization as a defense against paranoid fears and pure destructiveness
4	In the absence of partnered sexuality: Restriction of the ability to engage in pleasurable masturbation
5	Sexualized acting out without involvement of others, extent of risk-to-self and self-harming
6	Sexual assaults on other persons with a low level of harm
7	Sexualized sadism (against minors, other dependents, women, or men), nature and extent of harm
8	"Perverted" (i.e., sexualized-destructive) fantasy activity before or between offenses
9	Impulsive breakthrough or ego-syntonic planning
10	Progressive form of deviant development

Table 11.4 Dimensions of axis 1: Illness experience and treatment prerequisites

1	Current severity of the disorder or problem
2	Duration of the disorder/problem
3	Illness experience and presentation
4	Disease concepts of the patient
5	Change concepts of the patient
6	Change resources
7	Barriers to change

assessment of the offender and the prospects for treatment, information from criminal and court records must also be considered. To get legal access to them, the interviewer must first obtain the consent of the person concerned. To evaluate these data, psychodynamic diagnosticians must attempt to further systematize and formalize conceptual considerations. The information can then be used for rating criteria, which are organized below into six axes.

Axis 1: Illness Experience and Treatment Prerequisites (Basic Module)

The entry into the axis model proposed here is made with the basic module in axis 1 of the OPD-2[3] (including the so-called psychotherapy module). As with all other patients, it must be clarified how severe any mental disorder is at present, how long it has existed, how the patient experiences and presents this disorder, what the patient would like to change and what are the facilitating and hindering factors.

The dimensions of axis 1 (Table 11.4) are already broken down into several items in the OPD-2 [75], each of which can be rated in 5 levels (from "not/hardly" to "very highly").

Axis 2: Basic Forensic Module

In the case of forensic patients, it is important to establish whether there is a history of delinquency and, if so, what it is, what security measures are currently in place, and to what extent the offenses committed are seen by the patient as the consequences of purely external dilemmas or unfortunate circumstances or whether the patient accepts responsibility for them. The current attitude toward one's own offense and toward antisocial acts in general is, of course, important information for determining the indication for forensic psychotherapeutic treatment. In addition, the type of previous cooperation with care and therapy services should be recorded here, whether there are ideas for change regarding the patient's own propensity to commit an offense, but also how severe the social stress factors are and how well the problem-solving skills for social challenges are developed (Table 11.5).

---

[3] OPD-2: Operationalized Psychodynamic Diagnostic-2 [71]. OPD-2 is an originally German-language manual for establishing comprehensive psychodynamic diagnoses. It is based on a semi-structured psychodynamic interview and an ensuing expert-rating. Its evaluation rests on five axes: [1] Illness experience and treatment prerequisites, [2] Relationship, [3] Conflict, [4] Structure, [5] Mental and psychosomatic disorders.

Table 11.5 Dimensions of axis 2: Basic forensic module

1	Type and number of prior offenses, criminal history, and periods of incarceration
2	Age at first offense and first conviction
3	Safeguards currently in force
4	Internal or external attribution of offense responsibility, degree of insight into own pathological, offense-relevant patterns
5	Cooperation with probation services, in previous therapies, etc.
6	Attitudes toward antisocial behavior in general
7	Concepts of change in relation to delinquent behavior
8	Resources and barriers to change in relation to delinquent behavior
9	Social conditions, criminogenicity of the environment
10	Social competence

Table 11.6 Dimensions of axis 3: Offense analysis

1	Type and focus of offense (e.g., outcome-focused vs. process-focused; single offense or serial offense).
2	Relationship between fixation and regression; presence of particularly stressful life events leading up to the offense.
3	Dominant feeling in the context of the offense: Anger, revenge, feeling of power, sexual desire?
4	Number and gender of victims
5	Role of addictive substances in the offense
6	Degree of familiarity with the victim(s)
7	Degree of planning of the index offense and possibly previous offenses
8	Sadism signs, such as abduction, confinement, humiliation, torture, ritualization
9	In cases of child abuse or rape: Classification according to Knight & Prentky's offender typology [62, 76]
10	In cases of child abuse and rape: Classification according to Groth's, and Groth & Birnbaum's offender typology [60, 61]

Axis 3: Offense Analysis

The offense represents an aspect of external reality that must not be neglected in psychodynamic forensic diagnostics. In particular, aspects of the form and execution of the offense are rated here, based on empirical research, which are considered relevant for the assessment of the risk of recidivism. However, it is also a matter of the extent of objectifiable aggression as well as known offender typologies, which enable the determination of relevant subtypes, especially in the case of child abusers and rapists (Table 11.6).

Axis 4: Identity, Superego and Sexualization

Structural identity axis is broken down into three sub-axes, which represent the central psychopathological problem areas mentioned in Section "Descriptive Psychopathology and Offense-Analysis". As graded structural dimensions. Although they are by no means completely independent of each other, levels of integration can be achieved to variable degrees in the three dimensions:

- Identity integration and impulse control.
- Narcissistic regulation and superego development.
- Integration versus instrumentalization of sexuality.

Since these subaxes are conceptualized as discontinuous dimensions, their parameter-values are given as levels on a scale. In order to determine which level in each subaxis applies to a particular patient, the diagnostician has to look at the areas of disturbance characteristic for the three prototypes listed above (Tables 11.1, 11.2 and 11.3).

Subaxis 4.1—Identity Integration and Impulse Control

The examination of the integration of identity is primarily intended to determine the differentiation and integration of self- and object representations, as well as the quality of object relations that depends on them. Closely related to this are the abilities to control impulses and regulate affect (Table 11.7). The functionality of the ego depends to a large extent on identity integration [65, 68, 77]. Differentiation in this context means the structurally anchored ability to distinguish between inner and outer reality. *Integration* describes the structural and functional synthesis of the originally fragmented or split partial self and partial object representations. It presupposes the differentiation of inner and outer reality. *Fusion* means the absence or undoing of differentiation between the representations of inner and outer reality. The 10-level scale ranges from good integration without neurotic limitations to chronic loss of reality testing due to the permanent fusion of self- and object representations. Levels 1–3 belong to the normal/neurotic structural level; levels 4–8 and 9–10, respectively, the borderline and the psychotic structural levels.

Table 11.7 Levels of sub-axis 4.1: Integration of identity and impulse control

	Differentiation and integration of self and object representations	Ability to control impulses
1	Good integration without neurotic rigidity	Normal impulse control
2	Good integration with selective neurotic rigidity	Selectively overstressed impulse control
3	Good integration with comprehensive neurotic rigidity	General perfectionist impulse control
4	Sufficient integration (higher borderline level)	Good impulse control, but occasional impulse breakthroughs
5	Moderate integration (medium borderline level)	Habitual (but circumscribed) impulsivity
6	Low integration (low borderline level 1) and very unstable relationships	Chronic impulsivity, but limited inhibition of violent impulses
7	Low integration (low borderline level 2) in violent or only short-term relationships	Ego syntonicity of violence or other delinquency
8	Low integration (low borderline level 3) without any ability to relate (complete dehumanization)	No inhibition of object-hostile impulses at all
9	Temporary fusion of self- and object conceptions (psychotic personality organization without schizophrenia symptomatology)	Impulse control reduced due to stress-related lack of reality testing
10	Permanent fusion of self- and object conceptions (chronic schizophrenia or affective psychosis)	Impulse control reduced by chronic lack of reality testing

Subaxis 4.2—Narcissistic Regulation and Superego Development

Examination of self-value regulation reveals the subject's existing or lacking capacity to pursue (and at least partially achieve) the satisfaction of his or her most important needs and goals within the framework of a value system associated with normal self-esteem, appropriate respect for others, and a commitment to social challenges (mature value system). Unconscious conflicts in neurotic disorders often lead to regression not only to pregenital (meaning more primitive) drive tendencies but also to an infantile value system that is structurally anchored in a rigid superego. More severe narcissistic problems result in the formation of a pathological grandiose self, which—based on splitting, denial, and omnipotent control—achieves an artificial and structurally questionable stabilization of self-esteem, but at the same time increasingly affects superego development [78–80]. The degrees of the omnipotence of the projective mechanisms and the intensity of the aggression projected by them define the further degrees of severity of narcissistic and superego pathology (Table 11.8).

Table 11.8 Levels of sub-axis 4.2: Narcissistic regulation and superego development

	Narcissistic regulation	Superego development
1	Normal narcissism (mature self-esteem regulation)	Normal, differentiated, and abstracted superego: satisfaction of the most important needs possible within the framework of a mature value system
2	Conflict-induced regression to infantile narcissism	Neurotic superego: need satisfaction blocked by infantile value systems in individual conflictual areas
3	Character neurotic regression to infantile narcissism	Character neurotic superego: need satisfaction blocked by infantile value systems in all important areas
4	Pathological grandiose self (narcissistic personality disorder) with moderate projective tendency	Superego with weak points: coherent, sometimes perfectionist superego—with situationally activated "holes".
5	Pathological grandiose self (narcissistic personality disorder) with strong projective tendency	Dysfunctional superego with persistent "holes" (habitual but circumscribed antisocial traits with subsequent feelings of guilt)
6	Narcissistic personality disorder with chronic antisociality	Barely integrated superego with chronic antisociality: hardly any feelings of guilt, rather mood swings
7	Syndrome of malignant narcissism with ego-syntonic violence and paranoid worldview	Disintegrated superego with extensive absence of guilt: Ego-syntonic sadism associated with masochistic mechanisms
8	Destructive narcissism, completely dominated by own claim to power (psychopathic personality disorder)	Completely disintegrated superego with absence of guilt: Ego-syntonic sadism without masochistic mechanisms.
9	Self-esteem regulation requires temporary abandonment of reality testing (psychotic narcissism)	Superego function is undermined by temporary loss of reality testing
10	Self-esteem regulation requires chronic abandonment of reality testing (chronic psychotic narcissism)	Superego function is undermined by chronic loss of reality testing

Subaxis 4.3—Integration Versus Instrumentalization of Sexuality

The psychodynamic investigation of sexualityasks to what extent its genital and pregenital aspects have become integral components of mature internalized object relations and, subsequently, of personal identity, or whether important, especially pregenital aspects have been split-off and functionalized for identity-stabilizing and/or relationship-hostile purposes. In particular, the questions arise: How intense is the pregenital aggression, which the perversion is supposed to bind and bundle? And how pronounced is the disposition or compulsion/addiction to act out this aggression? Progressing perversions lead on the one hand to an increasing dehumanization of the other, on the other hand they can also contribute to the destruction of reality testing or occur together with it (Table 11.9).

Axis 5: Descriptive-Phenomenological Diagnoses

Here, the OPD-2 is used again, and axis 5 (mental and psychosomatic disorders) is adopted unchanged (Table 11.10).

Table 11.9 Dimensions of subaxis 4.3: Integration versus instrumentalization of sexuality

Structural diagnosis of sexuality	Level of integration and instrumentalization of sexuality
Normal sexuality	Perverse aspects as an integrated part of normal sexuality
Slightly neurotic sexuality	Individual pregenital (perverse) tendencies are repressed and recur as neurotic symptoms (e.g., simple bodily dysfunctions)
Character neurotic sexuality	Perverse tendencies are repressed and recur as severe neurotic traits (e.g., chronic anhedonia, compulsive systems, psychosomatic symptoms)
Benign perversion	Perversion is acted out in fantasy, masturbation, and consensual relationships
Transgressive perversion	Perversion is acted out in assaults against other (non-consenting) persons, but only a relatively minor harm is done
Ego-dystonic malignant perversion	Perversion is acted out clearly harming others, but leading to subsequent (ineffective) feelings of guilt
Ego-syntonic malignant perversion	Perversion is acted out harming others without causing significant feelings of guilt, although self-harm may occur
Perversion with complete demumanization Dedisobjectification	Perversion is acted out by harming others without causing feelings of guilt
Perversion with temporary loss of reality testing	Perversion is acted out ego-syntonically only when reality testing is lost, after that realistic self-reproach may occur
Perversion with chronic loss of reality testing	Perversion occurs ego-syntonically, but may alternate with periods of psychotic self-reproach and self-punishment

Table 11.10 Dimensions of Axis 5: Descriptive Phenomenological Diagnoses

5a: Mental disorders	ICD-10 (research criteria)	DSM-5 (optional)
Principal diagnosis:	F _ ____. _____	______. ____
Further diagnosis 1:	F_____. _____	______. ____
Further diagnosis 2:	F_____. _____	______. ____
Further diagnosis 3:	F_____. _____	______. ____
5b: Personality disorders	ICD-10 (F60xx or F61. x)	DSM-5 (optional)
Principal diagnosis:	F_____. _____	______. ____
Further diagnosis 1:	F_____. _____	______. ____
5c: Physical diseases	ICD-10 (not Chapter V [F]!)	
Principal diagnosis:	_______. _____	
Further diagnosis 1:	_______. _____	
Further diagnosis 2:	_______. _____	
Further diagnosis 3:	_______. _____	

Treatment of the Forensic Patient: From TFP to TFFP

Transference Analysis as the Central Mechanism of Action

The central idea of TFP as a treatment modality is that the split internalized relational representations are activated and restaged in all present relationships of borderline patients, including the therapeutic relationship. In this context, we refer to the re-enactment of internalized partial relational dyads as transference, or more precisely, split transference.

- A part of the dyad is regularly projected into the therapist, which may be a partial self or a partial object representation.
- The patient makes a temporary identification with the complementary part of the dyad.
- The therapeutic relationship very quickly takes on the shape and coloring of the dominant internalized relational images.

By working with these re-enacted, transferred relationship patterns, TFP essentially works with the basic building blocks of personality organization. The decisive therapeutic mechanism of action is the integration of one-sided positive and one-sided negative partial self and partial object representations leading to complete or "whole" self and object representations. This process then enables augmented ego functions, i.e., improved affect regulation, capacity for sublimation allowing for facilitation of thinking and expression of creativity, and impulse control.

These improved ego functions correlate with what Fonagy et al. [81] describe as improved capacity to mentalize [81]. Mentalization means the ability to distinguish between mental states and actions, to recognize the former as the causes of the latter, and to be able to reflect on this connection. The ability to think about mental states implies stable empathy with both self and others and requires whole, realistic, and multidimensional images of self and objects. Both are possible only when the originally separated positive and negative experiences of the self with others are integrated into some degree [82, 83].

Improvement of Reflective Function

Fonagy et al. also devised a method to operationalize the concept of mentalizing [66]. This method became known as the *Reflective Functioning Rating Scale* (RFRS). Levy et al. (2006) used this instrument to evaluate changes in reflective functioning in borderline patients using TFP in comparison with other treatment modalities [84]. In doing so, improvement in reflective function was understood as a measure of structural change.

The landmark 2007 study by Clarkin et al. compared TFP, dialectical behavioral therapy (DBT), and supportive psychotherapy (SPT). Measurements before the start of therapy showed that patients with borderline personality disorder had RF ratings of 2.8–3.3 points, which, as expected, is well below normal average values (which lie at +/− 5 points). RF measures after 1 year of treatment showed significant differences between the three treatment methods, with only the TFP-treated patients making statistically significant progress. The ability of TFP to produce structural changes in the personality of borderline patients was confirmed in a clear manner. Apart from the RF results, the study by Levy et al. [84] contains the following findings:

- TFP patients showed a significant increase in more secure attachment patterns after 1 year of therapy, while DBT and SPT patients did not.
- TFP patients showed a significant increase in attachment coherence, whereas such a result was not found in DBT and SPT patients.

Structural Level, Reflective Function, and Delinquency

It has often been pointed out that borderline personality disorder and antisocial personality disorder have many aspects in common and that the two diagnoses show a gender complementary distribution [85]. From a TFP perspective, both personality disorders exhibit a borderline personality organization (with splitting, identity diffusion, but preserved reality testing as central structural features), within which, however, a spectrum of superego disorders of varying severity can be identified (see Table 11.8 given earlier).

In a closer examination of similarities and differences between the “normal” borderline patients in private practices, those in psychiatric hospitals, and borderline delinquents in forensic institutions, the need to distinguish between different levels of severity of borderline pathology quickly emerges. From the beginning, Kernberg distinguished two, later three, levels within the borderline personality organization [65, 68, 69, 86] (i.e., higher, medium, and lower borderline levels). Severe superego disorders are regularly associated with the lower borderline structural level. For forensic diagnostics, a further subdivision of the low borderline level proved to be necessary to differentiate the manifestations of psychopathology and associated prognosis in subgroups of offenders ([53, 87] and Section "Forensic Patients and their Psychopathology" in this chapter).

It is important to examine one aspect of the differential diagnosis of patients across the spectrum of borderline pathology, specifically the different levels of mentalizing identified in "normal" borderline and prison populations. Levinson & Fonagy [72] applied the RFRS to a group of prison inmates, to personality-disordered patients in a psychiatric hospital, and to a "normal" control group. Whereas the RF of normal college students averaged five points on the RFRS scale (which ranges from −1 to +9), the RF of clinical borderline patients showed an average score of 3.77 (similar to the Levy et al. 2006 score in the New York-TFP study), and the average RF of prison inmates showed a score of 2.11, which was still far above the average RF of incarcerated violent offenders (1.4 points).

Levinson & Fonagy [72] also compared the above-mentioned groups in terms of the number of individuals in the so-called deficit range ("low scorers" with an RF score below 3). This group included 73% of the prison inmates and as many as 93% of the violent offenders, but no one from the control group. These data support the clinical impression that forensic (and particularly violent) patients are more impaired than ordinary borderline patients and that in forensic psychotherapy we are looking for a treatment approach that is able to work with and help those markedly low-scoring borderline patients [88–90].

What TFP principles might be of utility for the clinicians working with these patients?

Framework and Technical Procedure in TFFP

This challenge is taken up in TFFP on several levels. From the general TFP concept comes the distinction between diagnostics, the framework of therapy, strategy, tactics, and techniques. It is specified for the treatment of sex offenders as follows, done here in overview and with reference to other publications for additional detail [51–53, 91].

- *Diagnostics* take place in 2–3 diagnostic interview sessions before the start of therapy. The aim is to determine the specific subtype and severity of the borderline disorder, to clarify the level of mentalization, motivation for therapy and forms and risks of secondary gain from illness. In addition, it is necessary to assess for diagnostic exclusion criteria; these criteria are defined by levels 8–10 in all sub-axes 4.1.-4.3. (see Section "Forensic Patients and their Psychopathology" of this chapter), i.e., they pertain to (a) the presence of a psychotic personality organization, and (b) the absence of any capacity for relationship, guilt experience, or other inhibition of harm. In the case of sex offenders, a detailed examination of the sexual disposition, as well as clarification of the convicted offenses and the patient's subjective attitude toward these offenses, is crucial.

- *General conditions of treatment* are defined in the therapy contract, and a procedure in case of non-compliance is always discussed in advance. The contract includes the following:
  - General aspects such as timeliness and reliability in attending therapy sessions, financing, tasks of patient and therapist in therapy, implications of a forensic therapy instruction (obligation to report non-compliance), other limits of confidentiality vis-à-vis prison, court, and other forensic professionals (e.g., acute danger to self and others as well as possible risk of absconding), necessity of file inspection, etc.
  - Individual aspects, such as threats to therapy due to the specific risk of recidivism, e.g., violence, other violations of the law, drug use, etc., but also possible threats to therapy due to suicidality, self-injury, or self-harm (e.g., due to anorexia), dishonesty, etc.
- *Strategies* describe long-term goals to be achieved over extended periods of therapy, specifically the awareness, naming, and integration of split, oscillating, and mutually defensive object relation dyads and their development into triangulated, and therefore more mature, stable, and nuanced representations of relationships.
- *Tactics* are the terms of reference that guide the TFP therapist in shaping an individual therapy session. They include guidelines
  - For maintaining the therapy contract
  - For identification of those aspects of the material that should be addressed and, specifically, of those threats to the therapy setting that need to be prioritized before transference analysis proper can begin
  - For managing the intensity of the affect of the patient, as too little affect does not lead to activation of the problematic transference dyads, too much affect, on the other hand, endangers the receptivity for interpretations.
  - In TFFP, in addition to the usual TFP contract conditions, compliance with criminal laws, penitentiary rules, and forensic therapy agreements, must be prioritized before focusing on transference manifestations.
- *Techniques* guide the therapist's approach from moment to moment. They determine how material is explored and which interventions are selected in the therapeutic process. The general techniques of TFP are technical neutrality, interpretation, transference analysis, and monitoring of counter-transference [49]. There is an explicit possibility in TFP to temporarily deviate from technical neutrality in order to ensure the continuation of therapy. However, if the therapy is to be continued, the interruption of technical neutrality must be analytically processed (i.e., its meaning brought into the patient's awareness). "Interpretation" designates here the entire process of interpretation, which consists of the following components:

- Clarification of the conscious ideas
- Confrontation with conscious and preconscious contradictions
- Interpretation in the narrower sense (i.e., the formulation of hypotheses about unconscious or split-off motives)

By their nature, these technical notions also apply in TFFP. However, there are three additions:

- Technical neutrality is further limited by the fact that the forensic therapist must report to the prison or the court authorities whether therapy is actually occurring on a regular basis [51].
- The interpretation process shifts considerably toward the components of clarification and tactful confrontation, especially in the early and middle phases, since the mentalizing capacity of violent and sexual offenders is exceptionally low. In this phase of the interpretation process, elements of mentalization-based work might be indicated [56, 92] in order to adequately prepare for interpretation in the narrower sense.
- Transference analysis takes a special form, especially in transference-focused sex offender treatment, in that the patterns of transference found are also systematically applied to pre-offense development and, in particular, to the offense situation, and these experiences are related and interconnected [91]. This will be explained in more detail in the following sections.

TFFP Strategies

This section will focus on strategies in the application of TFP to offenders in general and sex offenders in particular. It will illustrate how TFFP incorporates both the general forensic issues and the specific challenges of the sexual offender patient population into the strategic design of treatment.

Strategy 1: Define the Dominant Object Relationship Dyad

The initial therapeutic situation in working with (sex) offenders shows similarities and differences to starting therapy with non-offending borderline patients. Some similarities include the following:

- The manifest chaos in the activated relational patterns, which reflects the underlying inner chaos in the self and object representations;
- The diffusion of identity, grounded in the strong use of splitting, projective identification, and denial as defense mechanisms;
- The tendency to use narcissistic fantasies of grandiosity as a defense against paranoid fears and intense envy.

Characteristics of (sex) offenders in the initial phase of therapy are as follows:

- The extent and importance of secrets that the patient feels he or she must protect from the therapist;
- The importance of split-off or narcissistically pseudo-integrated object relations dyads imbued with a destructive element;
- The importance of sadomasochistic sexualization as a defense strategy, which is itself defended against or concealed;
- The mechanism of adaptation to, or imitation of, the therapist, whereby the delinquent patient wants to avoid any real feelings in the therapeutic relationship;
- The extent of omnipotence in the application of the above-mentioned defense strategies, which entails, or is partly based on, the particularly low capacity to symbolize and reflect.

The first TFFP strategy will be presented as an example here in relation to the initial therapy situation with pedosexual offenders. Analogous to the general TFP strategy, the first goal is to "name" the dominant object relations dyads that the patient activates spontaneously and are initially outside of the patient's awareness of his relationship with the therapist. However, the chaotic emotional situation typically spreads instantaneously to the therapist as well and does not facilitate the naming of the dominant dyads immediately. Unnoticed (non-verbal) acting-in by the patient can trigger unusual emotional reactions in the therapist. Therefore, the therapist must first strive to be as tolerant as possible of his or her own confusion so as not to prematurely narrow perception of the relationship.

At the same time, the therapist must remember the typical strategies of pedosexual patients: adaptation, imitation, and the hidden, potentially sexualized power struggle. Are there signs of this? Where does a possible lack of symbolization show up in the form of veiled acting out? Uncertainty immediately arises as to whether the signs are interpreted correctly or whether the therapist is succumbing to his own prejudices. The therapist can only slowly move from tolerance of the chaos to cautious hypotheses regarding the currently dominant object relationship dyads, which he initially keeps to himself. Only when repeated confirmations for hypotheses are found, will the therapist tentatively explicate his perception of the current relationship patterns between him and the patient in the metaphorical form typical for TFP, for example:

Defensively overwhelmed child	Penetrating overstimulating mother
Submissive child who agrees to everything	Flattered and seduced father
Distrustful and anxious child	Dishonest and devious father
Fearful, needy, and grateful child	Incarcerating, sexual-sadistic, exploiting Nazi doctor
Sexually exploited guinea pig (or other pet)	Sexually assaulting child or big brother

"Tentative interpretation"means that the therapist offers a formulation without conveying certainty, pays close attention to the patient's reactions, and tries to evaluate them as either confirmation or refutation of his hypotheses. One could distinguish the following single steps within the context of the first strategy:

Step 1: Experience and tolerate your confusion.
Step 2: Pay attention to your unusual feelings, which may indicate unnoticed and unmentalized actions of the patient.
Step 3: Let your knowledge about the transference dispositions of pedosexuals (i.e., patterns of imitation, simulation, and masochistic submission, the "sneaking in", the unexpected "overwhelming", the "mother identification", the self-swapping, etc.), inform your thinking [53].
Step 4: Formulate the dominant object relation dyads first for yourself.
Step 5: Name the actors of the dominant dyads in metaphorical language.
Step 6: Observe and reflect on the patient's reaction.

This process of tolerating chaos, monitoring countertransference, reflecting on familiar patterns, tentative (at first silent, then spoken) naming, and considering the patient's reaction, must be repeated several times until the therapist slowly begins to feel increasing confidence.

Strategy 2: Recognize and Interpret the Role Reversals Within the Therapeutic and Offense Situations

While the therapist attempts to find a common language with the patient through examination of the most accessible elements of the current therapeutic relationship, a parallel effort should be made to explore the typical role reversals within the treatment relationship. The elaboration of current relationship patterns often cannot be separated from a discussion of role changes. For example, a pedosexual patient who feels victimized by a sadistic prison system and its apparently pseudo-friendly representative in the form of a therapist, will belittle the latter expressing accusations of incompetence or depravity. In doing so, the patient assumes a powerful position, with the therapist at the mercy of his attacks, obligated to put up with his accusations. Here the role of the sadistic attacker has changed from therapist to patient. However, the therapist can—in the patient's perception—quickly return to his original role, which is perceived as tormenting, if he points out the patient's instant identification with a sadistic father or simply points out the patient's difficulties. In TFP this is called the "oscillation of relational dyads."

Clinical Illustration

Mr. B. is a single, middle-aged man who had lived with his aging, mentally ill mother until her death. Mr. B.'s father had passed away years earlier, but his mother had insisted at the time that Mr. B. continue to live with her. During this period, Mr. B.'s mother had described Mr. B. as "the man of the house," but at the same time, she dominated him as she had previously dominated the father. Mr. B. had numerous privileges in the household, but he was not allowed to bring a girlfriend home, for example. He felt trapped in his role, since on the one hand, he was supported by his mother who cooked for him and spared him many expectable challenges of daily life, but on the other hand, he felt "kept" and tormented by his mother, as if he were a pet. This constellation reactivated for Mr. B. an older internalized dyad related to a history of painful phimosis surgery and aftercare and an abusive relationship with an aunt, which his mother insisted be kept secret.

Mr. B. was imprisoned for a crime of pedophilic sexual assault, which happened shortly after the death of the mother. Mr. B. had met a woman who had two small daughters and was looking for someone to watch the children when she wanted to go out in the evening. The patient took over this task but soon felt exploited by the woman, as she came home much later than agreed and did not pay him the established fee in full. Mr. B. believed she wanted to lure him into a relationship and assume responsibilities in her home, which Mr. B. did not want at all. Mr. B. grew hateful and preoccupied with revenge, which may have had to do with his former role as a partner substitute with mother. In the relationship with the daughters, he cared for, he finally enacted a characteristic role reversal we are dealing with in this section in assuming the role of the dominating and sadistic mother figure. The sadistic quality of the crime reflected his own experience of abuse as a child, while at the same time, the crime reflected an identification with the abuser. This identification allowed the patient to project his own feeling of being abused into the girls and at the same time to realize his unconscious wishes of revenge for all those situations where he had been the victim of women.

All these relational aspects were repeated in the transference. In pedosexual patients like Mr. B., a familiar transference pattern often observed will reflect the patient's experience of being simultaneously cared for and dominated by the therapist, as by a controlling mother. In this case, Mr. B. also felt taken care of by getting the therapy that he had wished for, but at the same time he believed that the therapist wanted to hold him down and infiltrate him (with echoes of both general domination and sexual penetration) and that the therapist might even derive advantages from this by making a career as an "expert" in pedophilia. As a result, a role reversal occurred in which Mr. B. provided a lot of material that seemed highly relevant to the therapist. The therapist was spellbound and showed restraint so as to encourage the material to continue emerging. However, the therapist also felt increasingly restricted in his freedom of thought and interpretation because Mr. B. progressively reacted to interpretations with punishing silence. The therapist nevertheless saw the patient as being on a good path and wanted to support his steps toward release from prison. The therapist was finally able to point out that Mr. B. sometimes felt dominated and abused by the therapist in a similar way as he had earlier felt dominated and abused by his mother, but that the reverse situation was also repeated, in which he (the patient) made the therapist dependent on him and controlled him for his own benefit. Situations had also occurred in which Mr. B. behaved in an openly boundary-violating manner toward the therapist.

A crucial step in the middle phase of the therapy with Mr. B. was the elaboration of the similarities between experiences in therapy (i.e., Mr. B.'s self-perception both as a victim of a sadistic therapist and as a perpetrator of attacks on the therapist) with the sadomasochistically structured relationship with his mother before the offense and the reversal of this pattern in the pedosexual act. Finally, the exploration of the observed subjective equivalence of important aspects of the patient's history and his ongoing relationship with his therapist could also be linked to a reflection on the real differences, for example, between his relationship with his mother, the abuse of the girls, and the events in therapy.

This short vignette from the treatment of Mr. B. is meant to describe only the basic structures of a recurring and protean object relations dyad. It was interwoven with several other dyads concerning the patient's relationship with his aunt, but also with his father and grandmother. All these core relationships contributed to pathological relational dyads in the personality organization of Mr. B. They had to be worked out separately but could only be overcome by elaboration of their systemic interrelation. In other words, the main internalized object relationship dyads stabilize each other and their omnipotent effect, meaning the tenacity of a powerful fantasy that is not corrected by reality testing, can only be broken through and dissolved commonly as a system.

Summarized and generalized, the steps of the second TFFP strategy can be formulated as follows:

1. Step: Work out a common language with the patient to describe the therapeutic relationship.
2. Step: Describe the typical role changes within the therapeutic dyad.
3. Step: Find the object-relations dyads in pre-criminal development.
4. Step: Find the role reversals in the offense situation.
5. Step: Show the subjective (i.e., psychological) equivalences between the role reversals in the therapeutic and the offense situation.

It is typical that the sexually delinquent patient with borderline structure will describe a self-representation that is clearly split into a victim side and a perpetrator side; the perpetrator side is usually downplayed or denied. The therapist is thus confronted with two potentially oscillating scenarios: a patient with completely unconscious splitting processes, or a patient with more ego-syntonic, psychopathic dissimulation, including deliberate lying.

The subjective awareness of having been a victim as a child is initially felt to be unbearable and, in the case of an adult borderline personality organization, mobilizes affects of hatred and revenge, in which the victim and perpetrator sides come close together and the patient's unconscious identification can oscillate. The therapist should always see the disavowed side as well and appreciate the power of splitting and projection. However, the patient can give up neither the denial nor the separation of the perpetrator and victim sides as long as the nameless fear and humiliation of his victim experience cannot be tolerated and the reality and extent of his hatred and destructiveness cannot be acknowledged. Integration of the two sides can succeed in the long run only if the patient's thirst for revenge is transformed into grief, grief which would reflect an acknowledgment of fear, humiliation, and hatred.

Strategy 3: Interpret Mutually Defensive Relational Dyads Within the Therapeutic and Offense Situations

In the longer term, therapeutic work brings to light that behind the dominant (albeit oscillating) object relationship dyads and their typical emotional coloring, other object relationship dyads with contradictory emotional coloring are hidden. This is an aspect in the dynamics of inner object relations that goes beyond the role reversals worked on in strategy 2 and brings to the surface deeper (i.e., more strongly defended) layers of psychic structure.

The hitherto dominant object-relations dyads, for example, were essentially characterized by fear, mistrust, and hatred, in both oscillating expressions. The emotional coloration was just as characteristic for the expression of the dyad in which the patient experienced himself as a victim as for the other expression in which he assumed the perpetrator role and made the therapist the victim.

In the advanced therapy phase, we can increasingly recognize that the negative emotional coloring of the entire prevailing relationship dynamic served the goal of warding off or protecting an idealized positive (e.g., a needy self/loving object) relationship dyad. These are relationship dyads separated, indeed split off, from each other, serving a defensive purpose of protecting the positive, idealized dyad (e.g., about longing and love) from destruction by the destructive-paranoid dyad.

This dynamic of defense against contradictorily charged emotional relationship dyads is thus first traced in the transference relationship. The therapist increasingly notices how the patient, behind his constant attacks and devaluations of the therapist, also hides his need to be a valuable and desired patient for him and, conversely, to be able to show him his recognition and admiration. The interpretation of this hidden relationship dyad can quickly bring it to light, usually with the immediate, albeit often transient, consequence that now the fearful-hateful dyad seems to have disappeared. The defensive relationship has then simply reversed without changing structurally. Now the therapist seems to be the most helpful and understanding person the patient has ever met. Negative feelings toward him seem completely unimaginable, there is no distrust and no deep fear toward him.

Like the oscillating perpetrator-victim role change within the originally dominant object-relationship dyad, this now advanced treatment phase is about interpreting and overcoming the extreme alternation between the positive and the negative relationship perceptions. At the same time, the issues touched upon in this process must also touch upon the patient's biographical relationship states, and it will turn out that a certain defensive constellation between affectively opposing relationship types was characteristic of the situations before the first and subsequent abusive offenses occurred in each case. The single steps of strategy 3 can be formulated as follows:

1. Step: Deepen the common language with the patient to be able to discuss more complex emotional and relational aspects.
2. Step: In the transference, trace out rejected relationship dyads with opposing emotional content and mutual defensive function.
3. Step: Discover mutually defending relationship dyads in the transference.

4. Step: Elaborate mutually defending relationship dyads in the pre-offense situation.
5. Step: Trace the mutually defending relationship dyads in the offense situation.
6. Step: Show the equivalence in the mutually defensive dyads of transference, and the pre-offense and offense situations.

In the treatment of Mr. B., three important object-relationship dyads appeared, each of which was defended by oppositely charged ones. They occurred in a certain order, reflecting increasingly deeper layers of the patient's complex defense organization. In abstract terms, the following defense constellations were involved:

- Deception and dishonesty should protect the patient from the onset of paranoid anxieties in the first phase.
- After that, sadomasochistic enactments functioned as a defense against desires for an idealizing-holding relationship.
- Finally, a sexual-sadistic transference emerged as a defense against aroused-fusing relationship expectations.

Psychopathic Transference

As usual in forensic psychotherapies, the therapy with Mr. B. began with the activation of narcissistic, relationship-avoiding, and even psychopathic forms of transference. Mr. B. concealed large parts of his pedosexual fantasies and skillfully adapted to the therapist's expectations. He managed to manipulate the therapist to a large extent and to appear as an engaged, cooperative patient. The therapist initially believed himself to be in a well-running therapy, while in fact everything of substance was kept outside. This can be understood as an expression of a dominant psychopathic transference. Its essential characteristics and the technical handling of it can be summed up as follows [68]:

- The patient attempts to deliberately deceive or defraud the therapist. Lying and manipulative or parasitic behavior occur.
- The patient is convinced that the therapist is dishonest, he projects his own tendencies into the therapist, i.e., he tries to corrupt him.
- Behind this is the deep, unconscious conviction that any kind of closeness and any attachment are untrustworthy.

Technical handling:

- All lies must be made explicit and confronted. They should be interpreted as protective mechanisms against the expectation of being deceived oneself.
- If the patient does not want to talk about "certain things", the reasons must be analyzed.
- The dissolution of dishonesty allows the previously averted paranoid tendencies to emerge.

Paranoid Transference

The therapist slowly noticed that the patient agreed with the therapist's interpretations too quickly and too often. He was submissive and finally, Mr. B's fear could be best understood as reflecting a concern that the therapist would send secret therapy reports to the court to be able to keep Mr. B in prison longer.

After the therapist had interpreted this fear as the reason for the patient's dishonesty, the patient felt better understood. Mr. B. was able to admit that he experienced his penal detention, particularly his unlimited "*special treatment order*" (i.e., the so-called "Maßnahmenvollzug" in Austria), as a sadistic rape in which the therapist had been involved. It strongly reminded him of the feeling of being held in his mother's house. Here, too, I summarize the essential characteristics as well as the TFFP handling of it in a punctuation:

- The patient experiences fear and distrust of the therapist.
- The therapist is perceived as dangerous and potentially harmful.
- The therapist is attacked and showered with accusations.
- Omnipotent projective identifications can potentially lead to corresponding reactions and behavior on the part of the therapist that may be outside the therapist's awareness.

Technical handling:

- Clarification of the facts and at least partial establishment of a common perception of reality.
- The apparently dangerous and harmful intentions of the therapist are interpreted as projections of the patient.
- Successful, even partial, resolution of sadistic projections leads to a new phase of typically sadomasochistic transferences.

The patient had indeed become more honest, and his fears of mistreatment by the therapist emerged more strongly as a result. Mr. B. often experienced the therapist's interpretations as attacks and as intrusions, and he himself attacked the therapist because of the latter's ties to the prison system. It was finally possible to establish that Mr. B. was constructing "facts" in order to have reasons for his mistrust and for his attitude of reproach; this was achieved by exploring the patient's fears about the therapist's confidential reports to the court. The patient was able to see, at least in some moments, that his own anger could be justified repeatedly in the context of these paranoid projections.

Sadomasochistic Transference

Mr. B. felt guilty at that moment and suffered from the feeling of having wronged the therapist. However, this did not last long. The consequence of working through the paranoid fears was a long phase of oscillation between new aggressiveness and guilty submissiveness.

At one point, when the therapist tried to get more details about the patient's sexual fantasies, Mr. B. believed the therapist was becoming aroused by these sexual stories himself. The therapist seemed to "penetrate" the patient and the sadomasochistic pleasure the patient associated with these fantasies seemed to be taken away from him by the therapist. On other occasions, Mr. B. turned the tables, so to speak. He was then himself intrusive and overpowering. For example, he did not wait by the door of the treatment room until the therapist opened it, but opened the door himself. Without asking, he put away documents that were on the table. On the one hand, it seemed that Mr. B was trying to force the therapist to enter a sadomasochistic roleplay, on the other hand, he did not seem aware of his boundary violations. The therapist felt overrun and deprived of his freedom, but Mr. B. experienced even cautious exploration of the assaults as deeply embarrassing and mortifying. In summary, the sadomasochistic transference and the TFFP approach to it can be depicted in this way:

- The patient's self-representation is split between a victim and a perpetrator side.
- The therapist becomes entangled in the sadomasochistic dynamic as the patient provokes situations in which the therapist seems to be able only to remain passive (masochistically silent) or to address the issue (mortifyingly sadistic).
- The experience of being a victim mobilizes desires for revenge, acting out on this impulse turns the patient into a perpetrator. Both experiences are initially experienced strictly separated by the split transference.

Technical handling:

- The therapist must always keep both sides in mind and tactfully address each denied side or interpret its projection onto the therapist.
- The patient can begin to grieve his history of victimization and perpetration only by acknowledging his own experiences of powerlessness and his own feelings of hatred.
- Integration can only succeed when the thirst for revenge has been transformed into mourning.

Idealizing Transference

Before the victim's and perpetrator's experiences of pedosexual patients can be truly mourned, further hidden layers of transference usually must be experienced and processed first. Primarily, after numerous role reversals in the sadomasochistic transference constellation, it turned out that Mr. B. seemed to hold on to the tormenting themes with a certain tenacity, even desperation. It seemed apparent to the therapist that an emotionally opposing dyad experienced by Mr. B. would be held unconscious or at least unnoticed at that point. The therapist responded to subtle communications from Mr. B. that suggested a longing for a special, even ideal, relationship with his treater. The therapist's observation led the patient to display a more relaxed disposition. He now said that the therapist was the first and only person who was genuinely interested in him as an individual; only he could help him.

Mr. B. developed fantasies in which he was adopted by the therapist and recognized as a son.

- The patient overcomes (at least for a time) his mistrust and sadism toward the therapist and reactivates an object relationship of primitive idealization.
- In this way, he avoids working through the conflicts with the therapist, especially the full truth about his perversion and delinquency.
- He tries to skip over the painful grief of both his own actions and his own experience of having been abused.

Technical handling:

- Before mourning becomes possible, there is often still a phase of overtly sexualized transference to negotiate, in which the original perverting relationship constellation is repeated.
- This phase is inevitably triggered by the interpretations the therapist offers to try to understand the idealizing transference as a defense against cruel violent fantasies.

Sexually Sadistic and Aroused-Fusing Transference

Mr. B. had often reported his interest in clitoral circumcision in Africa. This theme got reinforced strikingly when the therapist addressed the defensive function of Mr. B's adoption fantasies. Mr. B expanded on it with astonishing knowledge about the sexual exploitation that had been perpetrated by Nazi doctors in concentration camps. It was clear that he associated the therapist with this practice.

The investigation of these ideas again revealed an oscillating dyad, in which Mr. B. was at one point the victim of sexual-sadistic experiments (with links to his humiliating-painful phimosis treatment by mother and grandmother and the abusive acts of the aunt), while he was at another time immersed in fantasy as a clitoris-cutting or otherwise sexually mutilating man in Africa, who in this way cruelly took revenge on "the women" who had destroyed his childhood. A preadolescent suicide attempt, which Mr. B. had committed as a 10-year-old after his aunt had forced him to perform cunnilingus on her for the first time, also played a role. Neither father nor mother had believed him in the wake of the abuse by the aunt and continued to send him to her. Mr. B. had also developed the suspicion at that time that at least the father might have been privy to the abuse and had received money from the aunt for it.

Correspondingly, the therapist appeared to the patient either as a psychoanalytic "Mengele" or as a weak victim on whom he could take sadistic revenge by exposing him to his colleagues as a complete failure (i.e., as castrated).

In this extremely sadistically charged phase of the therapy, there also existed a defended counterpart, an emotionally oppositely-cathected relationship dyad with a positive but similarly primitive quality. Mr. B. developed in this phase the fantasy of not only becoming part of the therapist's private life but even of being able to invade his body and live there. This fantasy proved to be an expression of a long resisted excited and fusing mother transference. Since (in his fantasy) there were no father and no siblings, the mother's body was experienced as his own and sole legitimate possession. It seemed natural to relate this to the mother's narrative that she had experienced Mr. B's birth as if it were a magical redemption after a previous miscarriage. He had been breastfed for a long time, but as a result of a school failure in elementary school, he had been deported to a convent school where initial abuse by teachers and fellow students had taken place.

The excited-fusing transference had the significant function of saving a subjectively positive experience from its destruction by extreme feelings of fear and hatred. Allowing it to come to light, enabled Mr. B. to feel a sense of shock and to come closer to the numerous losses he had suffered in his childhood. The pain of being separated in the therapeutic relationship could be connected to these early experiences, and a first mourning process could begin.

Strategy 4: Working Through the More Mature Affective Experiences and Stabilizing the Mature, Triangulated Relationship Patterns that Have Emerged

The mourning processes in the wake of working through the different, successively emerging object-relations dyads initiate a fundamental restructuring of the patient's inner world. The overcoming of the splitting processes between the perpetrator and the victim side, which up to now had led to constantly oscillating role changes within the sadomasochistic object relationship dyad, allows the formation of more stable self and object representations. One's own weaknesses and dissocial fantasies no longer must be immediately denied, projected, or acted out. The integration of various mutually rejecting, affectively contrasting dyads allows for the alloying of the primitive affects involved into more mature feelings and thus the development of whole (at least relatively more complete) representations of self and object instead of the previous partial representations.

This is also associated with a maturation of the patient's defense structure. Splitting, which now loses importance, is replaced by repression as the central defense mechanism. The moderation and merging of the previous paranoid fears with the more mature feelings of guilt arising from the mourning process consolidate a stable, if partially perfectionist, superego. This means that several of the relational dyads experienced as dysfunctional and threatening are now relatively permanently relegated to the unconscious, allowing for a more stable, though still partially distorted, perception of self and object. The identity diffusion typical of borderline personality organization dissolves and gives way to a clearer identity. The following additional signs of integration become apparent:

- Psychopathic transference is resolved
- Increasing tolerance of the patient toward his inner turmoil
- Reduction of splitting and related defense mechanisms.
- Alternative memories of childhood
- The idealizing transference is partially processed
- The paranoid transference is essentially worked through

- Increasing consolidation of the integrated identity
- Decrease of acting out
- Increasing tolerance of guilt regarding antisocial tendencies
- Increasing the reflective capacity of the patient
- Capacity of attachment increases
- Capacity to tolerate separation and being alone increases

The dyadic relationship representations are gradually overlaid and restructured by triadic representations, i.e., by internalized conceptions of differentiated relationships to two parental objects that in turn have a relationship with each other. This structure prepares the acceptance of being separated from 'mother' and the internalization of bids and bans. Gradually, the patient develops increased self-control in relationships, now influenced by an emerging value system, while internalizing the limits of pursuits solely in his own interests. New and larger spaces for symbolization, mentalization, and complex thinking emerge, although the effects of repressed desires and ideas also impose new limitations on thinking. Since the personality is still marked by weaknesses of the ego function and permeated by (now rather depressive) anxieties, repression still shows traces of rigidity, and the inner world still shows substantial lack of freedom. Typically, even in the final phase of TFFP, forensic patients still show numerous neurotic symptoms as an expression of these personality weaknesses.

The therapist's task is to continue the therapy increasingly in the model of traditional psychoanalytic treatment. The individual aspects of the treatment contract lose importance, as do the thematic hierarchies because the patient's personality structure now permits his constructive cooperation in the treatment. On the one hand, it is now a matter of changing the rigidity of the defense system further in the direction of flexibility and permeability by interpreting repressed, unconscious desires and ideas about relationships. On the other hand, it is still a matter of perceiving, verbalizing, and interpreting split-off remnants of unintegrated relationship dyads, i.e., of continuing, refining and consolidating the work that has been achieved.

Recapitulatory Remarks

The purpose of this section was to show the ways in which psychodynamic psychotherapy of offenders has changed and how it has evolved, partly under the influence of the cognitive-behavioral turn in offender therapy in the 1990s. Criticisms of older depth psychological delinquency therapies, specifically that there had been little or no focus on the criminal offense, are addressed in TFFP by explicitly elevating the linkage of transference analysis to offense analysis to a strategic maxim. TFFP also addresses the allegation of a lack of stringency and systematics in the therapeutic approach by anchoring clear principles in the diagnostic process, as well as in the therapy contracts and the thematic hierarchies for the choice of focus in the individual sessions, which are intended to prevent and counteract possible manipulations of the delinquent patient as well as distortions of perception as a result of the therapist's countertransference.

At the same time, it should be evident that the psychodynamic understanding of the psychopathology of offenders, and the transference-countertransference currents induced by them, are of significant, even indispensable, value. The concepts of different levels of psychological structure, borderline personality organization, splitting, denial, projection, and projective identification are generally essential for working with severely personality-disordered patients. They are particularly valuable for therapy with offenders in that the disturbance of these patients is usually quite severe and the power of the defensive maneuvers mentioned is especially strong. Every therapist inevitably succumbs to some degree to the entanglements of the relational confusion that occurs when working with this population; the route out of this confusion toward effective intervention requires clear diagnostic and therapeutic principles, strategies, tactics, and techniques.

What is the source of institutional or government support for this initiative?

Institutional Contexts for the Treatment of Forensic Patients

Constraint Context and Projection

Forensic psychotherapies do not take place in a vacuum. In the vast majority of cases, they would not take place at all if state institutions did not provide them. Self-motivation of delinquent patients is almost never sufficient to initiate psychotherapy, on the other hand, forensic psychotherapy does not take place entirely against the will of those affected.

Offense, social coercion, and forensic psychotherapy stand in a dialectical relationship with each other, in which not least the specific psychopathology of offenders is reflected. By forcing society to intervene repressively to protect the victim, the offense activates a powerful mechanism that is the result of projective identification. Through his offense, the delinquent externalizes an intolerable and unassimilable part of himself. More precisely, it is a (more or less archaic) destructive object relationship that is acted out by the delinquent, which also involves affects that the delinquent cannot hold, cannot modulate, cannot "contain." In a way, this corresponds to the process of projective identification in the infant and toddler as described by Bion [93–95].

In delinquency, a partial regression to this early mechanism takes place, whereby the "maternal digestive function"is assigned less to the individual victim than to the "social body" as a whole (regression to a depersonalized „*global object*"in the sense of group analysis [96]). The offense does not only trigger reactions in the victim. Society as a whole is addressed and reacts with the help of its repressive apparatuses, which take up the projected affects in their own way. To what extent these can only repel the affects projected into them "undigestedly" (for instance in the form of the death penalty or of sadistic punishments) or transform them into a more mature form depends on the mentalization capacities in these institutions (see Sections "Prisons" and "Conclusion"). In any case, the delinquent delegates the container function almost entirely to society. Finally, forensic psychotherapy, if it is applied instead of, during, or after a prison sentence, is also determined by this offense-catalyzed projective identification. It is part of a social containment of projected delinquent affects and fantasies.

The forensic psychotherapist must be aware of this fundamental constellation of his therapeutic situation. In this respect, it differs significantly from usual psychotherapies, even from psychodynamic borderline therapies, with which it otherwise has much in common.

The extent of the delinquent patient's projective identification often necessitates a coercive context for conducting therapy. Many psychodynamic therapists believe that a lack of voluntariness makes it impossible to conduct psychodynamic psychotherapy. Without an available, healthy self-part, not only is a working alliance impossible but no therapeutic process can be initiated, because the healing dialectic of inner forces and fantasies must come to a standstill through the global externalization of fundamental parts of the personality.

However, this assumption, which at first seems plausible, has been empirically refuted (also in the case of substance abusers), not only because numerous studies show that therapy can reduce the recidivism rates of offenders (e.g., [97]). It is simply also a clinical fact of experience that despite a coercive context, workable transference processes do get underway. The reason for this is that the coercive context of forensic therapies is not simply a coercive structure entirely external to the patient's psyche, but that the coercion is triggered by projective processes and continues to be experienced as alien coercion only because of the externalization of certain parts of the self. For the unconscious, coercion may play a similar role here as the unequal distribution of power between children and adults does for adolescent children. In the optimal case, authoritative guidelines oscillate in their meaning between security-providing container function and autonomy-desire-stimulating freedom restriction. In the context of the severe superego-pathologies of delinquent patients, these functions appear of course partly grotesquely distorted. While some feel subjected to concentration camp-like ordeals, enslaved, or made guinea pigs of questionable medical experiments by their therapist, others experience therapy as the only place of safety and benevolence, fearing they will be expelled when the judicial therapy order expires.

In whatever way forensic patients subjectively experience the coercive context, in most cases the associated fantasies and acting out provide valuable material for examining the patients' inner world. The offense appears here again and again, reflecting the junction where the pathology of the patient's inner world spills over into the outer world in such a way that the latter absorbs the violence of the object relations thus externalized and transforms them, among other things, into forensic psychotherapy. The perpetrator would never have gone into this treatment without the coercive context, because the extent of pathology would not have permitted entering voluntarily into a dependent relationship.

The patient's engagement in forensic psychotherapy can thus be seen as a gradual (re)internalization of the coercive context in the sense of building up inner boundaries. If in the early stages often only the external coercion is seen, later a split between the benevolent therapist and the oppressive justice system in general often becomes visible. A sign of a relatively advanced therapeutic process is when the patient is able to understand the restriction of freedom in retrospect as a consequence of his own tendencies to act out and the related inability to take adult responsibility.

It is not claimed here that all delinquents are ultimately "*criminals from a sense of guilt*" as in the terms outlined by Freud [3], meaning that they unconsciously desired and brought about punishment by society. The projective identification described here is not about unconscious feelings of guilt, but about primitive destructive aggression and primitive envy. This aggression is directed not only against the integrity of the concrete victim, but also against the legal structure of society. It puts society as a container to the test. While "*criminals from a sense of guilt*" unconsciously want to be "caught", this does not apply to the primitively projecting criminals. They try to destroy the container. Nevertheless, there is something like an innate preconception that aims at containment of the projected primitive affects [94]. And when all options for containment have failed in a person's personal environment, the state repressive system is finally challenged.

Prisons

Patients most often begin forensic psychotherapy while in prison. In most countries, this possibility is limited to certain special prisons or forensic institutions, where those offenders are held who have been found by the court to show a clear involvement of a mental disorder in the causes of the offense. Prisons have a typical structure, and this is of course essential for the implementation of forensic psychotherapy. Three general points of view are decisive here:

First, there is a mix of occupational groups that work in a prison and are involved with the prisoners. The institutionally central occupational group is the guard officers, who are mainly responsible for the internal and external security of the institution, but in most countries are also assigned some educational function in relation to the inmates. In addition to the guard officers, there are a certain number of staff members in the therapeutic institutions to be discussed here who are responsible for the care and health services of the inmates (specialized services). As a rule, there are social tensions between the guard officers and the specialized services, which stem from the fact that neither professional group is sufficiently aware of, nor appreciates the function of, the other. Inter-professional tensions in prisons also reflect the social and political tensions of the surrounding society. They manifest themselves, among other things, as ideological oppositions between the goal of containing and suppressing crime versus the goal of (re-)socializing offenders. A sufficiently constructive relationship between the professional groups is indispensable for the success of therapeutic efforts, which is why it is necessary for the prison management to take care of this relationship and continuously promote exchange and mutual understanding of the different tasks and competencies.

This brings us to the second relevant aspect of the prison structure, the management structure. The prison director needs a second level of management where the various tasks of the prison are divided into clear areas of responsibility. Psychiatry, psychology, social work and others with psychotherapy training are cooperative professions in the area of care and need a clear division of tasks so that they are not burdened by territorial disputes and extraneous competition between members of the prison staff. Their cooperation with security staff must also be clearly regulated so that there is neither loose coexistence nor rivalry over responsibilities between specialist and guard services. Ideally, the professional groups are clearly delineated, feel valued, and supported by the management in a balanced way, and therefore develop neither envy for, nor devaluation of, each other. Under such conditions, the guard services can be a valuable enrichment of the therapeutic function of the prison, just as, conversely, the specialized services can become a recognized element of prison security.

The third structural aspect that is central to forensic psychotherapy in a prison concerns the function of the care services team. Depending on the size of the prison, this may have to be organized in a differentiated and hierarchical way, but the crucial function is that of case discussions. These case discussions facilitate the airing of the different perspectives and attitudes of the staff toward the individual inmates. Each perspective represents one of the many aspects of the patients' often very split mental structure and should not be ignored. The integrative and mentalizing capacity of the team or the entire team structure, including the management level, is ultimately the basis for reflecting on and overcoming the endemic processes of splitting that are continually engendered by the inmates to the institution and reflected by it. It is precisely this persistent working against the forces of disintegration and fragmentation that is the crucial institutional process required for therapeutic efforts to bear fruit.

Forensic Psychiatry

In most countries, the treatment of offenders with mental illnesses in the narrower sense is assigned to certain specialized psychiatric institutions. This usually concerns psychotic patients, but also certain groups of severe personality disorders and addictive disorders, depending on the legal situation.

Institutionally, psychiatry is structured differently than prisons, because it is part of the health care system and therefore usually under the direction of a physician. Moreover, in forensic psychiatry, there is a system of care, which is then also responsible for security, or there is a separate guard service in addition to care. Whatever the concrete professional administration of the institution, some basic structural problems of forensic psychiatry are quite similar to those of the prison.

Again, there are tensions between the professional groups, although, in this situation, tensions between nurses and physicians dominate. In addition, there may also be tensions between the physicians and the non-medical care services (psychologists, psychotherapists, art therapists, etc.) as well as between these and possibly other professional groups such as cleaning or technical staff. In all cases, the aim must always be to promote mutual appreciation and cooperation by ensuring that the tasks of the various groups are clearly defined and demarcated and that there is as much information shared as possible about the tasks and working conditions of the other groups, and that a systemic overall view is conveyed that makes the entire process visible as a necessary co-production of all professional groups. The potential benefits of mutual support can only be raised if inter-professional envy and jealousy can be explored and overcome.

This goal is also dependent on the transparency and the quality of the management structure in forensic psychiatry. The heads of department must be able to play their dual role, namely, on the one hand, to take up the activities of the staff and support them, and on the other hand, to implement the perspective and priorities of the institution as a whole. Furthermore, the heads of department, for their part, must cooperate and prepare all information for the medical director and concretize and implement the central decisions downwards. In order for this to work, the medical director is challenged to find the right person for the right position.

The points outlined about the functioning of the therapeutic team and of the team structure in general in prison can be applied without qualification to the specialized forensic psychiatry division. Even in a treatment setting dominated by psychiatric patients, the perception of the countertransference reactions of the various staff members is important, as is the team's ability to integrate different perspectives and opposing opinions.

Outpatient Follow-Up

In outpatient aftercare facilities, released prisoners or forensic psychiatric patients receive further treatment and are supported on their path to full autonomy. Such facilities do not exist everywhere, but they are particularly important for absorbing the shock that release means (at least unconsciously) for many inmates of forensic institutions and for psychotherapeutically processing the problems of the transition. Here, there is no guard staff but usually, a few nurses are present, so professional group tensions focus on those between physicians and therapists. The management of professional group tensions thus reflects to some extent the management of team tensions.

Nevertheless, a distinction must be made between the extent to which structural or institutional tensions are at issue, e.g., questions of differences in service law or professional competencies, and the extent to which different perceptions of transferences and group dynamics are the topic. While in the case of the former, management and the management structure are called upon to work out optimal solutions, in the case of the latter, it is more a matter of team competence, which may also have to be supported from outside through supervision or team development.

Outlook and Conclusion

Psychodynamic Diagnostics: Is a STIPO-F Coming?

It was shown in this chapter that TFP principles can be applied to a large extent in the treatment of forensic patients and that the modifications necessary for this in the form of the development of TFFP have already progressed significantly. Nevertheless, in some ways, TFFP is still in its infancy.

When considering diagnostics, Section "Forensic Patients and their Psychopathology" demonstrated that the TFP tradition has numerous foundational insights into personality organization and also offers relatively differentiated models of prototypes and structural axes that are relevant for forensic psychotherapy. But in this context, exact operationalization, systematization, and evaluation are still lacking.

In analogy to the development of a forensic supplement to the OPD-2 in Germany (OPF-F) [75, 98], it would also make sense to think about the development of a forensically supplemented structured interview on personality organization (STIPO-F). For this purpose, it would be necessary to operationalize the axis model presented in Section "Axis Model". By means of concrete questions and to link it to the existing STIPO. In a previous paper [87], this author proposed to elicit the meaning of the offense for the patient as an expression of and compensation attempt for his structural limitations elucidated by a series of offense-specific questions. In this sense, one can describe different structural levels specifically for the domains of property, violent, and sexual delinquency, which could potentially be made use of as measures of therapeutic progress but also as indications of the remaining risk of recidivism. It is clear that extensive research remains to be done on this.

A Manual for TFFP?

Similar considerations can be made regarding further deepening and systematizing the therapeutic approach according to TFP principles with delinquent patients. In this chapter, the focus was on the presentation of the four strategies and how they could be modified for forensic applications. It also described some forms of transference that play a major role in the treatment of pedosexual offenders and developed suggestions for a technical approach to dealing with this population.

This approach should be further extended in several respects. First, the repetitive forms of transference would need to be examined for a broader range of delinquency at different structural levels. It seems that there are indeed presentable types and degrees of severity of structural constellations that explain to some extent the different forms of property, violence, and sexual offenses, and at the same time make clear the patterns of internalized object relations of the offenders. These are repeated in individual but typical forms in therapeutic work as transference/countertransference dispositions and as such form the material to be worked on therapeutically. Such a system of delinquent transferences would certainly be a valuable building block for the training of forensic psychotherapists [55].

A systematic presentation of delinquent transferences, including an evaluation of corresponding countertransference reactions, would also be significant for the development of a TFFP group therapy concept. Building on the already elaborated transference-focused understanding of group processes and for TFP interventions in this context [99, 100], the necessary modifications for the forensic context are to be elaborated and presented.

Other topics that would be essential for a future manual for TFPP but require additional comprehensive clarification include the forensics-specific modifications of the therapy contract and the modifications of the tactical and thematic hierarchies as they are crucial in TFP. As far as the framework and the therapy contract are concerned, there is already preliminary work [51] addressing the numerous technical problems arising from offenders' tendency to deny and trivialize their offenses. It would also be necessary to differentiate the requirements for a therapy contract according to the different forensic regimes, such as normal penal detention, relaxed enforcement, and forensic aftercare. As far as the thematic hierarchies are concerned, particular attention should be paid to the numerous forms of behavior that are not yet punishable but increase the risk of recidivism, as well as to the tendency of delinquent patients to narrow and trivialize the therapeutic conversation. Finally, forensic psychotherapies usually differ from non-forensic ones in terms of termination, because the end of therapy often does not result primarily from the therapeutic process but from court-ordered deadlines (e.g., release from prison or lifting of measures).

Conclusion

To conclude, it might help to list the most important ways that TFP principles can help forensic professionals deal with the institutional contexts in which their work takes place:

- The fact that forensic institutions exist reflects to some degree a necessary containing function of the state. This containing function helps to embrace and mitigate the violent emotions of a group individuals who are not adequately held in check by their personal and community environments.
- Forensic institutions have the task to provide security for society both by detaining convicted offenders and by supporting their personality development.
- It is helpful to view the professional groups within forensic institutions as components of a complex system that need to work together in an integrative way but are in danger of coming into opposition and rivalry with each other.
- These problems may have organizational or ideological reasons, but they most often are also a reflection of primitive defense processes which are originating from, or involving, the inmates. Projective identification of dissociated affects can trigger regressive processes in staff members.

- It is the persistent working against such forces of splitting and fragmentation that is the crucial institutional process required for therapeutic efforts to bear fruit. This integrative work is also a process of mentalization in both staff and inmates.
- The management of the forensic institution has the responsible task of enabling and encouraging the cooperation of the professional groups and teams. In that task the management fulfils a triangulating function in regard both to regressive tendencies in the relation between the professional groups and in the relation between the staff and the inmates.

TFP principles can be of use in multiple spheres in forensic institutions. A transference-focused understanding of team dynamics considers the various group processes, especially in case discussions, as a mirror of the inmates' inner world. In this context, the specialist team should act as a "mentalization agency"and translate the conflicts between caregivers into thoughts and words. However, the mentalization task also exists for the conflictual relationship between inmates and the judicial authority as a whole. Inmates' transferences extend not only to the various individuals with whom they interact, but also to the correctional institution as a whole. It also affects the relationship between professional groups and that between the various hierarchical levels of a correctional institution. TFP principles can also help the management level in prisons to reflect on their "countertransference" to the inmates and the institutional conflicts and to avoid actions marked by impaired mentalization.

Finally, a TFFP manual would need to include considerations of the institutional framework of forensic therapies. TFP offers the opportunity to reflect psychodynamically on institutional reality at different levels. Reflection on unconscious communication in correctional settings can be helpful for staff as well as for the management levels of correctional institutions. In particular, it can be a boost to their resilience given the inevitable contagion of institutional communication by pathological projections.

References

1. Winnicott DW. The maturational processes and the facilitating environment. London: The Hogarth Press and the Institute of Psychoanalysis; 1965. 276 p
2. Kahr B. Sigmund Freud and the case of the pedophile. Psychotherapy Review. 1999;1:89–90.
3. Freud S. Some Character-types Met with in psycho-analytic work [1916]. The standard edition of the complete psychological works of Sigmund Freud, volume XIV. London: W. W. Norton & Company; 1990. p. 309–333.
4. Aichhorn A. Wayward youth. A psychoanalytic study of delinquent youth. Foreword by Sigmund Freud. Evanston: Northwestern University Press; 1984 [1925]. 206 p.
5. Alexander F, Healy W. Roots of crime. Psychoanalytic studies. Montclaire/N.J.: Patterson Smith; 1969 [1935]. 305 p.
6. Bowlby J. Forty-Four Juvenile thieves: their character and home-life. Int. J. Psycho-Anal. 1944;25:19–53–107–128.
7. Glover E. The diagnosis and treatment of delinquency. In: Institute for the Scientific Treatment of Delinquency. Mental Abnormality and Crime. London: Macmillan & Co; 1944. p. 269–299.

8. Glover E. The roots of crime. New York: International Universities Press; 1960. 422 p
9. Friedländer K. The psychoanalytical approach to juvenile delinquency. Theory—Case Studies—Treatment. New York: International Universities Press 1971 [1947]. 296 p.
10. Eissler KR, Federn P, editors. Searchlights on delinquency. New psychoanalytic studies. New York: International Universities Press; 1958 [1949]. 456 p.
11. Schmideberg M. The analytic treatment of major criminals: therapeutic results and technical problems. In: Eissler KR, editor. Searchlights on delinquency. New York: International Universities Press; 1949. p. 174–89.
12. Johnson AM, Szurek SA. The genesis of antisocial acting out in children and adults. PsaQ. 1952;21:323–43.
13. Winnicott DW. The antisocial tendency [1956]. In: Winnicott DW, editor. Through paediatrics to psycho-analysis. London: Tavistock; 1958. p. 306–15.
14. Winnicott DW. Deprivation and delinquency. London: Routledge; 1985. 304 p
15. Joseph B. Some characteristics of the psychopathic personality [1960]. In: Meloy JR, editor. The mark of Cain. Psychoanalytic insight and the psychopath. Hillsdale, London: The Analytic Press; 2001. p. 227–38.
16. Goudsmit W. Psychotherapie bei Delinquenten Psyche. 1964;17:664–84.
17. Goudsmit W. Bemerkungen zur Indikation der Psychoanalyse bei Tätern von sehr schweren Delikten. Psyche. 1974;28:684–705.
18. Menninger K. The crime of punishment. New York: The Viking Press; 1968. 305 p
19. Klüwer K. Die Delinquenten und ihre Behandlungsmöglichkeiten. In: Die Psychologie des 20.Jh., Tiefenpsychologie, Bd.2: Neue Wege der Psychoanalyse—Psychoanalyse und Gesellschaft—Die psychoanalytische Bewegung, Weinheim/Basel; 1982 [1976]. 728 p.
20. Schorsch E, Galedary G, Haag A, Hauch M, Lohse H. Perversion als Straftat. Dynamik und Psychotherapie. Berlin-Heidelberg: Springer-Verlag; 1985. 184 p
21. Berner W, Karlick-Bolten E. Verlaufsformen der Sexualkriminalität. Stuttgart: Enke Verlag; 1986. 200 p
22. Berner W. Das Selbstvertauschungsagieren Pädophiler. Psychotherapie-Psychosomatik-Medizinische Psychologie. 1985;35(1):17–23.
23. Berner W. Therapie sexueller Delinquenz unter institutionellen Bedingungen. In: Sigusch V, editor. Sexuelle Störungen und ihre Behandlung. Stuttgart: Thieme; 2001. p. 501–16.
24. Berner W. Perversion. Psychosozial Verlag: Gießen; 2011. 144 p
25. Glasser M. Psychodynamic aspects of paedophilia. Psychoanal Psychother. 1988;3:121–35.
26. Meloy JR. The psychopathic mind. Origins, dynamics, and treatment. Lanham, New York, Oxford: Jason Aronson; 1988. 474 p
27. Cordess C, Cox M, editors. Forensic psychotherapy. Crime, psychodynamics, and the offender patient. London, Philadelphia: Jessica Kingsley Publishers; 1995. 992p.
28. Morgan D, Ruszczynski S, editors. Lectures on violence, perversion and delinquency. The Portman papers. London: Karnac; 2007. 260 p.
29. Lackinger F, Dammann G, Wittmann B. Psychodynamische Psychotherapie bei Delinquenz. Praxis der Übertragungsfokussierten Psychotherapie. Stuttgart: Schattauer Verlag; 2008. 472 p
30. Lackinger F. Zur psychodynamischen Diagnostik antisozialer Störungen. In: Dulz B, Kernberg O, Briken, P, Rauchfleisch U (Hg.). Handbuch der antisozialen Persönlichkeitsstörung. Stuttgart: Schattauer; 2016. p. 219–238.
31. Lackinger F. Zur psychodynamischen Therapie von pädosexuellen Tätern. In: Stompe T, Laubichler W, Schanda H, editors. Sexueller Kindesmissbrauch und Pädophilie. 2nd ed. Wien: Medizinisch Wissenschaftliche Verlagsgesellschaft; 2017. p. 143–68.
32. Meloy JR, Yakeley J. Antisocial personality disorder. In: Gabbard GO, editor. Gabbard's treatments of psychiatric disorders. American Psychiatric Publishing, Inc.; 2014. p. 1015–1034.
33. Boer DP, Wilson RJ, Gauthier CM, Hart SD. Assessing risk of sexual violence: guidelines for clinical practice. In: Webster CD, Jackson MA, editors. Impulsivity: theory, assessment and treatment. New York: Guilford Press; 1996. p. 326–42.
34. Hanson RK, Bussiere M. Predicting relapse: a meta-analysis of sexual offender recidivism studies. J Consult Clin Psychol. 1998;66:348–63.

35. Redondo S, Sanchez-Meca J, Garrido V. The influence of treatment programmes on the recidivism of juvenile and adult offenders: a European metaanalytic review. Psychol Crime Law. 1999;5:251–78.
36. Schmucker M. Meta-Analysen zur Sexualstraftäterbehandlung. In: Berner W, Briken P, Hill A, editors. Sexualstraftäter behandeln mit Psychotherapie und Medikamenten. Köln: Deutscher Ärzte-Verlag; 2007. p. 13–31.
37. Quinsey VL, Lalumiere ML, Rice ME, Harris GT. Predicting sexual offenses. In: Campbell JC, editor. Assessing dangerousness: violence by sexual offenders, batterers, and child abusers. Thousand Oaks: Sage; 1995. p. 114–37.
38. Alexander MA. Sexual offender treatment efficacy revisited. Sexual Abuse J Res Treatment. 1999;11:101–16.
39. Rice ME, Harris GT. The size and sign of treatment effects in sex offender therapy. Ann N Y Acad Sci. 2003;989:428–40.
40. Harris GT, Rice ME, Quinsey VL, Cormier CA. Violent offenders: appraising and managing risk. 3rd ed. Washington, DC: American Psychological Association; 2015. p. 195–222.
41. Laws R, editor. Relapse prevention with sex offenders. New York: Guilford Press; 1989. 338 p
42. Laws R, Hudson SM, Ward T, editors. Remaking relapse prevention with sex offenders: a sourcebook. Thousand Oaks: SAGE; 2000. 559 p
43. Pfäfflin F. Rückfallpräventionsprogramme für Sexualstraftäter. Recht & Psychiatrie. 2001;19(3):140–51.
44. Fiedler P. Sexuelle Orientierung und sexuelle Abweichung: Heterosexualität—Homosexualität—Transgenderismus und Paraphilien—sexueller Missbrauch—sexuelle Gewalt. Weinheim, Basel: Beltz; 2004. 520 p.
45. American Psychiatric Association. Dangerous sex offenders: a task force report of the American Psychiatric Association. Washington, DC: American Psychiatric Press; 1999. 194 p
46. Urbaniok F. Der deliktorientierte Therapieansatz in der Behandlung von Straftätern—Konzeption, Methodik und strukturelle Rahmenbedingungen im Zürcher PPD-Modell. Psychoth Forum. 2003;11:202–13.
47. McGauley G, Yakeley J, Williams A, Bateman A. Attachment, mentalization and antisocial personality disorder: the possible contribution of mentalization-based treatment. Eur J Psychother Counselling. 2011;13(4):371–93.
48. Ware A, Wilson C, Tapp J, Moore E. Mentalisation-based therapy (MBT) in a high-secure hospital setting: expert by experience feedback on participation. J Forensic Psychi Psychol. 2016;27(5):722–44.
49. Clarkin JF, Yeomans FE, Kernberg OF. Transference-focused psychotherapy for borderline personality disorder: a clinical guide. Washington, DC: American Psychiatric Publishing; 2015.
50. Clarkin JF, Levy KN, Lenzenweger MF, Kernberg OF. Evaluating three treatments for borderline personality disorder. Am J Psychiatry. 2007;164:922–8.
51. Lackinger F, Dammann G. Besonderheiten der Behandlungsbedingungen bei der übertragungsfokussierten Psychotherapie (TFP) persönlichkeitsgestörter Delinquenten. Recht & Psychiatrie. 2005;23(3):103–15.
52. Lackinger F. Transference focused forensic psychotherapy (TFFP). Die Psychodynamische borderline-Therapie wird forensisch adaptiert. Forensische Psychiatrie und Psychotherapie—Werkstattschriften. 2007;14(1):61–103.
53. Lackinger F. Psychoanalytische Überlegungen zur Pädophilie. Psychotherapeut. 2009;54:262–9.
54. Lackinger F. Rahmen und Grenzen der ambulanten Täterbehandlung im Forensisch-therapeutischen Zentrum Wien (FTZW). Forensische Psychiatrie und Psychotherapie. 2011;18:93–109.
55. Lackinger F. Zur Dynamik von Übertragung und Perversion. In: Lackinger F, Dammann G, Wittmann B, editors. Psychodynamische Psychotherapie bei Delinquenz. Praxis der Übertragungsfokussierten Psychotherapie. Stuttgart: Schattauer Verlag; 2008. p. 197–217.

56. Lackinger F, Zimprichowa D. Zur Indikation von TFP bei Straftätern. In: Lackinger F, Dammann G, Wittmann B, editors. Psychodynamische Psychotherapie bei Delinquenz. Praxis der Übertragungsfokussierten Psychotherapie. Stuttgart: Schattauer; 2008. p. 66–80.
57. Dammann G, Yeomans FE. Antisoziale Persönlichkeitsstörung und Übertragungsfokussierte Psychotherapie. In: Dulz B, Kernberg O, Briken P, Rauchfleisch U, editors. Handbuch der antisozialen Persönlichkeitsstörung. Stuttgart: Schattauer; 2016. p. 399–417.
58. Lohmer M, Brem J. Abwehr und Gegenübertragung in der Therapie der Antisozialen Persönlichkeitsstörung. In: Dulz B, Kernberg O, Briken P, Rauchfleisch U, editors. Handbuch der antisozialen Persönlichkeitsstörung. Stuttgart: Schattauer; 2016. p. 418–27.
59. Dammann G. Psychodynamische Psychotherapie mit Menschen mit antisozialen und psychopathischen Störungen der Persönlichkeit. Forens Psychiatr Psycholog Kriminol. 2018;12:238–55.
60. Groth AN. Patterns of sexual assault against children and adolescents. In: Burgess W, Groth AN, Holmstrom L, Sgroi SM, editors. Sexual assault of children and adolescents. New York: Lexington Books; 1978. p. 3–24.
61. Groth AN, Birnbaum HJ. Men who rape: the psychology of the offender. New York: Plenum; 1979. 227 p
62. Knight RA, Prentky RA. Classifying sexual offenders: the development and corroboration of taxonomic models. In: Marshall WL, Barbaree HE, editors. The handbook of sexual assault: issues, theories, and treatment of the offender. New York: Plenum; 1990. p. 23–53.
63. Rehder U. Klassifizierung inhaftierter Sexualdelinquenten. 1. und 2. Teil. Monatsschr Kriminol Strafrechtsref. 1996;79:291–304, 373–85
64. Simkins L, Ward W, Bowman S, Rink CM, DeSouza E. Predicting treatment outcome for sexual abusers. Ann Sex Res. 1990;3:21–57.
65. Kernberg OF. Borderline conditions and pathological narcissism. Lanham: Jason Aronson; 2004 [1975]. 376 p.
66. Fonagy P, Target M, Steele H, Steele M. Reflective-functioning manual 5.0. London: University College London; 1998.
67. Meyer AE. Zur psychoanalyse der Perversionen. Theol Sex. 1976;5:169–76.
68. Kernberg OF. Severe personality disorders: psychotherapeutic strategies. New Haven: Yale University Press 1993 [1984]. 396 p.
69. Clarkin J, Caligor E, Stern B, Kernberg OF. Structured interview for personality organization—revised (STIPO-R). New York: Personality Disorders Institute, Weill Medical College of Cornell University; 2016. 61 p.
70. Caligor E, Stern B, Kernberg OF, Buchheim A, Doering S, Clarkin J. Strukturiertes Interview zur Erfassung von Persönlichkeitsorganisation (STIPO)—Wie verhalten sich Objektbeziehungstheorie und Bindungstheorie zueinander? Persönlichkeitsstörungen. 2004;8:209–16.
71. Hoerz-Sagstetter S, Caligor E, Preti E, Stern BL, Chiara DP, Clarkin JF. Clinician-guided assessment of personality using the structural interview and the structured interview of personality organization (STIPO). J Pers Assess. 2018;100(1):30–42.
72. Levinson A, Fonagy P. Offending, and attachment: the relationship between interpersonal awareness and offending in a prison population with psychiatric disorder. Can J Psychoanal. 2004;12:225–51.
73. Green A. Todestrieb, negativer Narzißmus, Desobjektalisierungsfunktion (aus: Le travail du négatif [1993]). Psyche. 2001;55(9–10):869–77.
74. Patrick CJ. Psychophysiological correlates of aggression and violence: an integrative review. Philos Trans R Soc Lond Ser B Biol Sci. 2008;363:2543–55.
75. OPD Task Force, editor. Operationalized psychodynamic diagnosis OPD-2: manual of diagnosis and treatment planning. (E. Ristl, Trans.). Cambridge: Hogrefe & Huber Publishers; 2008. 408 p.
76. Knight RA. Validation of a typology for rapists. J Interpers Violence. 1999;14:303–30.
77. Kernberg OF. Aggressivity, narcissism, and self-destructiveness in the psychotherapeutic relationship: new developments in the psychopathology and psychotherapy of severe personality disorders. New Haven: Yale University Press; 2014 [2004]. 288 p.

78. Kernberg OF. The almost untreatable narcissistic patient. J. Amer. Psychoanal Assn. 2007;55(2):503–39.
79. Kernberg OF. The narcissistic personality disorder and the differential diagnosis of antisocial behavior. Special issue: narcissistic personality disorder (ed. by OF Kernberg). Psychiatr Clin N Am. 1989;12(3):553–70.
80. Kernberg OF. An overview of the treatment of severe narcissistic pathology. Int J Psychoanal. 2014;95(5):865–88.
81. Fonagy P, Gergely G, Jurist EL, Target M. Affect regulation, mentalization, and the development of the self London: other press; 2005 [2000]. 592 p.
82. Yeomans FE, Clarkin JF, Diamond D, Levy KN. An object relations treatment of borderline patients with reflective functioning as the mechanism of change. In: Busch F, editor. Mentalization. Theoretical considerations, research findings and clinical implications. New York, London: The Analytic Press; 2008. p. 159–81.
83. Kernberg OF, Diamond D, Yeomans FE, Clarkin JF, Levy KN. Mentalization and attachment in borderline patients in transference focused psychotherapy. In: Jurist EL, Slade A, Bergner S, editors. Mind to mind. Infant research, neuroscience and psychoanalysis. New York: The Other Press; 2008. p. 167–201.
84. Levy KN, Clarkin JF, Yeomans FE, Scott LN, Wasserman RH, Kernberg OF. The mechanisms of change in the treatment of borderline personality disorder with transference focused psychotherapy. J Clin Psychol. 2006;62(4):481–501.
85. Dammann G. Antisoziale Dimensionen in der Pathologie von Borderline-Patienten. In: Dammann G, Wittmann B, editors. Lackinger F. Schattauer: Psychodynamische Psychotherapie bei Delinquenz. Praxis der Übertragungsfokussierten Psychotherapie. Stuttgart; 2008. p. 184–96.
86. Hoerz S, Clarkin J, Stern B, Caligor E. The Structured Interview of Personality Organization (STIPO): an instrument to assess severity and change of personality pathology. In: Levy RA, editor. Handbook of evidence-based psychodynamic psychotherapy. 3rd ed. New York: Humana Press; 2012. p. 571–92.
87. Lackinger F. Psychodynamische Strukturdiagnostik und Deliktanalyse bei persönlichkeitsgestörten Delinquenten. In: Lackinger F, Dammann G, Wittmann B, editors. . Stuttgart: Psychodynamische Psychotherapie bei Delinquenz. Praxis der Übertragungsfokussierten Psychotherapie, Schattauer; 2008. p. 3–37.
88. Fonagy P. The developmental roots of violence in the failure of Mentalization. In: Pfäfflin F, Adshead G, editors. A matter of security. The application of attachment theory to forensic psychiatry and psychotherapy. London, New York: Jessica Kingsley Publishers; 2004. p. 13–56.
89. Fonagy P. Persönlichkeitsstörung und Gewalt—ein psychoanalytisch-bindungstheoretischer Ansatz [2006]. In: Lackinger F, Dammann G, Wittmann B, editors. . Stuttgart: Psychodynamische Psychotherapie bei Delinquenz. Praxis der Übertragungsfokussierten Psychotherapie, Schattauer Verlag; 2008. p. 326–65.
90. Fonagy P, Target M, Steele M, Steele H. The development of violence and crime as it relates to security of attachment. In: Osofsky J, editor. Children in a violent society. New York: Guilford Press; 1997. p. 150–81.
91. Lackinger F. TFFP as a sexual offender treatment modality. Diagnostics, contract setting and treatment process; 2010. Unpublished lecture given at IATSO conference in Oslo 2010.
92. Bateman A, Bolton R, Fonagy P. Antisocial personality disorder: a mentalizing framework. Focus J Lifelong Learning Psychiat. 2013;11:1–9.
93. Bion WR. Learning from experience. Lanham: Jason Aronson; 1994 [1962]. 111 p.
94. Bion WR. Elements of psycho-analysis. London: Heinemann 2004 [1963]. 116 p.
95. Bion WR. Sexual behavior and the law (review). Int J Pychoanal. 1966;47:579–81.
96. König K, Lindner WV. 'Transference in groups'. In: König K, Lindner WV, editors. Psychoanalytic group therapy. Northvale, London: Aronson; 1994. 216 p.
97. Eher R, Lackinger F, Frühwald S, Frottier P. Beziehungsorientierte Psychotherapie bei entlassenen Straftätern und einer Gruppe von Sexualstraftätern. Ergebnisse einer 7-Jahres-Katamnese. Recht & Psychiatrie. 2006;24(2):83–90.

98. Arbeitskreis OPD-Forensik. Das Modul Forensik. Diagnostik und Therapieplanung in der forensischen Psychotherapie mit der OPD-2. Das Diagnostik Manual. Forensische Psychiatrie und Psychotherapie. 2015; 22(1):5–30.
99. Mattke D, Dammann G, Martius P. Der Transfer von einzeltherapeutischen Behandlungskonzepten auf Gruppenformate: Das Beispiel der Übertragungsfokussierten Psychotherapie (TFP). Vandenhoeck & Ruprecht—e-libray. Online veröffentlicht. Apr 2014. https://doi.org/10.13109/grup.2007.43.3.161.
100. Kernberg OF. Psychoanalytic individual and group therapy: the model of transference focused psychotherapy (TFP). In: Kernberg OF, editor. Love and aggression. Arlington: American Psychiatric Publishing; 2012. p. 31–56.

Using Transference-Focused Psychotherapy (TFP) Principles in the Treatment of Medical and Personality Disorder Comorbidities

12

Richard G. Hersh, Mark Petrini, Elisa Bergonzini, and Maria Moscara

Introduction

The complicated overlap of many aspects of medical care and certain fraught personality disorder (PD) presentations can pose unusual challenges to clinicians in various treatment settings. The broad continuum of clinical situations reflecting these challenges include: (1) medical complications arising directly from specific PD phenomena; (2) medical complications arising indirectly from specific PD phenomena or those conditions identified at higher-than-expected rates in PD populations; and (3) complications arising when PD patients access routine or acute medical services and the related, widely described frustrations experienced by the medical providers who care for these patients.

Parts of some paragraphs are slightly modified excerpts from: Moscara M, Bergonzini E. Integrating the principles of transference-focused psychotherapy with psychiatric consultation for patients admitted to a general hospital: A clinical application of a psychotherapeutic tool. Int J Appl Psychoanal Studies. 2020:1–12. https://doi.org/10.1002/aps.1661

R. G. Hersh (✉)
Department of Psychiatry, Columbia Vagelos College of Physicians & Surgeons, New York, NY, USA
e-mail: rh170@cumc.columbia.edu

M. Petrini
Departments of Psychiatry and Medicine, Columbia Vagelos College of Physicians & Surgeons, New York, NY, USA
e-mail: mp19@caa.columbia.edu

E. Bergonzini
Department of Mental Health, Modena Health Agency, Modena, Italy
e-mail: e.bergonzini@ausl.mo.it

M. Moscara
Modena, Italy

R. G. Hersh, C. De Panfilis (eds.), *Implementing Transference-Focused Psychotherapy Principles*, https://doi.org/10.1007/978-3-031-68062-5_12

The goal of this chapter is twofold: (1) to present a survey of the complex interface of medical and PD pathology and to place the utility of applied transference-focused psychotherapy (TFP) principles in that context, and (2) to focus on two specific applied TFP implementation strategies aimed at addressing the thorny situations referenced. The many possible ways of working with TFP principles in this arena are based on the theoretical underpinnings of TFP as an extended, individual psychotherapy, but with notable adjustments made for the significantly different environments outlined. The two specific initiatives examined are: (1) a consultation-liaison (CL) service where the integration of TFP principles in work with general hospital (GH) patients has been introduced to complement the standard approach offered, and (2) a TFP-informed teaching intervention as part of a standardized curriculum for trainees in internal medicine. These initiatives were developed in their respective contexts, but their roots are clearly identifiable in the basic tenets of TFP as outlined in the treatment manuals and informed by the evolving movement of applied TFP.

Interventions for the Overlap of Health-Related Concerns and Personality Disorder Pathology Where does a discussion of the implementation of TFP-informed interventions fit in the broader topic of managing co-occurring medical and PD disorders? What is known about this pattern of co-occurring disorders? What guidance has previously been offered to mental health and general medical professionals? A discussion of co-occurring medical concerns and PD pathology will largely be based on the literature focusing on patients with borderline personality disorder (BPD). BPD is the most extensively studied of the personality disorders, and a number of investigators have rigorously examined many facets of medical health and well-being in BPD patients. In addition, the interplay of other PD presentations and medical health and service utilization patterns have also been explored, although less extensively.

The following areas of investigation and associated references included provide background for discussion of the efforts highlighted:

Epidemiology:

- Patients with PD pathology are seen frequently in primary care medical settings. In one study, 24% of patients in a primary care setting met criteria for a PD diagnosis [1].
- The prevalence of BPD in primary care populations has been noted to be four times higher than that found in community samples. The lifetime prevalence of BPD in a sample of an urban primary care practice was 6.4%. Of note, half the patients with BPD had not had mental health treatment in the past year, and half were not identified by their primary care physicians as having a mental health problem [2].
- An examination consultation-liaison patients indicated that 20% met criteria for a PD diagnosis. The study referenced reviewed records of over three thousand patients hospitalized over nine years in the GH setting [3].

Healthcare utilization patterns:

- Patients with BPD were identified as having increased frequency of referrals to medical specialists at visits to primary care clinicians [4].
- Patients with BPD were noted to have patterns of non-adherence with: (1) instructions from clinicians, (2) completing requested testing, and (3) overall medication compliance [5].
- The presence of a PD diagnosis correlated with increased healthcare utilization in one study, particularly in the primary care setting [6].
- A PD diagnosis has been associated with a wide range of adverse health outcomes and with high rates of healthcare utilization [7].

Medical comorbidity:

- An examination of the physical health, lifestyle choices, and use of medical care in remitted and non-remitted female patients diagnosed with BPD at index hospitalization found the following: Non-remitted patients were found to significantly more likely to report syndrome-like conditions, obesity, osteoarthritis, hypertension, back pain, or urinary incontinence. Non-remitted patients also were more likely to endorse regular smoking, daily consumption of alcohol, lack of regular exercise, daily use of sleep medications, and frequent use of pain medications [8].
- Multiple medical sequelae have been linked to a diagnosis of antisocial PD [9].
- A national household survey in Great Britain concluded that people in the community at risk for a PD were also at increased risk for cardiovascular disease, suggesting personality traits may have a direct role in the contribution to cardiovascular disease. Specifically, psychological characteristics such as negative affectivity, affective instability, and hostility can make PD patients more vulnerable to cardiovascular diseases [10].
- The comorbidity of BPD and physical health conditions in a nationwide sample suggested that the presence of BPD symptoms was significantly associated with multiple medical conditions including arteriosclerosis, hypertension, hepatic disease, arthritis, venereal disease, gastrointestinal disease, and arthritis [11].
- Narcissistic disorders were identified as having an impact on medical care [12].
- One study concluded that the presence of disordered personality was an important risk factor for impaired function *regardless of actual health status.* This study looked at middle-aged adults and specific indices such as medication use and pain level [13].
- The bidirectional effects of narcissistic disorders and medical conditions were considered [14].

Attitudes of medical personnel in different services:

- Guidance to obstetricians and gynecologists in their work with patients with BPD was offered by a team of clinicians. They suggested specific interventions informed by an attitude of support, limit-setting, and judicious psychiatric referral [15].

- The frequent requirements for high levels of time and energy required for the primary care clinician when providing medical care for the patient with BPD were outlined by one group of medical clinicians. They emphasized the need for improved education about BPD for primary care providers and specific skills training [16].
- The benefits of identifying those patients on an acute care medicine unit with PD pathology, given the ramifications of the hospitalization for the patient and the hospital staff, were emphasized [17].
- An overview for neurologists of the issues associated with the management of their patients with co-occurring BPD underscored the necessity for recognizing and prioritizing the contribution of BPD symptoms and recommended an approach anchored by collaboration with others involved in the patient's care, attention to boundaries, monitoring of countertransference, and close attention to clinician consistency [18].
- An assessment of the patients in a prospective study of the course of BPD concluded that failure to recover from BPD seemed to be associated with costly health services utilization including increased emergency room visits and inpatient medical hospitalization [19].

Overarching strategies:

- A proposal to consider the "difficult" patient as one likely to have a PD was proffered. This proposal suggested that the family practice physician: (1) explore the patient's sense of identity and interpersonal relationships; (2) use validation, promote mentalization, and manage countertransference; and (3) recommend medications only as adjunctive to psychotherapy and targeted for specific symptoms. This eclectic approach for the primary care clinician included dialectical behavioral therapy (DBT), mentalization based therapy (MBT), and TFP elements [20].
- A comprehensive review of personality pathology in primary care emphasized screening, collaboration, psychoeducation tools, and intramural psychologic services as effective solutions [21].
- A study of the attitudes of general practice physicians in Australia in their efforts to care for patients with BPD yielded recommendations. Strategies endorsed included: setting up boundaries, using management contracting, and identifying both short-term and long-term goals [22].
- A review of BPD in patients with medical illness includes discussion of the empirically validated treatments for BPD and their possible benefit for health care professionals, i.e., avoiding fruitless power struggles between patients and caregivers [23].

This review underscores the following: (1) patients with PD pathology are well represented in primary care and consultation-liaison services; (2) patients with PD pathology will, on average, have higher rates of healthcare utilization of different kinds; (3) patients with a variety of PD diagnoses will have higher rates of medical comorbidity; (4) clinicians in multiple medical subspecialties have described their distinct concerns about developing skills managing patients with PD pathology; and (5) proposed approaches to the quandaries evident in the overlap of somatic illness and PD pathology have drawn on the applicable parts of the evidence-based individual and group treatments.

Addressing Medical Comorbidities in TFP

In TFP as an extended, individual psychotherapy, contingencies are described for the commonly occurring introduction of medical comorbidities in the treatment of patients with BPD. These co-occurring conditions are sometimes a direct result of the BPD symptoms, such as assessment of sequelae of non-suicidal self-injurious behavior (cutting, burning, head-banging) or overdoses, or injuries related to expression of intense anger or unstable relationships from physical altercations. Medical conditions directly related to BPD diagnostic criteria can include results of impulsive behaviors such as metabolic instability from bulimia nervosa or obesity from binge eating. In addition, a number of other medical syndromes have been identified as more frequently associated with BPD, including chronic pain and sleep disorders. The TFP treatment contract will proactively address any of these medical concerns in advance of starting treatment. In general, the TFP clinician will be alert to the risk of any medical comorbidity that might in some way undermine the stability required for consistent exploration in psychotherapy. Therefore, extensive discussion in advance of those medical concerns directly related to the BPD criteria (e.g., a process for evaluating wounds from self-injury), or those indirectly related to BPD criteria (e.g., ongoing adherence to a prescribed medical program to address chronic pain), would be required.

The standard TFP approach in preparation for an individual psychotherapy would proceed in a deliberate and orderly way. This deliberate approach would automatically probe important material related to a patient's state of health. Attention to medical comorbidities would be addressed by: (1) conducting a diagnostic assessment integrating both standard DSM-5 nosology and the structural interview as described by Kernberg [24], including questioning about physical and/or somatic symptom disorders; (2) sharing the clinician's impression of diagnoses, including pertinent medical comorbidities and/or somatic symptom disorders; (3) identifying the patient's personal goals and treatment goals, including those related to health concerns, when indicated, (4) contacting key current and prior treaters, including medical specialists, when relevant, (5) offering, or in some cases requiring, a family meeting to review diagnoses and treatment options, including discussion of medical comorbidities, when pertinent; and (6) outlining in detail a treatment agreement that would require appropriate management, with expected adherence, of co-occurring medical conditions. All of these elements would be required to be in place before the actual exploratory psychotherapy would begin. The psychotherapy would proceed informed by: (1) "strategies" or organizing goals of integration of those aspects of the patient's behaviors not fully or consistently in the patient's awareness; (2) "tactics" or those pre-conditions, those steps in the assessment process outlined above, required for safe and fruitful psychotherapeutic exploration, and (3) "techniques" or the moment-to-moment interventions. All three elements, strategies, tactics, and techniques, would require added dimensions when matters related to medical conditions or complaints are central in a clinical presentation.

TFP as an individual psychotherapy, while developed initially for patients with BPD, has since been adapted for use with patients with other PD presentations and for certain higher-functioning patients. The basic tenets of a TFP-informed exploration of medical and health topics would apply to this wider group of patients with diagnoses other than BPD.

The Evolution of "Applied TFP" and Topics Related to Medical Care

Zerbo et al. in 2013 described the introduction of TFP as an empirically validated extended individual treatment for patients with BPD to psychiatry residents at New York University [25]. They traced the subsequent modification of TFP principles for working with patients in settings including the consultation-liaison service, the general inpatient psychiatry service, and the forensic inpatient psychiatry service. This account emphasized the adaptability of TFP principles and their use in shorter-term, higher acuity, medical model sites. This modification of TFP principles directly addressed three important observations: (1) patients with PD pathology are well represented in most mental health settings staffed by trainees, *even when clinicians in those settings are not inclined to either diagnose or treat PD pathology;* (2) despite the valiant efforts of a small group of investigators motivated to develop useful, inclusive approaches to treatment of patients with suspected or documented PD pathology in general psychiatry settings, many, perhaps most, clinicians remained easily overwhelmed or flummoxed by PD patients outside of specialized psychotherapy situations*;* and (3) clinicians in these different settings can benefit from having a coherent and flexible overarching approach when seeing patients with PD pathology, *even if they are not offering an extended individual or group treatment.*

Hersh, Caligor, and Yeomans in *Fundamentals of Transference-Focused Psychotherapy: Applications in Psychiatric and Medical Settings* [26] built on the work of Zerbo et al. by considering the wider applicability of TFP principles, including in inpatient psychiatry and outpatient pharmacotherapy. They offered a preliminary examination of the interface of medical and psychiatric conditions, outlining the following familiar scenarios:

- BPD symptoms including recurrent self-injury or parasuicidal behaviors, impulsive sexual activity, binge eating, and recurrent physical fights leading directly to medical sequelae

- Medical conditions identified at higher-than-expected rates in BPD populations studied including chronic pain, sleep disorders, and irritable bowel syndrome
- Iatrogenically-induced medical conditions frequently associated with polypharmacy including metabolic syndrome (obesity, hypercholesterolemia, hypertriglyceridemia, elevated fasting glucose levels), diminished libido or anorgasmia, or sedative-hypnotic dependence
- Poor health-related choices including high rates of smoking, alcohol, and recreational drug use, and avoidance of regular physical exercise
- Specific medical conditions or complaints that can contribute to a passive or parasitic lifestyle
- Complications associated with routine or acute medical care including treatment avoidance, lack of adherence, or treatment overuse
- Complications associated with routine or acute medical care including patterns of alienating or over-involving staff and clinicians

This discussion detailed above was clearly rooted in the recommendations for management of medical concerns in TFP as an extended individual psychotherapy, but as TFP principles were applied in other psychiatric settings, it followed that some of the same interventions related to medical topics could be used in alternative situations, albeit with important adaptations. Examples might include how the psychiatrist whose role is limited to prescribing only might employ TFP principles when managing medication side effects. In this scenario, the prescriber using an atypical antipsychotic agent for a BPD patient with intermittent paranoid thinking might negotiate in advance a treatment contract detailing expectations for laboratory testing and appropriate exercise. In another vein, the inpatient psychiatrist working with a patient with BPD and chronic sleep disturbance that has contributed to nightly dependence on sedative-hypnotic agents might integrate details of improved sleep hygiene into a treatment contract. This contract could address patient responsibilities while staying as an inpatient and then extend for continued use as an outpatient following discharge.

Specific Applied TFP Initiatives in the Treatment of Medical and Personality Disorder Comorbidities

Use of TFP Principles in a Consultation-Liaison Service in a General Hospital

CL services in the GH have developed over decades in several countries with very different organizations, resources, and structures [27]. They share the mission of providing psychiatric consultation for patients hospitalized with physical illnesses in the GH, and ensuring a liaison function with the medical staff who treat these patients [28]. In this section, we use the biopsychosocial concept of "liaison" [29] to refer to the relationship between the consultant psychiatrist and the medical staff of each ward.

Liaison in psychiatric consultation is a well-established practice [27] recommended by the European guidelines [30]; it requires a collaborative relationship between clinicians of varying medical subspecialties and psychiatrists to integrate the necessary medical and psychiatric interventions for each unique patient. Moreover, liaison requires the psychiatrist to highlight the patient's prevailing needs in the hospitalization experience, and the underlying, often unconscious, dominant affects in evidence. Recognition of the psychic needs related to the experience of illness and hospitalization, and the associated dominant affects, allows psychiatrists to have effective communication with patients with PD pathology, and to build a therapeutic alliance with these patients.

Within this framework, we will illustrate how TFP principles may help consultant psychiatrists in their liaison work for patients with PD pathology who are hospitalized in the GH.

The use of TFP principles in the CL service of Modena (Italy) is a tool added to interventions as ususal [31, 32].

Who Are the Clinicians?

The psychiatric consultation in the GH takes place in a complex and atypical setting [31].[1] The consultant psychiatrist is required to have specific skills and in-depth knowledge of various interviewing techniques in order to be flexible and meet the needs of patients. Consultation is required by a GH physician when he or she believes it is necessary to make a psychiatric diagnosis or confirm or rule out a psychiatric diagnosis made in another health care setting. The psychiatrist evaluates the indication for prescribing psychopharmacologic therapy; the GH physician may also request psychiatric consultation when he or she has a particular difficulty in establishing and maintaining an alliance of care with the patient and such difficulty is likely to compromise the patient's health, if the patient delays or does not agree to significant diagnostic examinations or is poorly adherent to recommended care.

As the request for psychiatric consultation is made by a GH physician, this setting does not require the consultant psychiatrist to enter into a direct therapeutic contract with the patient; it is customary for the GH physician to inform the patient that he or she has requested a psychiatric consultation [33]. In this context, the consultant psychiatrist must have the expertise to establish a working alliance with the patient in a short period of time. At the same time, in order to fully evaluate the presence and impact of personality pathology on the patient's current clinical status, the consultant psychiatrist will need to thoroughly interview the patients to evaluate

[1] The paragraphs "*Who are the clinicians?*", "*Who are the patients?*" and "*What TFP principles might be of utility for these clinicians working with these patients?*" are slightly modified excerpts from: Moscara M, Bergonzini E. Integrating the principles of transference-focused psychotherapy with psychiatric consultation for patients admitted to a general hospital: A clinical application of a psychotherapeutic tool. Int J Appl Psychoanal Studies. 2020:1–12. https://doi.org/10.1002/aps.1661

important dimensions of personality [34, 35]; particularly the stability of the sense of self, the quality of object relations, the defensive style, the management of aggressiveness and reality testing. Relevant factors to be assessed are also the coping strategies with which the patient has faced previous illnesses, adherence to prescribed treatments, relationship with previous treaters, and the nature of prior treatment alliances.

Who Are the Patients?

The liaison between the consultant psychiatrist and medical staff is particularly important for patients with PD pathology hospitalized in the GH for physical illnesses. The relationship with these patients must take into account their difficulties in decoding the patient's complex communications regarding their health and lifestyles. For PD patients, physical health represents an area of conflict in which reality testing can become more compromised, and thinking tends to be more concrete, often"with a parallel decline in the capacity to reflect on internal states in self and other [36].".

When communicating, clinicians must consider the particular difficulty that patients with PD pathology may have in correlating their symptoms or illness with their lifestyle and problematic behaviors. This difficulty is likely due to the activation of primitive defense mechanisms including denial, splitting, and projection; the prominent use of these defense mechanisms involves a blurring of the capacity for reality testing.

The massive activation of denial can manifest itself with both a verbal adherence to prescribed diagnostic examinations and simultaneous behaviors that contradict this adherence (e.g., patients who give consent to perform gastroscopy, but then fail to comply with the pre-test fasting prescribed). Denial, projection, and splitting can also lead to other contradictory behaviors, for instance, a patient's agreement to adhere to a prescribed medication regimen and to perform diagnostic examinations, without being able to follow the healthier lifestyle interventions prescribed (e.g., attending rehabilitation programs aimed at quitting smoking, making an appropriate diet, maintaining abstinence from alcohol or drugs, etc.). Finally, projection can manifest itself by attributing unconsciously to the treaters who prescribe diagnostic examinations and pharmacological treatments an intention to dominate or control the patient's life.

The presence of these primitive defense mechanisms may affect the quality of the communication between the clinician and the patient with a PD. Clinicians may find it difficult to explain to patients with PD diagnoses that the prognosis of their medical disease is correlated and influenced by the presence of unhealthy lifestyle behaviors, a history of fluctuating adherence to medical therapies, and non-adherence with follow-up investigations. For instance, it could be hard to inform patients with exotoxic and dysmetabolic liver pathology that their prognosis is affected by their ability to maintain abstinence from alcohol and drugs, to regularly take medications, and to follow a proper diet. The difficulty in communicating this information to the patients with PD pathology is related to the fact that they may experience these communications as harsh criticism.

Furthermore, medical hospitalization itself poses unique challenges to PD patients. Hospitalization is aimed at making a diagnosis and prescribing complex therapeutic pathways and represents a high-activation affective situation [37]. Affective activation and the patient's need for a therapeutic relationship with the medical professionals create a regressive emotional context which, whether consciously or not, activates internalized object relations. Patients who are first diagnosed with a medical condition during hospitalization may, in particular, have the subjective feeling of suddenly turning from a condition of health to one of physical illness; only after being admitted to a GH will some patients experience themselves as physically ill.

As a consequence, patients have to face a dual stimulus, both environmental, related to hospitalization, and internal, related to the conflicts that hospitalization activates; together this dual stimulus stresses the functioning of the structure of personality. Patients with a sufficiently flexible personality structure activate the most adaptive behaviors, while those with a more rigid structure can activate more maladaptive behaviors and their underlying primitive defense mechanisms.

As Zerbo et al. [25] emphasize, "different internal object relations will be activated in different contexts so that at any given moment a particular object relation will organize an individual's subjective experience. In the setting of severe personality pathology and especially during crises, these dyads tend to be especially highly affectively charged, extreme and unstable." These internal dynamics may affect patients' capacity to think clearly and accurately evaluate their treatment situation, thereby preventing them from full adherence to the proposed treatment. Thus, when medically hospitalized, PD patients require sensible, specific psychological interventions to support their treatment alliance and ensure that they are not penalized for receiving standard medical treatment, as compared to patients without a PD. For this clinical population, the use of TFP principles in psychiatric consultation may help in illuminating patients' personality structure and their relational dynamics with the GH staff. The assessment made during the psychiatric consultation can also be used to provide guidance to the patient about the utility of further structured psychological interventions, which can be carried out after the discharge from GH, aimed at facilitating self-observation and understanding of the unconscious mechanisms underlying poor or ambivalent self-care.

The Beginning of the Psychiatric Consultation

The GH clinicians request the psychiatric consultation and inform the patient. The psychiatrist typically begins the interview by exploring the concerns that prompted the referring physician to request the consultation, and by asking the patient whether or not the patient agrees with these concerns. When the patient concurs with the referring physician, psychological distress becomes the focus of the consultation. When the patient does not concur with the referring physician, their disagreement becomes the focus of the consultation. The analysis of this disagreement allows the clinician to identify and address the impasse in the therapeutic relationship between the patient and the medical staff, which could hinder the diagnostic and therapeutic processes [31]. The aim of the interview with the patient with a PD with associated maladaptive behavior is both to make a diagnosis and to overcome any rupture in the therapeutic alliance, providing the medical staff with the relational tools to manage patients that are perceived as "overwhelming". In fact, the medical staff often requests psychiatric consultation for the "difficult" patient who likely has an undiagnosed PD [38]. In most cases, the psychiatrist does only one consultation, but there are patients for whom more consultations are needed, especially in the case of lengthy hospitalizations. The setting of the consultation in GH is complex due to the numerous sources of clinical information and relationships the patient has with different members of the staff (clinicians, nurses, physiotherapists, etc.), and it differs from a standard psychiatric assessment. The psychiatrist assesses the patient's relationship with the medical staff and the emotions that he or she arouses among members of the staff, that is, the countertransference that the patient engenders.

What TFP Principles Might Be of Utility for the Clinicians Working with These Patients?

Hospitalization is a specific and highly demanding context for the patient due to meal times, administration of drugs, diagnostic exam planning, sharing the room with other patients, etc. Adaptive coping skills require the development of integrated object relations, allowing the patient to face the current relational context in a flexible way. The hospital triggers an attitude of dependence on the clinicians and induces regression in the patient [39]. Patients with a more flexible personality structure will experience the regression of the medical hospitalization as egosyntonic, essential for the goals of the intervention. Patients with PD pathology may experience the hospital mainly in a conflictual manner. Difficulty in relying on clinicians and thus regressing functionally can negatively affect the therapeutic alliance and adherence to care.

For instance, in patients with BPD, the hospitalization may activate an all-good object relation in which there is a representation of the self as content and satisfied in relation to a representation of the other who is able to perfectly provide for all his or her physical and emotional needs. The affects connected with this internal dyad are closeness, warmth, and gratitude. The opposite dyad in the split internal world of these patients, also not fully conscious, is an all-bad object relation in which the representation of the self is that of a victim of the aggression by the other, who is experienced as neglecting, harming, or abusing. Feelings of fear, anxiety, and rage are associated with this negative dyadic representation. Both idealized and persecutory self-other representations are based on splitting and are equally pathological. Importantly, these opposite sets of object relations can oscillate in the relationship with the medical staff. Conversely, for patients with narcissistic PD (NPD), the experience of being in need of care at the conscious level may activate a passive-needy self-representation toward which the patient defends himself through the denial of this need at the unconscious level. The GH setting activates a representation of a vulnerable self in relation to the representation of a caring other. Nevertheless, when this caring setting shows inevitable shortcomings (delays, organizational difficulties, problems in daily communication, etc.), the opposite object representation gets activated. Of note, both BPD and NPD patients find it difficult to tolerate frustrations. When frustrations arise during the hospitalization, then the deeper, defended-against, and unconscious pair of opposite object relations may be activated in a defensive and automatic way and may manifest as an angry and devaluing attitude toward the medical staff. The greater the rigidity of the personality structure, the more rapidly the two opposite pairs of object relations oscillate. This rapid oscillation can manifest as a role reversal in the dominant object relations dyad; for example, subjectively the patient feels like a victim of an inadequate treatment but behaviorally reacts by attacking the ward staff. Such kind of role reversal can indicate to the consulting psychiatrist the presence of a significant personality pathology that can lead to poor treatment adherence. In fact, patients with difficulties in tolerating the regression and the temporary dependence required by the hospitalization may fail to maintain adaptive coping skills and a successful diagnostic/therapeutic alliance.

In one scenario, a psychiatric consultation may be requested for a male patient who, after several days of hospitalization, manifests verbal aggression toward the clinicians; the consultant psychiatrist learns, during the interview, that the patient had been prescribed a coronary angiogram. When the clinician informed him of the date of the diagnostic examination, the patient perceived this date as too delayed given the seriousness of his cardiac symptoms and his concerns for his health.

Despite the clinician informing him that his symptoms did not require urgent intervention, the patient was not reassured and maintained an attitude of distrust. In the psychiatric consultation, it emerges that the patient perceives himself as a victim of inadequate treatment and manifests distrustful behaviors toward the clinician, whom he experiences as insufficiently solicitous. His difficulty in trusting the clinician does not allow him to have a temporary regression and adaptive behavior to the situation, and this undermines the therapeutic alliance. The patient would likely experience the clinician as caring only if the intervention could be scheduled as the patient had desired, and any deviation from the timetable he expected is felt to be excessive and the result of a lack of concern and attention.

A psychiatric consultation in the GH also assesses whether the patient shows consistency in relationships with significant others in his or her life and in the relationships with the staff. Exploring interpersonal relationships with significant others in different areas of life allows the psychiatrist to infer assumptions about the patient's habitual functioning and underlying object relationships. In some cases, a gap is revealed between the patient's every day relationships and the ones activated by the illness, the hospitalization, and the meeting with the psychiatrist. An adaptive pattern may be observed when the patient has flexible behavior, promoting accommodation to his or her illness condition. However, a non-adaptive pattern may be in evidence when the patient presents an uncharacteristically rigid attitude toward staff and hospital requests. The comparison between the patient's habitual functioning and his/her functioning during hospitalization allows the psychiatrist to identify whether the patient has the capacity for resilience and flexibility.

Promoting Provision of Optimal Medical Care by Identifying the Transference and Countertransference Dynamics Between PD Patients and the GH Staff

PD patients are at risk of not accessing, or having delayed access to, complex diagnostic processes, medical care, and surgery [26, 31]. This may happen because of both their dysfunctional communication patterns and the intense reactions that they evoke in the medical staff.

For instance, PD patients may exhibit oscillating attitudes toward the need to provide informed consent to access different diagnostic tests and treatments. When the patient refuses to undergo a diagnostic test, despite having previously given consent, a TFP framework may help the consultant psychiatrist to assess whether the patient had previously given consent in a transient phase of idealization of the medical staff. Idealization may then collapse as a result of some difficulties in communicating with medical staff or because of the patient's perception that his or her needs have not been fully met. A refusal of care, or a rapid oscillation in consent, may conceal the patient's unconscious need to defend him or herself against the fear of being totally dependent on an object that may prove to be unreliable. It may be difficult for clinicians to understand that the patient's uncooperative behavior is based on an unconscious internal conflict that is more about the fear of dependence than, for instance, of the diagnostic examination itself.

GH doctors may also require consultation for patients who, after having previously verbally consented to a diagnostic examination, then do not comply with the necessary procedures to get ready for it. This refusal, expressed through behavior but not through words, may be conveyed by different kinds of acting out. For instance, the consultant psychiatrist may visit a patient who had eaten before a scheduled colonoscopy or a gastroscopy, while they had been expressly asked to fast as part of the lengthy preparation required to perform such examination. Ultimately, this behavior prevents the execution of the diagnostic procedure. These behaviors that undermine the patient's appropriate medical care, wholly or partly unconscious, highlight the splitting between opposite parts of the self: a needy part of the self that verbally agrees to prescriptions and relies totally on doctors who are perceived as competent and caring, and an omnipotent part of the self that through actions refuses prescriptions and does not rely on doctors because they are perceived as threatening or incompetent. In evaluating these patients, the consultant psychiatrist can use a TFP framework to clarify the opposing dyads that have been unconsciously activated and underlie the oscillating behaviors of (verbal) acceptance and (practical) refusal of treatment. We can hypothesize that facing a necessary diagnostic examination may nullify the effect of the defense mechanism of denial and, in particular, leave the patient vulnerable to the anguish of being sick and depending on others.

Moreover, patients with PD pathology may respond in different and contrary ways to various staff members or to the same clinician at different times. These communication patterns are challenging and can produce division and conflict in the medical staff. In these situations, TFP principles can assist the consultant psychiatrist in investigating whether the patient's inconsistent communications are conscious or unconscious and, in the latter case, if making clarification and confrontation interventions to explore the underlying split self-other representations can be of benefit.

Considering the previous example of a patient who is ambivalent in consenting to a prescribed diagnostic examination (e.g., a patient who verbally gives consent and then behaviorally boycotts it), the consultant psychiatrist reconstructs, during the interview, the different phases of the therapeutic alliance between the patient and the treaters, and makes some clarifications to better understand the patient's experiences. When split representations of the self and the treaters emerge, the consultant psychiatrist makes confrontations to elucidate that the consent was given in a phase of idealization of the treaters, while the refusal to perform the diagnostic examination emerges in a phase of devaluation. In the first phase of the idealization of the treaters, the patient relies on the clinicians whom he experiences as competent and caring, while in the second phase of devaluation, the patient perceives the clinicians as incompetent and neglectful. Only during the phase of idealization, is the patient aware of needing diagnostic examination to receive the necessary care. In formulating the confrontation, the consultant psychiatrist emphasizes that the behavior that leads to a boycott of the examination can stem from fear of the examination itself as well as distress given the dependence on the caregiving staff.

Importantly, such typical challenging behaviors when exhibited by patients negatively affect the treatment milieu, posing risks to both the patient's health and the clinical performance of the staff. The risk for patients with a PD diagnosis is that they receive treatments that do not correspond to the expected standards for the physical disorder for which they are hospitalized in the GH because, as previously described, they may interrupt complex diagnostic pathways and fail to adhere to recommended therapies or to carry out medical check-ups within the indicated timeframe. In a similar vein, the medical staff also run the risk of unconsciously conveying an attitude of neglect that prevents them from maintaining their usual standards of care when treating PD patients. Clinicians might not be confident that they will be able to build an alliance that will facilitate the patient's adherence to treatment. For instance, the medical staff may engage in neglectful behaviors in prescribing medications and diagnostic examinations because the staff members share, unconsciously, a devalued representation of the patient as someone who is incapable of honoring the commitments made to look after his or her own health. In such cases, the staff run the risk of failing to pursue care goals for the patient as they are not fully appreciative of the patient's unconscious motivations that underlie disregarding and challenging behaviors. The medical staff could also run the risk of counteracting the patient's challenging behavior by distancing themselves or conveying avoidant attitudes; this occurs when there is an identification with the patient's devalued representation of treaters that the patient projects onto them. Finally, the staff may also identify with the dissociated and devalued part of the patient, which induces a more primitive, all-or-nothing mode of thinking. This regression leads to the loss of awareness of the complexity of the patient who enacted the challenging behaviors, and protects the medical staff from the painful internal conflict between adherence to their mission of care and defensive, reactive distancing from the patient.

Ultimately, all these problematic attitudes exhibited by the GH staff can impede the delivery of optimal medical care when treating PD patients with physical comorbidity. The use of TFP principles may help to illuminate and contain such potentially counter-productive reactions. By using a TFP framework, the consultant psychiatrist assesses the relational dynamics between the GH staff and the patient, aims to provide insight, and allows for the identification of internal conflicts within the staff, linking it to the maladaptive relational characteristics of the patient with PD pathology.

The consultant psychiatrist in the liaison with GH staff shows how the patient's oscillating attitude, for example, on providing consent to a diagnostic examination, can activate different emotional reactions in staff members; some clinicians may have a more sympathetic attitude about the patient's difficulties in complying with prescriptions (e.g., observing fasting), others may have a less nuanced perspective about the recommendations given to the patient in order to undergo the examination. The consultant psychiatrist shows how both attitudes can be related to countertransference reactions: clinicians with a more sympathetic attitude unconsciously identify with the split representation of the patient as needy, while the others identify with the split representation of the patient as self-governing and capable of deciding autonomously when and how to treat themselves. The consultant psychiatrist shows how the splitting of the medical staff represents a countertransference response to the splitting of the patient's self-representations, whereby some clinicians manifest a concordant countertransference and others complementary countertransference [40].

Promoting Adherence by Enhancing the Patient's Capacity to Reflect on His/Her Problematic Behavior

TFP principles may help the consultant psychiatrist to formulate a thorough psychopathological and structural diagnosis of personality by integrating the information he or she receives from several sources: the interview with the patient, the staff's reasons for seeking consultation, and joint interviews with the patient and family members to develop "clear goals of intervention, even when there is a complex combination of physical, psychological and social factors contributing to the problem" [30].

A TFP-oriented assessment provides insight into the patient's personality structure, and overall level of personality functioning, in specific domains [41]; this has clear implications for understanding patents' behaviors during the hospitalization. Patients with healthy, neurotic, or high-level borderline personality structure react to the experience of illness and hospitalization by implementing flexible, adaptive coping strategies, appropriately managing the frustration of being in need, and especially the experience of relying heavily on medical staff [42]. Conversely, in patients with low-level borderline personality organization, the experience of hospitalization can activate, as previously described, two contrasting dyads. These dyads reflect a split between the representation of a vulnerable self, aware of the need to derive support from those involved, and the representation of an omnipotent self, signaling an independence of necessary external supports.

TFP-oriented psychiatric consultation helps to highlight how the coexistence of both the competence and the neglect in taking care of themselves reveals the presence of unconscious conflicting aspects of the patient. These two opposing dyads reveal the patient's contradictory states: one dyad is a defense against the other, particularly, the dyad in which the patient sees himself as not needing care and caretakers, which protects him against the opposite and deeper dyad in which he sees himself as needy, fragile, and devalued. A TFP-oriented formulation of these conflicting aspects of the self can be used to show the patient how his or her ambivalent behaviors, apparently opposite, have a psychological basis, in part unconscious. This promotes the patient's awareness of his communication patterns with the doctors in the here-and-now as well as in the past. To this end, the consultant psychiatrist makes clarifications and uses the consultation as an opportunity to facilitate the patient's self-observation, promoting recognition of the different parts of himself or herself activated by hospitalization and the need for care. Then, the consultant psychiatrist can confront the patient on the conflicting unconscious motivations that lead him to acting out and the refusal of behavior ensuring care. These interventions will promote patient's awareness of the representations of the needy self, ultimately helping the patient to establish an alliance of care with the medical staff and to undertake the appropriate treatment pathways for the somatic disorder.

What Are the Goals for Imparting to These Clinicians the Principles of TFP for Working with These Patients?

The consultant psychiatrist makes use of TFP principles to help the medical staff: (1) to observe the patient's verbal and non-verbal behaviors and communications as an expression of his or her inner world; (2) to assess the patient's relational patterns, of which he or she is not fully aware; (3) to understand the unconscious motivations underlying the patient's behaviors that led to the request for psychiatric consultation; and (4) to help professionals to understand the issues of transference/countertransference in the relationship between physicians, staff and patient.

Applying a TFP framework in liaison psychiatry provides the consulting psychiatrist with the theoretical and technical tools to assist medical staff in understanding the countertransference triggered by the relationship with the patient, which in turn could negatively impact treatment planning and delivery. TFP principles encourage clinicians to recognize that the devalued representation that some members of the medical staff, or the staff as a whole, may have of the patient (as irresponsible and therefore unreliable); this devalued representation of the patient can potentially invalidate the therapeutic alliance and, therefore, the diagnostic and therapeutic plan for treatment of the physical illness and, at the same time, can put staff members in conflict about the goals to be pursued.

What TFP Principles Might Be of Utility for the Clinicians Working with These Patients?

The understanding of countertransference allows the medical staff to be aware of certain negative representations that the patient may have projected onto them; some members, or the staff as a whole, run the risk of responding to this process of projection by conducting themselves in uncharacteristic, and sometimes unproductive, ways. Understanding the countertransference dynamics allows the staff to be aware of the splitting processes that they are confronted with when they are caring for a patient with moderate and severe personality borderline organization. Another important task of the TFP-oriented consultant psychiatrist is to bring to light the devalued representations that the medical staff has of its own competence when facing the challenge of treating certain "difficult" patients. These patients are perceived as poorly collaborating, ambivalent in the therapeutic alliance, erratic in the adherence to treatment and follow-up and, therefore, "overwhelming". The exploration of countertransference phenomena is necessary to enable the medical staff to conduct themselves professionally and proactively in order to make all possible efforts to promote adherence to medical care for patients with severe PD pathology.

The clinical vignettes in this chapter are a composite and do not reflect actual specific cases; this has been done to protect patient privacy.

Clinical Illustration

Ms. V. is a 50-year-old woman who is known by her primary care physician's (PCP) office to be a "difficult patient" who routinely expresses many complaints about her care and the ways she feels she is mistreated during her office visits. She is obese, with very limited functioning that is compromised by her dependence on sedative-hypnotic agents for sleep and her chronic complaints of poor mobility related to osteoarthritis. Ms. V. has a distant past history of non-suicidal self-injury by cutting; when she was asked by her PCP about her well-healed wrist scars, she indicated that she was not comfortable providing information about her history of self-harm.

Ms. V. is admitted to the neurology ward of the hospital with a new-onset complaint of dizziness and syncope and she is assigned a doctor whom she does not know. Within 24 hours of admission, the medical staff requests a consultation with the CL psychiatry service because of escalating difficulties experienced by the assigned nurses and doctors in providing Ms. V. with standard care. Ms. V. became angry and threatening on the first night of her admission because the sedative-hypnotic medications provided, while the same agents she had been taking daily for many months, appeared to be unfamiliar in color and shape. She was verbally abusive to a student nurse who needed to take her vital signs, suggesting that she was being unnecessarily bothered, and she refused to speak with one of the neurology residents who was attempting to screen her for an essential neuroimaging study.

The consulting psychiatrist did not consider herself to be an "expert" in personality disorders, but she had familiarity with TFP principles and often integrated these principles into her standard bedside evaluation. She approached Ms. V. with some basic TFP concepts in mind: (1) an openness to making a PD diagnosis, even with incomplete information, (2) an expectation that she would initially be required to "tolerate the confusion" generated by the patient, (3) a prioritization of the emerging dominant object relations dyad in evidence and the goal of "naming the actors," (4) an expectation of role reversals, and (5) a likely benefit of using "therapist-centered" interpretations to manage periods of the patient's heightened affective state.

After meeting with the patient and collecting parallel information from those involved, the consultant psychiatrist met with the team of medical providers and ward nurses. She reviewed her preliminary thinking about the likelihood of a contribution of PD pathology, using simple language. She explained the distinction between symptoms of major depression (Ms. V. had repeatedly told the staff that she was "depressed" being in the hospital), and the dysphoria frequently associated with moderate to severe PD pathology. She described the patient's use of lower-level or splitting-based defenses, particularly denial and idealization/devaluation; she also underscored the likely emerging paranoid transferences in evidence that were closely associated with Ms. V.'s disruptive behavior.

The consultant psychiatrist did not offer her observations as a panacea for the staff, rather she aimed to convey certain limited goals. These goals included: (1) initially tolerating the confusion generated by Ms. V. and avoiding taking a defensive, and likely futile, position of appealing to the patient's logic; (2) actively monitoring countertransference reactions including an impulse to distance the patients or deviate from standard care by acquiescing to all of the patient's request and demands; (3) putting into words the observed dominant object relations dyad along the lines of "I'm guessing you're feeling vulnerable and powerless as a patient in the hospital and see me, as a clinician, as possibly indifferent or neglectful"; and (4) listening for role reversals and judiciously interjecting an observation of this pattern. The neurology resident participating in the group asked the consultant for guidance about how to manage Ms. V.'s hostile reactions to his communication about required testing. The consultant offered a version of the "therapist centered therapist-centered interpretation" used in TFP, suggesting the resident put into words how he imagined the patient was feeling. The consultant framed a comment such as: "Ms. V., my sense is that you see me now as an imposing doctor who is making you do these tests without appreciating the stress it causes you" as a containing intervention. The staff remained challenged by Ms. V.'s behavior during the remainder of the hospitalization, but using some of the consultant's insights helped them avert counterproductive power struggles. Moreover, because the medical team appreciated the contribution of PD pathology in this case, they were able to limit the expectable spitting within the team and avoided feeling deskilled or ineffectual in managing Ms. V.'s care.

Conclusion

In summary, applying TFP principles in CL psychiatry can: (1) facilitate the diagnosis of a PD by identifying object relations and role reversals; (2) help the medical staff to maintain their usual standard of care by focusing and managing their countertransference reactions; and (3) help to improve patients' adherence to treatment by augmenting their awareness of the internal motivations of their behaviors.

Using a TFP framework, the psychiatric consultation in the GH setting can become an opportunity to open new possibilities, for both PD patients and the medical staff. Central to the benefits of a TFP-informed approach is the effortful understanding of the psychological suffering associated with PD pathology. Two fundamental elements of the use of TFP principles in this context are: (1) promoting self-observation in the patient, and (2) developing the capacity to grasp the unconscious motivations of the patient's verbal and non-verbal communications by the medical staff. Moreover, the understanding of how PD pathology affects treatment and treatment alliance allows the medical staff to manage the inevitable frustration arising from the difficulty in pursuing their clinical goals.

Maintaining the ability to recommend the appropriate diagnostic and treatment pathways without being overwhelmed is paramount for every clinician and the medical staff as a whole. This process can be undermined when the patient projects onto them idealizing representations (i.e., as perfect providers), or devaluing representations (i.e., as incompetent and callous clinicians), that are often rapidly shifting. The overarching goal of a TFP-informed liaison role would be the elaboration of these unconscious representations, making it possible for the staff to monitor the risk of counterproductively distancing themselves from these patients while maintaining an internally competent and cohesive sense of professional identity.

Use of TFP Principles for Training in Internal Medicine

Patients with primary or co-occurring PD pathology are well represented in most settings in medicine [43]. Often, patients with PD diagnoses or traits will be described as "difficult" patients, when providers in these medical settings are either unfamiliar with PD diagnostic criteria or not disposed to making or documenting PD diagnoses. While most mental health providers receive only rudimentary education and training about PD assessment and treatment, medical providers, including physicians and nurses, may have negligible or no exposure to these topics [44, 45]. As a result, periodically there have been impassioned pleas for guidance from different medical specialists, all with similar expressions of confusion and distress. In a pilot program in the Department of Medicine at the Vagelos Columbia College of Physicians and Surgeons, a module on topics related to psychiatric co-morbidities in medicine clinic patients has been expanded to integrate certain key TFP principles [46]. The goals of this didactic initiative directly address the expectable presentations in general outpatient medical practice related to co-occurring personality disorder traits or personality disorders. This initiative moves beyond a standard introduction to management of common psychiatric disorders in general medicine, to a psychodynamically informed overview of practice management.

Who Are the Clinicians?

The audiences for this program are all second-year internal medicine residents treating patients in a weekly outpatient general medicine clinic. These clinics manage high-volume services, treating many patients with limited resources and multiple psychosocial stressors. The model of this clinic balances educational needs and a service requirement for the community. For most of these clinicians, exposure to information about PD diagnoses has been limited to a rare medical school lecture. While management of specific psychiatric disorders (anxiety, depression) in the general medicine clinic are standard part of some medicine residency programs, this application of TFP principles aims to go beyond usual circumscribed didactics.

Who Are the Patients?

The demographic distribution of the patients in this general medical clinic represents the local community of racial and ethnic minorities with relative socioeconomic disadvantages. A significant portion of the clinic population uses government-sponsored health insurance for access or falls into a group of uninsured individuals. Many of these patients are challenged by common chronic diseases (hypertension, diabetes, osteoarthritis), compounded often by poor lifestyle decisions including tobacco use, alcohol and substance use disorders, poor nutrition and limited exercise.

What Is the Contemporary Standard of Care for Clinicians Treating These Patients?

In general, almost all medical professionals, including trainees in general medicine, receive scant education about personality disorder pathology, including methods of assessment and intervention. While there is an extensive literature on the subject of managing the "difficult" patient in medical practice, there is less focus generally on linking patients described as such with specific personality disorder profiles. While risk management education may address concerns about patient boundaries and the risk of patient abandonment, these topics are not customarily linked to a discussion of PD symptoms. "Difficult" patients or patients with documented PD diagnoses will frequently be the source of complaints or the subject of clinic-wide review of untoward outcomes.

What Are the Goals for Imparting to These Clinicians the Principles of TFP for Working with These Patients?

The outline for this didactic program stresses certain central elements of TFP adapted for medical professionals who likely will have limited motivation or time to focus specifically on mental health concerns. Nevertheless, these clinicians in general medicine appreciate that co-occurring PD pathology can often undermine their attempts to provide consistent, standard medical care. The goals include helping with managing that subset of patients whose behavior is marked by poor adherence or disruptive actions. Along with patient management, guidance for effective, protective documentation is also offered. In addition, other objectives include increased clinician satisfaction and a reduction in splitting among clinic employees.

What Is the Source of Institutional or Government Support?

This teaching opportunity is financially supported by the Department of Medicine's residency training program. The introduction of a curriculum on psychiatric disorders with associated supervisory time dedicated to management of patients with PD presentations is considered integral to the training of a well-rounded and effective internist.

What TFP Principles Might Be of Utility for The Clinicians Working with These Patients?

The curriculum introducing medicine residents to TFP principles includes the following:

- Information about PD nosology and epidemiology
- Special consideration of PD patients with co-occurring substance use disorders, treatment avoidance or overuse, and risks for polypharmacy
- An openness to consideration of a PD diagnosis, even without complete background information
- Guidance about sharing with the patient the clinician's diagnostic impression using straightforward language
- Comfort with an expectation for obtaining permission to contact key active or prior treaters or family members, even when that might not be the patient's initial preference

- Initiation of a discussion about a treatment contract or agreement outlining in advance the respective responsibilities of both the patient and the provider that goes beyond the standard review of office policies
- Use of interventions including "naming the actors," identification or role reversals or clinician-centered interpretations during periods of heightened affect
- Monitoring three channels of communication: what the patient says, how the patient behaves, and how the medical professional feels
- Prioritizing the requirement for safety as a prerequisite for the clinician's capacity to think clearly and provide optimal care

What Are the Targets for Measurement to Gauge the Effectiveness of Instruction About the Application of TFP Principles?

Measuring the benefits of this training intervention could be achieved through:

- Clinician and staff satisfaction surveys
- Clinician and staff retention
- Patient satisfaction surveys
- Patient retention
- Tracking of costs associated with well-documented, problematic polypharmacy in certain patient populations
- Tracking costs associated with medico-legal complications

What Are the Didactic Materials Required to Impart TFP Principles to This Target Group of Clinicians?

Essential articles on the difficulties treating patients with PDs in medical settings, reviews of the topic of the "difficult patient" in medicine, and presentation of material making accessible and relevant aggregated information from research findings.

What Is the Format for the Instruction of TFP Principles to This Audience?

Assigned reading, PowerPoint presentations, group discussion with case presentations, and role-playing.

Clinical Illustration

Dr. A. is a second-year resident in internal medicine treating a 40-year-old divorced woman in his clinic. When Dr. A. took over care for this patient, Ms. M., he was told by the graduating resident that Ms. M. was a "difficult patient, probably the most frustrating" of the patients on his roster. Dr. A. was told that Ms. M.'s behaviors included alternating between periods of non-adherence and marked neediness. Ms. M.'s conduct was notable for missing follow-up meetings and failing to have recommended laboratory testing done, with other periods of marked escalating demands in the clinic, causing disruption for the staff and requiring the former resident to take extra time when Ms. A. did come for her appointments, given the requirements to manage her various complaints and frequent outbursts.

Taking over Ms. M.'s care, Dr. A. felt comfortable with the medical issues at hand, Ms. M.'s hypertension and Type II diabetes mellitus, but Dr. A. was aware of his mixed feelings of fear and resentment. After a first challenging meeting with Ms. M., who was late, demanding, and devaluing of Dr. A.'s recommendations for a new diabetes regimen, Dr. A.'s chief resident suggests he present Ms. M. in their behavioral medicine course taught by Dr. P., a practicing psychiatrist who had previously trained in internal medicine. Dr. P. lectured on a few specific topics related to treating psychiatric conditions like depression and anxiety in primary care, but he focused mostly on using TFP principles in practice management, including with those patients known to have personality disorder diagnoses or those simply described in the clinic as "difficult" patients.

Dr. A. presented Ms. M.'s history, highlighting her past patterns of ER visits after "accidental" medication overdoses following arguments with her former husband, her well-documented disruptive anger identified in her exchanges with office personnel, and her marked mood reactivity with prior residents in the clinic, vacillating between belligerence and pleas for special attention. Dr. P. as supervisor used the case of Ms. M. to elucidate for the residents these key points about using TFP principles in their work:

- *The benefits of considering a PD diagnosis when indicated, even with only partial information*
- *Using countertransference as a guide to diagnosis and interventions*
- *Standardizing a treatment approach and remaining alert for deviations in practice*
- *Creating and maintaining a treatment contract beyond standard clinic policies*
- *Documenting in a thoughtful and protective way*

Dr. P. used role-playing with Dr. A. to demonstrate these points for the residents. Dr. P. modeled a series of questions that helped to elucidate Ms. M.'s history of those elements evident that suggested a primary or co-occurring PD diagnosis. Dr. P. helped Dr. A. to explore his countertransference, specifically his feelings of fear, frustration, or anger, and how this impacted his appointments with Ms. M. By stressing the benefits of standardizing a treatment approach, Dr. P. was able to explore how deviations from standard practice should alert the residents to the possibility of specific PD pathology exhibited by the patient and associated reactions by the resident. The creation and maintenance of a treatment contract was introduced as a novel and practical way for Dr. A. to address certain of Ms. M.'s behaviors including her non-adherence, her devaluation of the resident's time when missing appointments or coming late, or her disruptive expressions of aggression when verbally abusive with clinic staff. Rethinking documentation required for the particular challenges arising when managing patients with PD pathology helped address Dr. A.'s concerns about liability.

The following week when presenting the case again, Dr. A. was able to speak about his ongoing countertransference reactions including feeling devalued, deskilled and, at times, in danger, in his dealings with Ms. M. Dr. P. reviewed again some of the elements of TFP available to Dr. A. These included scripts such as the following:

- *"Naming the actors" of identifying the dominant object relations dyad in evidence: "In these situations my guess is that you feel vulnerable and invalidated, seeing me as indifferent to your needs and that makes you panicked and angry."*
- *Identifying the possible role reversal in play: "You've been accusing me of pushing you around because I'm requiring you get this lab test before our next appointment, but I'm aware in this situation you're the one with the power. You're raising your voice and controlling our discussion, and I'm left a bit helpless and at your mercy."*
- *Using therapist (or clinician)-based interpretations during an affect storm: "I can understand that you'd feel enraged when you experience your doctor as harmful and uncaring because of a limit to the number of Xanax pills prescribed at this time."*
- *Reinforcing points of the treatment contract: "I've said that I can't focus on you as much as I would like when you're late; can we agree again to a plan to have you come on time so that I can give you the care you deserve?"*
- *Over time, Dr. A. made adjustments in his treatment contract with Ms. M. as problems emerged. For example, Ms. M. disclosed at an appointment that she feared her overuse of alcohol could be complicating her attempts at dieting, leading to fluctuations in her blood sugars. In their session, they added to their treatment agreement the stipulation that Ms. M. would meet with the motivational interviewing counselor working in their clinic. At every meeting, Dr. A. would check on this aspect of their agreement and explore Ms. M.'s reaction to Dr. A.'s expectation that she would commit to working actively with the counselor on alcohol use moderation.*
- *In summary, Dr. A.'s integration of TFP principles allowed him to feel as though he had a toolbox of skills to use, rather than just feeling a mix of either angry and authoritarian or powerless and worried. The changes over time allowed Dr. A. to use more of his energies with Ms. M. on addressing her concerns, rather than making their time together feel wasteful and depleting.*

Conclusion

The interface of medical conditions and personality disorder pathology is often a complex and uncertain terrain. This chapter has introduced two inventive initiatives aimed at employing knowledge and skills honed in the world of PD research over decades for use in these novel formats. Both initiatives underscore the tremendous challenge faced by those clinicians with limited psychiatric or psychological training who nevertheless are charged with caring for patients with significant PD pathology in settings that are not designed specifically for that purpose. While TFP principles are derived from the psychoanalytic tradition, the modification of these traditional ideas has contributed to a growing movement that aims to rework these theories for contemporary use in settings other than the standard, individual outpatient psychotherapy.

The application of TFP principles in CL psychiatry and in the training of medical residents adds a robust dimension to the evolving field of applied TFP. As with the other projects in this emerging field, the clearly articulated needs of clinicians, patients, and families fuel the impetus for innovation and creativity. The well-documented sequelae to undiagnosed and untreated or under-treated PD conditions have created an urgency for fresh approaches in this field.

References

1. Moran P, Jenkins R, Tylee A, Blizard R, Mann A. The prevalence of personality disorder among UK primary care attenders. Acta Psychiatr Scand. 2000;102(1):52–7.
2. Gross R, Olfson M, Gameroff M, Shea S, Feder A, Fuentes M, et al. Borderline personality disorder in primary care. Arch Intern Med. 2002;162(1):53–60.
3. Diefenbacher A, Golombek U, Strain JJ. Personality disorders in consultation-liaison psychiatry—an empirical investigation. Eur Psychiatry. 2009;24(S1):1.
4. Sansone RA, Farukhi S, Wiederman MW. Utilization of primary care physicians in borderline personality. Gen Hosp Psychiatry. 2011;33(4):343–6.
5. Sansone RA, Farukhi S, Wiederman MW. Disruptive behaviors in the medical setting and borderline personality. Int J Psychiatry Med. 2011;41(4):355–63.
6. Quirk SE, Berk M, Chanen AM, Koivumaa-Honkanen H, Brennan-Olsen SL, Pasco JA, et al. Population prevalence of personality disorder and associations with physical health comorbidities and health care service utilization: a review. Personal Disord. 2016;7(2):136–46.
7. Dixon-Gordon KL, Berghoff CR, McDermott MJ. Borderline personality disorder symptoms and pain in college students: the role of emotional suppression. J Personal Disord. 2018;32(2):277–88.
8. Frankenburg FR, Zanarini MC. The association between borderline personality disorder and chronic medical illnesses, poor health-related lifestyle choices, and costly forms of health care utilization. J Clin Psychiatry. 2004;65(12):1660–5.
9. Compton WM, Conway KP, Stinson FS, Colliver JD, Grant BF. Prevalence, correlates, and comorbidity of DSM-IV antisocial personality syndromes and alcohol and specific drug use disorders in the United States: results from the national epidemiologic survey on alcohol and related conditions. J Clin Psychiatry. 2005;66(6):677–85.
10. Moran P, Stewart R, Brugha T, Bebbington P, Bhugra D, Jenkins R, et al. Personality disorder and cardiovascular disease: results from a national household survey. J Clin Psychiatry. 2007;68(1):69–74.
11. El-Gabalawy R, Katz LY, Sareen J. Comorbidity and associated severity of borderline personality disorder and physical health conditions in a nationally representative sample. Psychosom Med. 2010;72(7):641–7.
12. Magidson JF, Collado-Rodriguez A, Madan A, Perez-Camoirano NA, Galloway SK, Borckardt JJ, et al. Addressing narcissistic personality features in the context of medical care:

integrating diverse perspectives to inform clinical practice. Personal Disord Theory Res Treat. 2012;3(2):196–208.
13. Powers AD, Oltmanns TF. Personality disorders and physical health: a longitudinal examination of physical functioning, healthcare utilization, and health-related behaviors in middle-aged adults. J Personal Disord. 2012;26(4):524–38.
14. Kacel EL, Ennis N, Pereira DB. Narcissistic personality disorder in clinical health psychology practice: case studies of comorbid psychological distress and life-limiting illness. Behav Med. 2017;43(3):156–64.
15. Ricke AK, Lee MJ, Chambers JE. The difficult patient: borderline personality disorder in the obstetrical and gynecological patient. Obstet Gynecol Surv. 2012;67(8):495–502.
16. Dubovsky AN, Kiefer MM. Borderline personality disorder in the primary care setting. Med Clin North Am. 2014;98(5):1049–64.
17. Riddle M, Meeks T, Alvarez C, Dubovsky A. When personality is the problem: managing patients with difficult personalities on the acute care unit. J Hosp Med. 2016;11(12):873–8.
18. Hall K, Moran P. Borderline personality disorder: an update for neurologists. Pract Neurol. 2019;19(6):483–91.
19. Keuroghlian AS, Frankenburg FR, Zanarini MC. The relationship of chronic medical illnesses, poor health-related lifestyle choices, and health care utilization to recovery status in borderline patients over a decade of prospective follow-up. J Psychiatr Res. 2013;47(10):1499–506.
20. Kealy D, Steinberg PI, Ogrodniczuk JS. "Difficult" patient? Or does he have a personality disorder? J Fam Pract. 2014;63(12):697–703.
21. Huprich SK. Personality pathology in primary care: ongoing needs for detection and intervention. J Clin Psychol Med Settings. 2018;25(1):43–54.
22. Wlodarczyk J, Lawn S, Powell K, Crawford GB, McMahon J, Burke J, et al. Exploring general practitioners' views and experiences of providing care to people with borderline personality disorder in primary care: a qualitative study in Australia. Int J Environ Res Public Health. 2018;15(12):2763.
23. Doering S. Borderline personality disorder in patients with medical illness: a review of assessment, prevalence, and treatment options. Psychosom Med. 2019;81(7):584–94.
24. Kernberg OF. Structural interviewing. Psychiatr Clin North Am. 1981;4(1):169–95.
25. Zerbo E, Cohen S, Bielska W, Caligor E. Transference-focused psychotherapy in the general psychiatry residency: a useful and applicable model for residents in acute clinical settings. Psychodyn Psychiatry. 2013;41(1):163–81.
26. Hersh RG, Caligor E, Yeomans FE. Fundamentals of transference-focused psychotherapy: applications in psychiatric and medical settings. Cham: Springer International Publishing; 2016.
27. Laugharne R, Flynn A. Personality disorders in consultation-liaison psychiatry. Curr Opin Psychiatry. 2013;26(1):84–9. https://doi.org/10.1097/YCO.0b013e328359977f.
28. Marchi M, Magarini FM, Mattei G, Pingani L, Moscara M, Galeazzi GM, Ferrari S. Diagnostic agreement between physicians and a consultation–liaison psychiatry team at a general hospital: an exploratory study across 20 years of referrals. Int J Environ Res Public Health. 2021;18:749. https://doi.org/10.3390/ijerph18020749.
29. Engel G. The need for a new medical model: a challenge for biomedicine. Science. 1977;196:129–36. https://doi.org/10.1126/science.847460.
30. Sollner W, Creed F. European guidelines for training in consultation-liaison psychiatry and psychosomatics: report of the EACLPP Workgroup on Training in Consultation-Liaison Psychiatry and Psychosomatics. J Psychosom Res. 2007;62(4):501–9. https://doi.org/10.1016/j.jpsychores.2006.11.003.
31. Moscara M, Bergonzini E. Integrating the principles of transference-focused psychotherapy with psychiatric consultation for patients admitted to a general hospital: a clinical application of a psychotherapeutic tool. Int J Appl Psychoanal Stud. 2020;18:18.
32. Rigatelli M, Ferrari S. The Modena consultation-liaison psychiatry service. Italy Br J Psychiatry. 2004;184(3):268–9. https://doi.org/10.1192/bjp.184.3.268.

33. Radcliffe J, Yeomans FE. Transference-focused psychotherapy for patients with personality disorders: overview and case example with a focus on the use of contracting. Br J Psychother. 2019;35(1):4–23. https://doi.org/10.1111/bjp.12421.
34. Kernberg OF. Severe personality disorders. New Haven/London: Yale University Press; 1984.
35. Yeomans FE, Clarkin JF, Kernberg OF. Transference-focused psychotherapy for borderline personality disorder. A clinical guide. Washington, DC: American Psychiatric Publishing; 2015.
36. Caligor E, Kernberg OF, Clarkin JF, Clarkin JF. Psychodynamic therapy for personality pathology. Treating self and interpersonal functioning. Washington DC: American Psychiatric Publishing; 2018.
37. Kernberg OF. Object relations, affects, and drives: towards a new synthesis. Psychoanal Inq. 2001;21(5):604–19. https://doi.org/10.1080/07351692109348963.
38. Carsky M, Yeomans F. Overwhelming patients and overwhelmed therapists. Psychodyn Psychiatry. 2012;40(1):75–90.
39. Balint M. Thrills and regressions. New York: International Universities Press; 1959.
40. Racker H. The meanings and uses of countertransference. Psychoanal Q. 1957;26:303–57.
41. Lingiardi V, McWilliams N. The psychodynamic diagnostic manual. 2nd ed. New York: Guilford; 2017.
42. Caligor E, Kernberg OF, Clarkin JF. Handbook of dynamic psychotherapy for high personality pathology. Washington DC: American Psychiatric Publishing; 2007.
43. Schneider RK, Levenson JL. Psychiatry essentials for primary care. Philadelphia: American College of Physicians; 2008.
44. Ghatavi K, Waisman Z. Teaching medical students about personality disorders and psychotherapeutic principles: a resident pilot initiative. Acad Psychiatry. 2006;30:178–80.
45. Freilich L. A curriculum for training medical faculty to teach mental health car... and their responses to the learning. J Clin Outcomes Manage. 2020;27:166–73.
46. Petrini M. Management of personality disorders in primary care. New York: Pri-Med; 2015.

Using Transference-focused Psychotherapy (TFP) Principles in a Family Intervention for Adolescents with Personality Disorders

13

Alfons Icart and Teresa Ribalta

Introduction

This chapter illustrates the application of transference-focused psychotherapy (TFP) principles within a family-focused intervention named “TFP for parental functions” (TFP-PF). TFP-PF has been specifically developed for certain adolescent patients with severe personality disorder (PD) pathology, i.e., with mid- to low- borderline personality organization (BPO) according to Kernberg’s classification of personality pathology [1]. Our hypothesis is that pathological family functioning has fostered a “blocking” of the process of differentiation and development of the adolescent’s identity. As a result, the adolescent patients come to treatment with a limited appreciation of their difficulties and of the consequences of their behavior on their environment. The patients might deny having difficulties or claim to be able to solve them without any help. A typical response of the adolescent patient at the first consultation may be: “There is nothing wrong with me!” Contrary to the patient’s view, the people in their environment are usually well aware of their severe problems. Patients develop increasing acting out behaviors and relational problems, which often seriously affect their family and social environment, as well as their academic performance. Additional problems such as sexual promiscuity or substance use disorders may also be frequent.

These adolescents feel neither conflicted nor distressed by their behavior and most of them show partial or total reluctance in committing to individual treatment. They do not make an explicit request for help, but their family or significant others in their environment become increasingly concerned about their problematic

A. Icart · T. Ribalta (✉)
Grup TLP Barcelona, Barcelona, Spain

Fundació Orienta, Barcelona, Spain
e-mail: aicart@fundacioorienta.com; tribalta@fundacioorienta.com

R. G. Hersh, C. De Panfilis (eds.), *Implementing Transference-Focused Psychotherapy Principles*, https://doi.org/10.1007/978-3-031-68062-5_13

behavior and attempt to refer them to treatment; however, many of these adolescents reject this proposal. This adolescent patient group, thus, differs from adult PD patients with similarly externalizing patterns and equally severe problem behaviors who, conversely, exhibit extensive use of mental health services [2].

The TFP-PF initiative described in this chapter was developed in the Fundació Orienta in the southern metropolitan area of Barcelona, Spain. Fundació Orienta (FO) has worked for almost 50 years as an institution specializing exclusively in child and adolescent mental health. It provides both outpatient and day hospital treatments. As such, the FO also receives treatment requests from the families of the above-described subgroup of adolescents with PD. In the FO, these adolescents historically have been offered different types of individual psychotherapies, including TFP for adolescents (TFP-A) [3]. However, these attempts were often marked by failures in treatment adherence (e.g., non-attendance, delays, or interruptions). The therapeutic intervention proposed in this chapter represents a novel attempt to prevent therapeutic failures in this subset of adolescents functioning at a medium-low level of BPO.

Importantly, the TFP-PF initiative described here differs from other public mental health approaches that defer entirely to the preferences of the adolescent patient [4]. Our approach to initiating treatment also differs from the view of Fisch and Schlanger [5], who posit that "if there is no complaint, there is no treatable problem." Treating those adolescents who claim that they do not need any help requires incorporating the family into the therapeutic process [6]. This model has required an expanded and specific adaptation of the strategies, tactics, and techniques of TFP to a brief intervention for families. This TFP-PF model complements the work of the FO outpatient treatment unit, which is specialized in individual TFP-A.

Who Are the Clinicians?

The FO includes more than 100 mental health professionals (psychiatrists, psychologists, social workers, educators, and nurses). Clinicians are distributed in six outpatient centers and three day hospitals for adolescents, all within the local public health system.

The TFP-PF program was developed by six therapists trained in TFP-A and in family therapy. The public health system in the Barcelona catchment area allows for the implementation of innovative pilot programs. When their effectiveness is empirically demonstrated, these novel programs are then included in the portfolio of public services of the State Department of Health. Currently, the TFP-PF program is still in the evaluation phase of its effectiveness.

The FO Centres for Child and Juvenile Mental Health focus on the early detection and intervention of psychiatric disorders in general and, in particular, in patients who show evidence of a mid- to low-level BPO. As already highlighted by Paulina Kernberg [7], it is possible and advisable to detect PD pathology in children and adolescents. Current empirical evidence also points out that, given the malleability of BPD symptoms in adolescence, prevention and early intervention of personality disorders in young people can help to successfully modify the trajectory of developing borderline personality disorder (BPD) pathology [8–11].

Who Are the Patients?

TFP-PF is indicated for families with adolescents who predominantly present as functioning at a mid- to low-level level of BPO, according to Kernberg´s model [1]. The Diagnostic and Statistical Manual of Mental Disorders, fifth edition (DSM-5) [12], states that "personality disorder categories may be applied with children and adolescents in relatively unusual cases in which the individual's particular maladaptive personality traits appear to be persistent and pervasive and are unlikely to be confined to a particular developmental phase of devolopmental maturity or other mental disorder." Specifically, "To diagnose a personality disorder in an individual under 18 years of age, the features must have been present for at least one year." (page 648). The FO approach to diagnosis has also been additionally informed by the studies of Sharp et al. [8, 9], which show that the DSM criteria for BPD are indeed applicable to adolescent patients aged 12 years and older, supporting the idea that a diagnosis of BPD is indicated when those criteria are met, even in adolescents.

This group of adolescents typically shows a developmental block in the process of differentiation and integration of identity, thus leading to identity diffusion and an infantile mental organization. Primitive defense mechanisms, such as projection and denial, impair their self-awareness and appreciation of their problems and symptoms, and these attitudes are strongly ego-syntonic. Adherence to individual psychodynamic psychotherapy under these conditions is often impossible or may be marked by frequent interruptions from the initial stages of the treatment.

Optimal parental functions, which include providing support, setting boundaries, and modeling healthy behavior, promote children's autonomy and independence and play a key role in preventing this kind of blockage in the development of self, and specifically, of identity. In fact, the separation-individuation process described by Mahler [13] may be viewed as a developmental trajectory toward autonomy that begins in childhood but consolidates in adolescence, which unfolds naturally in the absence of mishaps. Developmental psychology research also demonstrates the influence of parental mental, social, and emotional health on a child's ability to establish secure relationships throughout life, as described by Erikson [14].

In keeping with this view, recent models of the etiology of BPD recognize that the disorder emerges from an interactive web of genetic, neural, behavioral, family, and social pathways, many of which converge within the parent-offspring relationship. As such, this interaction is an important context for the pathogenesis of BPD [15]. In BPD, the formation of a healthy parent-child relationship may be impaired. Conversely, positive parenting, such as that characterized by a careful equilibrium or parental warmth and regulatory control, is associated with lower risk of mental illness in youths [16, 17]. According to current scientific conceptualizations of parenting, several factors impact parenting behavior, such as parental traits (i.e., personality and developmental history, cognitive-affective processes, parental psychopathology, gender), child characteristics (i.e., temperamental styles), and family and social environment (i.e., socio-economic status, social support, marital quality, family structure) [18].

Of note, the model considers parenting as a buffered system: a risk factor might be compensated for by other positive or supportive influencing factors across domains. Conversely, a predominance of risk factors coupled with insufficient resilience factors may prevent the development of positive parenting [16].

If parental functions (PF) are well structured, they constitute a protective factor for the child's ability to continue to functioning well despite major environmental stressors, including family traumas (i.e., death of a parent, parental divorce, etc.). The basic PF can be summarized as follows:

a) The function of loving, caring, and providing for basic needs. A child's survival depends on other people taking care of his or her physical and mental needs.
b) The containment and educational function. This limit-setting function helps the child to differentiate the internal world-their thoughts, feelings, and personal experiences-from the external world, which includes their surroundings and the people in it. It provides a sense of reality and helps to prevent the child from becoming emotionally out of control. This normative function generates security because it helps the child to contain his or her aggression and to self-regulate. It also facilitates the introjection of authority, autonomy, and responsibility. It contributes to the development of a general ethical-moral dimension (Super-Ego) that will govern the adolescent's future relationships, not only with the family.

This conceptualization is closely aligned with research on positive parenting, which emphasizes the importance of the balance between expressing warmth and exercising discipline toward the child. Parents who exhibit this balance are responsive to their child's needs, respectful of the child's autonomy, but also set reasonable expectations and rules [17]. Extensive clinical observations within the FO practice suggest that, among some adolescents with medium-low BPO, the parents found it difficult to perform these PF and therefore did not adequately foster the child's differentiation. Rather, such inconsistent PF can impede the expectable process of the adolescent's identify integration by promoting, maintaining, or enhancing pathological manifestations in the relational bonds between the adolescent and parents.

These types of conflict could lead to several different clinical pictures, along a continuum of severity:

1. Parents may continue to take over the psychological functions tipically associated with their children's ego when they become pre-adolescent and adolescents. This dynamic means that children remain subject to their parents´ projections. In these circumstances, the parents may reflexively ascribe to their children wishes, motivations, and reactions that reflect their own point of view, and may not accurately correspond to the child's perspective. Thus, the children may be overly submissive by identifying with their parents' projections of how they should be

and act. The pre-adolescent may not be able to overcome this stage and become trapped in a dependency on the family environment [19, 20]. Some of them maintain an undifferentiated relationship with their parental figures, a dynamic described as a "parasitic relationship" by Bleger [21]. Clinically, according to Bleger's theory, some adolescents may exhibit a kind of fusion with their parents, thereby minimizing contact with the outside world and limiting their relationships to the family of origin or childhood friends, thus leading to clinical features consistent with an avoidant personality disorder.
2. Other adolescents with low-level borderline organization may show more severe narcissistic PD features. They try to avoid dependency and may feel attacked in any kind of relationship; they may show extreme rebelliousness and varying aggressive behaviors.
3. At the highest level of severity, a subset of adolescents show antisocial PD features: they act as defiant, do not respect boundaries, are often sexually promiscuous, and may initiate substance use.

In short, adolescents functioning at a medium-low level of BPO may present a wide range of manifestations, similar to what Cancrini [22] describes as the "borderline ocean", ranging from a clinical picture close to avoidant PD (more internalizing and submissive) to others close to narcissistic and antisocial PD.

The objective of a focal and brief family therapeutic intervention is based on the improvement of the PF in the relationship between the parents and the adolescent patient. The therapist will focus on the sequelae of inconsistent roles that undergird the challenges between parents and adolescents and will use clarification, confrontation, and therapeutic interpretation to make these difficulties clear to the family.

What Is the Current Standard of Care for Clinicians Treating These Patients?

Several evidence-based therapeutic approaches for adult BPD patients have been shown to be effective among adolescent patients as well, either in an individual or group format. However, differences between these specialized interventions and their comparators are clinically modest and scarcely sustained at follow-up. Furthermore, specialist treatments for adolescent BPD do not seem to lead to greater improvement in psychosocial functioning than general youth mental health care. This indicates that effective early intervention for BPD is possible even when BPD-specific therapies are not available [23]. However, low treatment retention rates have been reported among adolescents with BPD receiving general mental health care [23]. Specialist treatments seem to be associated with greater attendance, but evidence also indicates that more severely impaired patients with BPD (e.g., with lower reflective functioning) are more likely to drop out from specialist treatments [24]. Thus, for adolescents with severe disturbances who are reluctant to adhere to generalist or specialist treatments for BPD, involving the parents in a focused therapy represents a useful first step toward engaging them in treatment.

When including parents in the treatment intervention is necessary, the strategies, tactics, and techniques we use in our family therapeutic intervention on parental roles are different from those used in regular family psychotherapy. In fact, research has generally pointed out that often family members of individuals with BPD may show considerable levels of psychopathology themselves [25], and classical family therapy for adolescents with BPD may have a less than optimal course, with frequent impulsive acting out and relational difficulties [26]. These findings, over time, have encouraged the development of multimodal therapeutic approaches for adolescent BPD patients and their families, which focus on the psychopathology assessment and treatment of both the patient and the family and on the need to integrate medication and psychotherapeutic individual interventions with family psychoeducation and family therapy [27]. Currently, there is indeed much stronger evidence for the efficacy of family psychotherapy in adolescent BPD than for any pharmacological intervention [28]. For instance, family group therapy including both adolescents with BPD and their family members was found to increase motivation for treatment [29].

To date, several forms of interventions specific to families of BPD patients have been proposed.

The "Family Guidelines" proposed by Gunderson and colleagues [30] uses psychoeducation first to explain the diagnosis of BPD to the family without the patient being present and then to treat the whole family (including the patient) by means of a multi-family group intervention.

Hoffman and colleagues [31] proposed treating the adolescent BPD patient with individual dialectical behavior therapy (DBT) and the whole family (including the patient) within a DBT skills training group. DBT-based psychoeducational family and parenting skills groups have also been developed and can be performed with or without the patient being present [32], and in a multi-family format [33].

Other approaches are centered solely on the family members of the individuals diagnosed with BPD. Fearon et al, in 2006 [34] suggested the utility of group treatments with the patient's relatives aimed at promoting "mentalization" skills. Finally, the well-known family connections program (FC) [35] is not a form of family therapy but aims to support family members of patients with BPD. As compared to optimized treatment-as-usual, FC is more effective in decreasing carers' sense of burden, grief, and depression and in improving the family members' sense of mastery [36].

In sum, available evidence strongly supports the inclusion of family members in the treatment of BPD patients, but existing strategies differ with respect to the specific type of care delivered and its modality. Furthermore, to our knowledge, no study has focused explicitly on the type of intervention that could be better suited, specifically, for adolescents with BPO who had not responded to or had previously refused individual treatment.

What Are the Goals for Imparting TFP Principles to the Clinicians Working with These Patients?

The general objective of Transference-Focused Psychotherapy for Families TFP-PF is to facilitate the resolution of the adolescent patient's identity diffusion.

More specific objectives include identifying, confronting, and interpreting the pathological relational dyads that interfere with the necessary differentiation between parents and adolescents. [37–39]. The challenges for the adolescent's development are directly related to their relationship with their maternal and paternal caregiving figures.

TFP-PF begins with the assessment of the adolescent patient's and the family's difficulties. Then the therapist shares, in a joint session, his/her understanding of the existing conflict within the family group. During the following sessions, the therapist clarifies his/her view of the family's organization and dynamics, as well as the goals for treatment.

The initial objective is to show the current confusion of the roles within the family and the consequent challenges in the differentiation between parents and child.

Examples of problems related to role confusion include the following:

a) The child is treated as an extension of the parental self (i.e., the parent talks about the child in terms of his or her own needs, feelings, or desires). These projections may ultimately impair the adolescent's ability to make independent decisions. Therefore, to make it possible for the adolescent's differentiation process to evolve, parents need to learn how to avoid these projective patterns and stop functioning as a "substitute self" for the adolescent.
b) The adolescent has grown up as one part of a relational dyad with one of the parents (i.e., as the "partner" of one parent), and in this process, the parent in question has given up his/her parental role and relates to the adolescent more like a substitute spouse than as a parental authority figure.
c) One of the parental figures psychologically or verbally abuses the child and devalues him/her.
d) A parental pattern of heightened projection, but low bonding. In this scenario, the parent may exhibit excessive attention to, and concern for, the adolescent's developing autonomy, often marked by excessive control, which is inappropriate, given the adolescent's stage of development. At the same time, the parent may not provide a necessary level of care, despite this pattern of excessive control.

TFP-PF addresses these pathological dyads between the adolescent and the family. This allows many of these adolescents to begin to recognize their difficulties and therefore engage in individual treatment. Having undertaken TFP-PF often reduces the duration of individual treatment. The individual treatment indicated may be TFP-A, dialectical behavioral therapy (DBT) or psychodynamically oriented supportive therapy. In our clinical practice, we evaluate the adolescent's personality organization through a structural personality interview, their IQ level, and their ability to commit to a specific treatment framework [40]. TFP-A requires a normal IQ, a diagnosis of personality disorder excluding antisocial personality disorder, and the ability to commit to the treatment framework. DBT has a shorter treatment program and is indicated for highly dysregulated and acting-out adolescents who cannot commit to a longer treatment. Supportive therapy is an alternative if the adolescent is not highly dysregulated but cannot commit to the TFP-A treatment setting. Therefore, the indication depends on the clinical assessment and the commitment of the adolescent and his or her family to a particular treatment setting.

It is generally recommended to start TFP-PF and the individual therapy simultaneously (usually one individual session and one family session per week). The adolescent patient may find it easier to accept the need for individual treatment when it is openly acknowledged that the adolescent's difficulties reflect co-occurring parental difficulties. In the few cases in which the adolescent totally rejects the individual therapy, we start with TFP-PF only, aiming to initiate individual treatment as soon as possible. Once the family sessions are completed, the adolescent patient continues with the individual treatment only: either a weekly session, if it is a supportive modality, with a weekly individual session, plus a skills training group, in the DBT model, or with two weekly individual sessions in the case of TFP-A.

It is important that the patient´s family support their child's individual treatment, even during the initial phase of family therapy. When this support is missing or insufficient (due to the parents' severe mental illness or lack of motivation, parental conflict, etc.), therapists should consider partial hospitalization in the adolescent day hospital or, in the most severe cases, admission to the inpatient psychiatric hospital.

What Principles of TFP Might Be Useful for the Clinicians Working with These Patients?

Strategies

Our main objective in TFP-PF is to facilitate the development of the adolescent patient's autonomy within the family unit, thus favoring his or her process of separation and individuation.

The main strategy consists of making family members aware of the activation, within the family, of important patterns of object relations (dyads) and certain pathological family roles.

In TFP-PF, dyads are systematically defined and observed: (1) between the adolescent and the parents, (2) between the parents, (3) between each family member and the therapist, and (4) between the whole family and the therapist. Dyads can be explored in the "here-and-now" of family sessions. This work also includes identifying role reversals. The goal is to gradually improve parental functioning. Family participants may experience a different relational pattern developing as the treatment unfolds.

Tactics

Therapeutic Contract

Once the therapist and the parents have explored the key aspects of the conflict experienced in the family, a therapeutic plan is proposed. The family is asked to commit to a treatment contract, which involves open communication between family members but also the need to refrain from aggressive behavior. At the beginning of therapy, the expression of feelings may lead family members to episodes of affective storms during the session, which the therapist should interpret by helping them to mentalize. At the same time, the therapist and the parents need to come to an agreement to promptly recognize and proactively address anything the adolescent might verbalize, or concerning behaviors the adolescent might act out, which could endanger those involved during the session or jeopardize the continuity of treatment. The adolescent agrees to attend both the individual and the family sessions. The therapist clarifies that in the event that the individual treatment is actively compromised, or the adolescent's safety is threatened, the parents will be informed about that.

The family is informed when the adolescent patient has apparent challenges with engagement in a therapeutic process. It is emphasized—and anticipated— that the adolescent may act capriciously, and may want to interrupt either the individual or family therapy at any time. In this way, the family is forewarned in advance to help contain the adolescent's impulsive behavior.

Maintaining the Treatment Contract

If the adolescent is reluctant to attend and participate in the family sessions, the therapist will attempt to explore the relationship between this reluctance and the identifiable problematic aspects of family functioning and the adolescent's place in this family constellation. The therapist will proactively engage the patient in an exploration of these issues with the goal of offering him/her a non-judgmental dialogue.

Choosing the Priority Theme in Each Session

TFP-PF follows the same order of thematic priorities as in the TFP-A. The therapist monitors the three channels of communication regarding all family members, both in the context of their relationships with each other and with the therapist.

In each session, the economic principle (attention to the dominant affect), the dynamic principle (exploration of drive and defense, with emphasis on the transference), and the structural principle (elements of the patient's conflicts and specific related dyads) are applied.

The dominant affect of each family member is analyzed in the context of the relationship between family members and the group dynamics that emerge in each session. The central theme is chosen in accordance with the treatment goal, that is, by prioritizing the objective of fostering the adolescent's differentiation and independence.

Maintaining Technical Neutrality

The TFP-PF clinician aims to maintain technical neutrality in sessions with both the adolescent and their parents. In individual TFP, technical neutrality means not taking one side of the patient's internal conflict. In TFP-PF this also includes avoiding taking sides in conflict between family members. This is especially difficult in the initial treatment phase as family members may have different personal expectations and goals for the sessions. The therapist should keep in mind the overarching goal of the process, to address those patterns of interaction between the adolescent and parents that may contribute to impediments in the adolescent's development of autonomy. The therapist is mindful to avoid taking a side in emerging conflicts in sessions, even when there is overt pressure to do so, as is often the case, despite the risk of provoking expectable negative transference reactions when not taking sides.

Regulating the Intensity of Emotional Expression

Managing the intensity of emotional expression within the family group may lead the therapist to set limits at different points during the treatment, i.e., when chaos or aggression arise. Managing the emotional storms that often occur in the initial phases of a family intervention is also paramount. This tactic is important in fostering the family's ability to think; it serves as a model for family members in emotional containment and regulation.

There are two situations that require specific management tactics. The first is when the family members make extensive and predominant use of projective identification. This generates confusion among all the members and the therapist because it distorts reality and introduces a destructive element that threatens communication. The clinician should apply the tactic of clarifying the respective roles of those involved. The second situation is when the dominant affect in the interaction among the family members is aggression. Family members do not listen to each other, and their communication is under attack because words are used to offend rather than communicate a message. In this case, the therapist makes it a priority to stop this kind of interaction among family participants by explaining to them that it impedes proper communication within the session.

Techniques

The techniques applied by the TFP-PF family intervention are the same as those used in individual TFP-A but adapted for this specific format. The specific elements of TFP-PF are outlined below, in addition to the basic techniques of: (1) technical neutrality, (2) interpretation, (3) transference analysis, and (4) monitoring of countertransference.

The clinician should be clear about what the normal adolescence characteristics are and compare the problematic behaviors observable between the parents and the adolescent to normative adolescent behaviors. The TFP-PF therapist operates from a position of technical neutrality. At the same time, the therapist is alert to those situations that would require a deviation from this position, such as when the adolescent's behavior might endanger health or safety, or when there is substantive risk posed to the adolescent's personal, academic, or career future.

In the initial phases of TFP-PF, the therapist makes extensive use of clarification and confrontation and then proceeds slowly and carefully with the interpretation process. Preference is given to interpretations related to the transference in the here-and-now and to current relational patterns within the family and between the family and the therapist. The therapist must also be attentive to the development of reactions within the family, both among its members and between the family and the therapist. At the same time, the therapist should continuously monitor his own countertransference, which could, for instance, reveal as an identification either with the adolescent's rebelliousness or with the parents' suffering.

In TFP-PF, in order to promote differentiation, the therapist must work especially on elucidating and interpreting those primitive defense patterns that increase confusion and aggression in the family's everyday functioning, as well as during the sessions. In this regard, one major defense mechanism is the projection of one family member's guilt onto another family member, who then can become identified with these aggressive impulses by means of projective identification. Being attentive to parents' anxieties and grief can promote progressive differentiation between the parents and the adolescent patient. At the same time, the adolescent patient faces anxiety and grief during the transition from childhood to adolescence and early adulthood.

Phases of the TFP-PF Approach

Initial Treatment Phase

Frequently the clinician is faced with questions from all sides, with expressions of concern about the efficacy of the treatment. This is often accompanied by tests of the therapist's ability and challenges to the treatment frame. Adolescents with narcissistic features openly show their difficulty in trusting the treatment, especially if they have undergone unsuccessful treatments in the past. The therapist addresses this initial resistance and negative transference by interpreting this lack of trust and hope. We describe below three different attitudes toward the therapy, which vary according to the type of clinical presentation of the adolescent:

a) *Those coming with a clinical picture close to the avoidant personality disorder* tend to remain silent. When asked what they think, they usually answer "nothing is wrong with me, and I don't want to come." They try to persuade their parents that treatment is a waste of time because it will not lead to any useful results, just like the previously failed treatments with psychologists and psychiatrists.
b) *Those presenting a clinical picture close to antisocial personality disorder* express their opposition to coming; they even try to leave the consultation room, attack, or discredit the therapist. They may say: "You think you are so smart, but you are not going to make me change, I already know what I want to do and neither you nor anyone else is going to tell me what I have to do. You are all useless. Now I want to live my way, why don't you all just leave me alone? I'm sick and tired of all of you. You're all shit." At this point, the parents may become upset, ask the teenager not to speak this way, and even scold the patient, asking

for more polite behavior with the therapist. Under such circumstances, the clinician makes it explicit to everyone that the adolescent is precisely expressing what he feels. At the same time, the therapist makes it clear that the contract also included an agreement on limiting abusive language while maintaining the expectation that the patient will speak freely. As described by Winnicott [41], here the therapist exercises the function of sustaining. Over time, the parents would learn to contain the adolescent's challenging affects and learn to focus on, and to talk about, both positive and negative aspects of themselves and of their child, thus promoting identity integration.

c) *Those not tolerating limits and rebelling against them.* Some adolescents may present with a clinical picture consistent with infantile narcissism, which can be observed in BPD patients and is distinct from a pathological narcissistic personality disorder. They might have grown up without the experience of limit setting and/or have been overprotected.

   In these cases, at the beginning of the treatment, the therapist would point out the need to set boundaries. This helps the parents to realize that they must establish some minimum rules. After observing that the therapist has pointed out the need for limits, the adolescent may say, "No one is going to change me and you are not going to convince me of anything!" These situations will test the therapist's assertiveness and capacity to reinforce the family's ability to bring order to their interactions. The therapist must help by promoting tolerance and patience and accepting attacks on cooperation, by tolerating this initial confusion in the session. The therapist performs sufficient containment so that the family work can continue.

Intermediate Treatment Phase

The intermediate phase of TFP-PF aims to start promoting identity integration. This process is not linear but is characterized by episodes of regression. Over time, this integration may help the patient to develop a greater capacity for affective regulation, especially of negative feelings. This therapeutic work is reflected in evolving transference patterns; the initial transference stance, often marked by mistrust, will evolve, and a more nuanced and three-dimensional experience of the clinician will emerge. The goal over time would be the identification of elements of a more nuanced transference, one that integrates positive and negative experiences, which characterizes a healthier and more flexible personality presentation.

In our TFP-PF model, dyads of pathological relational functioning between parents and children and between the family and the therapist are interpreted. For example, a mother may maintain a role in which overprotection predominates, while the adolescent identifies with the role of an excessively reliant and weak person. In this case, the dyad would be represented by an overprotective mother/weak child. At the same time, in this family, a relational dyad between a powerful, devaluing father and a weak, devalued child can also be observed. The family as a whole may appear weak and dependent in front of the therapist as if expecting the therapist to protect them from their difficulties. As in individual TFP, in TFP-PF there are dyads of pathological functioning that can be interpreted in the relationships between the various family members. In TFP-PF relational dyads between the family group and the clinician can also appear and therefore be interpreted.

Changes in the interactions of family members also occur and are noticed by the therapist. There may be a strengthening of the organization of the parental functions in the family, which favors the integration of the family. This new organization of parental functions helps to transform the family group into a "working group" according to Bion's theory [42]: group members start thinking together while maintaining their own perspectives. The process of differentiation of family members begins. As the family intervention progresses, the adolescent and the family will be more capable of thinking, tolerating anxiety, and frustration, and reaching agreements as a family. When this occurs, it indicates that we are entering the final phase of this family intervention.

The intermediate phases of the TFP-PF family intervention are marked by the following:

a) Through the development of a limit-setting function in the family, the parents or caretakers themselves can contain the adolescent's regressive functioning and associated turmoil. For example, the father of a troubled teenager may have assumed a "traditional" role marked by limited involvement in day-to-day activities. When this father assumes a parental role with greater clarity, this may have an impact on the adolescent who might not have recognized parental authority in the same way before. Now the more engaged father begins to play a role of containment when the adolescent exhibits verbally aggressive behavior during therapy or threatens to walk out of a session or even drop out of treatment. Often the adolescent continues to rebel against parental authority, sometimes even against the therapist, but reactions of this kind greatly diminish as treatment progresses.
b) The ability to contain the paranoid and aggressive aspects of the adolescent and the family is developed. This is in sharp contrast with what can be appreciated during the initial stage of treatment, which is characterized by intense acting out and aggressiveness. Over time, helping family members to integrate the aspects of projected aggression decreases the frequency and intensity of mutual attacks. At the same time, it makes it possible for family members to experience and tolerate emerging feelings of guilt.

Parents are encouraged to intervene in some areas less frequently and to control their own fears. For instance, parents are advised to forgo protecting the adolescent when there is a risk of certain types of behavior. Parents may comment, "*How can I let my child go out if there is a chance that he or she will get drunk?*" or "*How can I avoid worrying about my child's studies*?" When parents can tolerate relinquishing total control over their child, the adolescent can gradually learn to take more responsibility. Often, toward the end of the intermediate phase of family treatment, many parents may recognize: *"Now that I am not worried about his studies, my child has begun to worry about his studies and is studying on her own."*

During the middle phase of treatment, if the adolescent had started a specific medication, the question of the advisability of withdrawing the medication is often raised and discussed with the family. When the adolescent demonstrates, during the treatment sessions, a greater capacity for self-control and increased self-reflection, it may be possible to begin to reduce medication in a safe and supervised manner. The family will need guidance on the role and limitations of pharmacological treatments. They will also need support in monitoring the patient's response to changes in medication patterns. The therapist should explain to the caretakers that isolated episodes of emotional dysregulation do not necessarily pose a serious risk or inevitably mean a need to restart the medication.

As the patient's difficulties with behavioral dysregulation decrease in the sessions, so do the problems at home, and the group begins to organize itself as a family. This is often reflected by the fact that family members initiate some activities together.

Additionally, progress in the differentiation between family members becomes noticeable.

The adolescent patient's overall functioning begins to improve. The patient achieves greater self-awareness, and develops a greater ability for self-direction, planning, and staying committed to goals. For example, a patient at this stage may ask a social worker or educator for help in finding resources that may be helpful for his/her aims.

At the same time, many uncertainties and fears may arise in the adult caregivers as a result of the challenge of letting go of their unconscious wish for the child to be dependent on them. In addition, up to this stage of treatment, parents have had little hope that their child could change and may find it difficult to observe and value their child's changes. At this stage of treatment, the therapist is facing a particularly difficult task. While the adolescent is excited about the new possibilities that are opening up, caregivers, on the other hand, may feel less optimistic because they fear that this may be just another failed attempt. This adult view may discredit the adolescent's progress or even slow down new projects or initiatives. The parents and the adolescent may have opposite views. At this juncture, the family may interject all sorts of problems, highlight the drawbacks of the patient's initiatives, or devalue these advances. The therapist is often in a difficult position; on the one hand, there is a need to appreciate the adolescent's progress and help him to continue to differentiate and separate from his parents; on the other hand, the therapist has the mission to help the parents understand their difficulties in seeing the adolescent's progress. The therapist strives to remain neutral in this situation, by balancing the feelings expressed by both the teenager and the parents.

In the penultimate session of the family treatment, the son shows the changes that have taken place in the family and says: "Now we can talk, because we respect each other, and we can come to an agreement. I want to tell you that I have been thinking that smoking is not good for me, and I want to quit."

The father dismisses him by saying, "Well, what you say is very nice, but you are addicted to tobacco, and what you say is not easy. I'm telling you because I know from my own experience." The son is surprised by the father's reaction and replies,

"Wow, you don't trust me at all! "This remark shows that the father finds it difficult to fully appreciate the developmental changes that the adolescent is making. He cannot conceive that his son can change so quickly. He still does not see his son as sufficiently different from him but sees him through the prism of his own experiences. The father and son have different views of the situation. By making this clear, the therapist can help differentiate the adults from the child. The goal for each family member is to develop their own identity and way of thinking, which may be different from that of the other members.

Final Treatment Phase

The goals set at the beginning are reviewed during the final phase of treatment with a collective dialogue as to whether they have been achieved satisfactorily. Basically, there should be a sufficient degree of parent-child differentiation and an improvement in the adolescent's functioning and autonomy. In this phase of treatment, parents should have become aware of the impact of their own emotional expressions and behaviors on the adolescent's process toward autonomy.

Adolescents begin to be more independent. They show greater self-direction, i.e., an increased capacity to set goals, make appropriate decisions, and carry them out. They also exhibit better self-awareness and emotion regulation and are more likely to take responsibility for their actions. They are more proactive and, above all, autonomous. There are more moments when they find themselves experiencing themselves and others in a more complex and nuanced way. They may begin to mourn a wished-for, idealized parental figure, and become more accepting of their parents' positive and negative attributes. At this time, they also begin to defend their identity and their way of thinking. Parents need to accept that this increased independent stance, to allow it to unfold and to accompany their child on this new path in life. However, although family members may rationally understand this process, not all of them emotionally experience it in the same way or with the same intensity.

On the one hand, the adolescent patients tend to experience this evolving process with more enthusiasm and an increasing desire to figure out their future. This may be accompanied by greater emotional flexibility, and better coping strategies in the face of environmental challenges. On the other hand, in this final stage of treatment, parents might be highly concerned about the adolescent's future, as well as about the changes that their child's increased independence will bring to their future as parents and as a couple (i.e., similar to the developmental changes that have been described as "empty nest syndrome" [43]. The positive attitude of the therapist, which reinforces the progress in the adolescent's increased identity integration and thereby transmits confidence, will help the parents to face this final moment of the treatment. Below different potential clinical situations are presented:

A. The Adolescent Wants to Drop out from the Family Treatment and the Family Agrees The therapist picks up on this desire and reflects on whether the initial goals have been achieved. If so, the therapist suggests that the TFP-PF family intervention should come to an end and that the adolescent can continue with his or her individual therapy.

In this brief example, the family sessions were held only with the mother and daughter (there were no other family members). The mother says: *"I have even thought about creating a brand-new future life for myself, I have caught up with old friends. I have been worrying about my daughter for all her life, about her doctors, her treatments, her studies, and it has not done any good. Now that she is starting to care about herself, everything is going better. She has stopped smoking, she cares about her own future, and she has started working. She has good friends. I see her doing much better".*

In the next session, the daughter says she wants to end these family sessions. *"My individual therapy is enough for me."* When asked what had made her come to this conclusion, she replied, *"Before, I didn't think, I wasn't aware of what was happening to me, and I didn't feel anything. I didn't worry or care about anything, about taking pills, drinking alcohol, smoking, having sex. It was a way to make me feel something,* (She becomes sad.). *I did what my friends told me to do, or whatever came to my mind at the time. Now I feel like everything has changed."* She looks at her mother, smiles briefly, and continues, *"Now my mother no longer drives me crazy with her stuff, and now I think about my actions and consider what is right or wrong. It's hard because I still have a lot of bad moments, I feel a lot of anguish, but now I have good friends who help me. I am taking a course and then I will try to continue working."* She looks at her mother and they both smile.

B). The Adolescent Feels Ready and Affirms his or her Identity, but the Parents Doubt that it Is Time to End Family Therapy The separation-individuation process has progressed. Nonetheless, the parents often would like to continue treatment. The therapist then reminds them that the therapy with the family should end once they achieved the goal of the adolescent´s independence, autonomy, and separation. Two different scenarios might arise.

B1) Parents Doubt that the Adolescent Is Sufficiently Prepared for Life This concern might be driven by overwhelming anxiety for the separation from their child. In this case, the therapist must pay attention to addressing separation anxieties and fears of change that may arise from parents' doubts about whether or not the treatment objectives have been achieved. The therapist helps the parents to become aware of the changes made by the adolescent and of the anxiety produced by the fact that he/she is ready to finally separate from them. One mother was able to verbalize that she and her husband experienced the separation of their adolescent son as a "tearing apart."

Parents' fear that their children are not prepared to defend themselves in life might be heightened and reinforced by their constant awareness of various dangers that exist in the modern society.

For instance, a mother asked for a private interview, claiming that it was very important for her to have it. During the interview, she said, *"Even though going out is already normal for her age, I can't let my daughter go out at night because I can´t forget that some boys tried to rape me at a party, when I was her age."*

She was helped to understand that her problem should not be a reason to hinder her daughter's autonomy; actually, if she did not accept her going out with her friends, her interpersonal problems, formerly characterized by isolation and social avoidance, could increase. Depriving her daughter of her social life because of her own fears was neither rational nor helpful. To address this risk of undermining the adolescent's progress, the mother was referred to professional help to address her trauma history. This clarification and her referral to therapy were key in resolving the conflict between her and her daughter.

B2) Parents Misinterpret the Adolescent's Assertion of his or her Own Identity and Autonomy as Defiance The adolescent's way of thinking, different from their parents, is sometimes confused with the tantrums that the adolescent had had before starting the treatment or just at the beginning of it.

In this case, the therapist should help parents, especially those who have projected their own desires onto their children, to tolerate and accept that their children´s way of thinking and acting are different from theirs. The therapist helps them understand that their doubts have to do with their difficulty in letting their child live in his/ own way, not as they had wished or planned for; this intervention is done to help them face this final phase of the therapeutic process.

C) The Parents Begin a New Stage as a Couple Once the Son/Daughter´s Independence Is Achieved The couple has been intensely dedicated and devoted for years to the child's upbringing. When the adolescent begins to make strides towards independence and autonomy, the parents might suddenly experience that they now have their private space, previously occupied by worries about their child. In most cases, the couple's relationship begins to improve. In other circumstances, a couple's crisis can become apparent at this stage. This is usually because when the children's difficulties diminish significantly, the relational difficulties between the partners become more evident or because they find out that they have different personal and life goals, which were previously obscured by their joint focus on parenting that until then had sustained them as a couple. In the case such issues arise, the TFP-PF therapist should be prepared to refer the couple to proper specialist treatment for couples.

What Is the Format for the Instruction of TFP Principles to this Audience?

The training curriculum for the TFP-PF psychotherapists includes sections on both theory and practice.

The section on theory emphasizes the acquisition of knowledge about the following topics relevant for youth mental health:

- How the child's and adolescent's personality is structured, as described by Paulina Kernberg [7]
- The main stages of child and adolescent development, i.e., of the age-related levels of differentiation and autonomy expected at each stage, particularly in adolescents, as outlined by the work of Malher [13]
- Melanie Klein's object relations theory [44]
- The fundamentals of family functioning [45]
- The structuring of the children-parental links (i.e., [41]
- The functioning of Bion's group dynamics [42]

The practical training includes the following:

- Participating as co-therapist in a TFP-PF family group. This therapy is led by an accredited TFP therapist with training and experience in family or adolescent parent group therapy.
- Attending as an observer supervision group of TFP-PF therapists using video-recorded clinical material.
- Carrying out two supervised TFP-PF family treatments.

What Is the Source of Institutional or Governmental Support for this Initiative?

As previously mentioned, TFP-PF is one of the innovative pilot programs accepted by the public mental health system of the Barcelona catchment area. Once this family intervention is deployed to a substantial number of patients and demonstrated as empirically effective, it will be proposed as a regular, long-term treatment project to be included in the public services portfolio of the State Department of Health.

What Are Possible Measurement Objectives for Gauging the Effectiveness of Instruction on the Applications of TFP Principles?

Drawing from our clinical expertise in the application of TFP-PF in the public health system, we developed a research protocol to evaluate the effectiveness of the TFP-PF intervention.

We are in the data collection phase at present, with the goal of using measurement tools to assess the efficacy of our family treatment intervention.

When an adolescent patient is referred together with his or her family for TFP-PF, in addition to a thorough psychiatric evaluation, a series of tests are performed to comprehensively assess his or her mental state. All these tests are administered not only prior to the start of treatment but also after 6, 12, and 36 months of treatment.

The Clinical Global Impression (*CGI*) *-BPD* [46] is an adaptation of the CGI scale [47], which assesses both the baseline severity of BPD and its changes over the treatment course. It consists of 10 items, scoring the nine relevant psychopathological domains of the disorder (fear of abandonment, unstable relationships, identity disturbance, impulsivity, suicidality, affective instability, chronic feelings of emptiness, anger, and paranoid ideation) and an additional global score.

The *Borderline Personality Questionnaire* (BPQ) [48] is an 80-item dichotomous response questionnaire developed for the diagnosis of BPD based on DSM-IV criteria. It has a total of nine subscales: impulsivity, affective instability, abandonment, relatedness, self-image, suicidality/mutilation, emptiness, intense anger, and quasi-psychotic states. The BPQ has been specifically accredited for use in the screening of BPD in young people [49].

*The Barrat's impulsiveness scale (*BIS-11) [50, 51] assesses levels of impulsivity and consists of 30 items that are grouped into three subscales: cognitive impulsivity (attention), motor impulsivity, and unplanned impulsivity. Finally, the *Self Harm Questionnaire* (SHQ [52]) assesses the presence of self-harming thoughts and behaviors in adolescents.

Clinical Illustration

Maria is a 16-year-old girl who began exhibiting symptoms of affective dysregulation at age 14. When she was age 15, she began cutting herself and periodically threatening suicide, which understandably alarmed her parents, leading them to bring her first to their pediatrician, who made a diagnosis of depression and recommended treatment with antidepressant medication. When this medication trial did not stem Maria's evolving pattern of intense anger and unstable relationships, she was then evaluated by a local mental health clinician who shared with Maria and her parents the clinician's diagnosis of BPD. Maria's six months of supportive psychotherapy did not significantly help with the severe behavioral problems she had, including failing to complete any schooling, and being repeatedly expelled after confrontations with teachers. Maria was only marginally committed to this individual treatment, often missing sessions or threatening to quit. At this point, Maria's distraught parents were made aware of Fundacio Orienta's TFP-PF intervention, and they initiated an evaluation.

At the outset of the TFP-PF treatment, Maria was made aware that, as agreed in the contract outlined by the TFP-PF clinician and Maria and her parents, she was expected to stay engaged in the treatment and postpone making important decisions without discussing them first during the family sessions. Once, early in the treatment, Maria decided on her own to stop attending the pastry assistant course that she had just started and simultaneously expressed vague threats of dropping out of the TFP-PF program; she rapidly got angry at her parents in this context, who did not agree with this decision to stop her studies. The parents convinced her to postpone this decision until discussing it in the family session. In the session with the family, they all expressed distress; they had had multiple arguments about these issues at home, in the period before the scheduled family intervention appointment. The therapist asked the patient how she understood the chain of events that had led her to consider abandoning her studies and her treatment. The patient explained that her pastry teacher had scolded her and that she had found this humiliating. As she spoke, her parents listened attentively. The therapist waited and, after a few moments, asked the parents to express their point of view.

The father replied, "That's how it always starts. No one can stop her. She's a capricious child."

The patient angrily stood up: "No one tells me what to do and no one stops me!" She added getting up, "So I'm leaving!"

The therapist reminded her of her commitment to refrain from making important life decisions without talking about them in the session. The therapist also suggested to her father that he shouldn´t allow his daughter to leave. The father warned the patient that he would call an ambulance if she tried to leave the session impulsively. It was a very tense moment for everyone. The father, feeling supported by the therapist, maintained his position with determination including the threat that he would call the ambulance should she elope, while the mother tried to calm her down with reassuring promises.

Maria was able to stay engaged in the TFP-PF treatment for six months. During this time, the therapist continued to address those challenges to the treatment agreement as they emerged. For example, he would comment immediately on those occasions when Maria was late to their meeting and to invite exploration of the meaning of this non-verbal communication, given their detailed treatment contract that had included timeliness for all meetings. The therapist monitored those evident dyads that included the recurrent pattern of Maria feeling "victimized" by her parents' routine requests, like that she keeps her room clean, alternating with Maria's "victimizing" of them, such as when she would stay out after her curfew in response to their request, knowing it would unnerve them. Because Maria initially had adamantly refused to engage in individual treatment, the TFP-PF therapist conducted weekly sessions until Maria tentatively changed her mind. Maria was then referred to a DBT treatment with one weekly skills session and one weekly individual meeting. At this juncture, another important dyad was observed, as Maria and her parents expressed mistrust of the DBT therapist, expressing concerns that the DBT interventions introduced would not help Maria if she were at the mercy of an overly critical instructor at her pasty-making school. Together they devalued the DBT treatment, undermining Maria's investment in the tools offered. The TFP-PF therapist used this scenario as an opportunity to describe the dyad he observed of "vulnerable family" and "indifferent therapists" thereby exploring a possible paranoid transference experienced by both the patient and her parents.

Over time, Maria grudgingly stayed in the DBT treatment, and became more conscientious about the TFP-PF meetings, to the point that she expressed some gratitude for the opportunity to explore in an environment that felt secure the challenges of living with her parents. Eventually, Maria and her parents determined that Maria's symptoms had diminished to the extent that if felt appropriate to end the family intervention as Maria would continue in DBT treatment only. This process occurred only with the TFP-PF therapist's help, as the parents expressed concern that Maria was moved to end the family work only as a gesture of defiance. When this was fully explored and when the parents felt sufficiently comfortable with this next phase, the TFP-PF treatment was ended.

Conclusion

As adolescent mental health professionals, we may face serious difficulties in treating some adolescent patients with mid-to low-level BPO, who may show a limited awareness of their difficulties and, thus, poor motivation for treatment. We have proposed a novel therapeutic family intervention aimed at enhancing the level of personality functioning of this patient group. This family approach applies the principles of TFP to improve parental functions. The goal of TFP-PF is to facilitate the process of differentiation and individuation of adolescent patients with BPO, foster their identity integration, and promote their adherence to individual psychotherapy. This treatment model is particularly useful for ameliorating their interpersonal functioning. Based on the positive clinical experience in applying TFP-PF, we have started an ongoing research initiative aimed at providing empirical evidence on its effectiveness.

References

1. Yeomans FE, Clarkin JF, Kernberg OF. Transference-focused psychotherapy for borderline personality disorder: a clinical guide. Arlington: American Psychiatric Publishing; 2014.
2. Bender DS, Dolan RT, Skodol AE, Sanislow CA, Dyck IR, McGlashan TH, et al. Treatment utilization by patients with personality disorders. Am J Psychiat. 2001;158:295–302.
3. Normandin L, Ensink K, Weiner A, Kernberg O. Psicoterapia focalizada en la transferencia para adolescentes con trastornos graves de la personalidad. Bilbao: Desclée de Brouwer; 2022.
4. Freixas J. A propósito del modelo de asistencia sanitaria. Actuaciones médicas lesivas para la salud mental. In: Tizón JL, Rosell MT, editors. Trabajo y salud mental. Barcelona: Laia; 1983.
5. Fisch R, Schlanger K. Therapy with intimidating cases: changing the unchangeable. San Francisco: Jossey-Bass Publishers; 1999.
6. Icart A, Freixas J. La familia. Comprensión dinámica e intervenciones terapéuticas Barcelona: Herder; 2013.
7. Kernberg P, Wenwe AS, Bardenstein KK. Trastornos de Personalidad en niños y adolescentes. México: El Manual Moderno; 2002.
8. Sharp C, Ha C, Michonski J, Venta A, Carbone C. Borderline personality disorder in adolescents: evidence in support of the childhood interview for DSM-IV borderline personality disorder in a sample of adolescent inpatients. Comp Psych. 2012;53:765–74. https://doi.org/10.1016/j.comppsych.2011.12.003.
9. Sharp C, Steinberg L, Michonski J, Kalpakci A, Fowler C, Frueh BC, Fonagy P. DSM borderline criterion function across age-groups: a cross-sectional mixed-method study. Assessment. 2019;26(6):1014–29. https://doi.org/10.1177/1073191118786587.
10. Chanen AM, Jovev M, Jackson HJ. Adaptive functioning and psychiatric symptoms in adolescents with borderline personality disorder. J Clin Psychiatry. 2007;68(2):297–306.
11. Chanen AM, McCutcheon LK, Jovev M, Jackson HJ, McGorry PD. Prevention and early intervention for borderline personality disorder. Med J Aust. 2007;187(7):18–21.
12. American Psychiatric Association. Diagnostic and statistical manual of mental disorders. 5th ed. Washington, DC: American Psychiatric Association; 2022.
13. Mahler M, Pine M, Bergman A. The psychological birth of the human infant. Nueva York: Basic Books; 1975.
14. Erickson N, Julian M, Muzik M. Perinatal depression, PTSD, and trauma: Impact on mother-infant attachment and interventions to mitigate the transmission of risk. Int Rev Psychiatry. 2019;31(3):245–63.

15. Steele KR, Townsend ML, Grenyer BFS. Parenting and personality disorder: an overview and meta-synthesis of systematic reviews. PLoS One. 2019;14(10). https://doi.org/10.1371/journal.pone.0223038.
16. Seeger FR, Neukel C, Williams K, et al. Parental mental illness, borderline personality disorder, and parenting behavior: the moderating role of social support. Curr Psychiatry Rep. 2022;24:591–601. https://doi.org/10.1007/s11920-022-01367-8.
17. Chen Y, Haines J, Charlton BM, et al. Positive parenting improves multiple aspects of health and well-being in young adulthood. Nat Hum Behav. 2019;3:684–91. https://doi.org/10.1038/s41562-019-0602-x.
18. Taraban L, Shaw DS. Parenting in context: revisiting Belsky's classic process of parenting model in early childhood. Dev Rev. 2018;48:55–81. https://doi.org/10.1016/j.dr.2018.03.006.
19. Icart A. Tratamiento del niño hiperactivo a través de la familia. Psicopatol salud ment. 2007;M2:31–42.
20. Icart A, Ribalta T. Intervención precoz en la prevención del trastorno hiperactivo. Una modalidad de psicoterapia familiar breve. Psicopatol salud ment. 2005;6:85–96.
21. Bleger J. Simbiosis y ambigüedad: estudio psicoanalítico. Buenos Aires: Paidós; 1984.
22. Cancrini L. L'oceano borderline. Racconti di viaggi. Milano: Raffaello Cortina Editore; 2006.
23. Chanen AM, Betts JK, Jackson H, et al. Effect of 3 forms of early intervention for young people with borderline personality disorder: the MOBY randomized clinical trial. JAMA Psychiatry. 2022;79(2):109–19. https://doi.org/10.1001/jamapsychiatry.2021.3637.
24. Jørgensen MS, Bo S, Vestergaard M, Storebø OJ, Sharp C, Simonsen E. Predictors of dropout among adolescents with borderline personality disorder attending mentalization-based group treatment. Psychother Res. 2021;31(7):950–61. https://doi.org/10.1080/10503307.2020.1871525.
25. Sansone RA, Sansone LA. The families of borderline patients: the psychological environment revisited. Psychiatry (Edgmont). 2009;6(2):19–24.
26. James AC, Vereker M. Family therapy for adolescents diagnosed as having borderline personality disorder. J Fam Ther. 1996;18:269–83. https://doi.org/10.1111/j.1467-6427.1996.tb00050.x.
27. Glick ID, Dulit RA, Wachter E, Clarkin JF. The family, family therapy, and borderline personality disorder. J Psychother Pract Res. 1995;4(3):237–46.
28. Marcinko D, Bilić V. Family therapy as addition to individual therapy and psychopharmacotherapy in late adolescent female patients suffering from borderline personality disorder with comorbidity and positive suicidal history. Psychiatr Danub. 2010;22(2):257–60.
29. Santisteban DA, Muir JA, Mena MP, Mitrani VB. Integrative borderline adolescent family therapy: meeting the challenges of treating adolescents with borderline personality disorder. Psychol Psychother Theory Res Pract. 2003;40(4):251–64. https://doi.org/10.1037/0033-3204.40.4.251.
30. Gunderson JG, Hoffman PD. Understanding treating borderline personality disorder. Guide for professionals and families. Arlington: American Psychiatric Publishing; 2005.
31. Hoffman PD, Fruzzetti AE, Swenson CR. Dialectical behavior therapy-family skills training. Fam Process. 1999;38(4):399–414. https://doi.org/10.1111/j.1545-5300.1999.00399.x.
32. Fruzzetti A, Shenk C, Hoffman P. Family interaction and the development of borderline personality disorder: a transactional model. Dev Psychopatol. 2005;17(4):1007–30. https://doi.org/10.1017/S0954579405050479.
33. Miller J, Rathus JH, Linehan M, Swenson CR, Ivanoff A. Dialectical behavior therapy with suicidal adolescents. New York: The Guilford press; 2007.
34. Fearon P, Target M, Sargent J, Williams LL, McGregor J, Bleiberg E, Fonagy P. Short-term mentalization and relational therapy (SMART): an integrative family therapy for children and adolescents. In: Allen JG, Fonagy P, editors. The handbook of mentalization-based treatment. New York: Wiley; 2006. p. 201–22.
35. Hoffman PD, Fruzzetti AE, Buteau E, Neiditch ER, Penney D, Bruce ML, Hellman F, Struening E. Family connections: a program for relatives of persons with borderline personality disorder. Fam Process. 2005;44(2):217–25. https://doi.org/10.1111/j.1545-5300.2005.00055.x.

36. Flynn D, Kells M, Joyce M, Corcoran P, Herley S, Suarez C, Cotter P, Hurley J, Weihrauch M, Groeger J. Family Connections versus optimised treatment-as-usual for family members of individuals with borderline personality disorder: non-randomised controlled study. Borderline Personal Disord Emot Dysregul. 2017;4:18. https://doi.org/10.1186/s40479-017-0069-1.
37. Icart A, Freixas J. Atención al adolescente bordeline mediante las intervenciones sobre las funciones parentales. Psicopatol. salud ment. 2020;36:65–76.
38. Icart A, Freixas J. A mí no me pasa nada. Barcelona: Editorial Octaedro; 2020.
39. Sánchez JA, Icart A. Simbiosis y narcisismo en la adolescencia. A propósito de un caso. Psicopatol salud ment. 2018;32:57–65.
40. Normandin L, Costa X. Trabajando con los padres en Psicoterapia Focalizada en la Transferencia para adolescentes. Psicopatol salud ment. 2016;28:45–54.
41. Winnicott D. Group influences and the maladjusted child. El aspecto escolar en el desarrollo familiar e individual. London: Tavistock; 1965.
42. Bion WR. Experiencias en grupos y otros trabajos. Londres: Routledge; 1961.
43. Norris JE, Tindale JA. Among generations. The cycle of adult relationships. New York: W. H. Freeman and Company; 1994.
44. Klein M. A contribution to the psychogenesis of maniac-depressive states. Int J Psychoanal. 1935;16:145–74.
45. Meltzer D, Harris M. The educational role of the family: a psychoanalytical model. London: Karnac Books; 2013.
46. Pérez V, Barrachina J, Soler J, Pascual JC, Campins MJ, Puigdemont D, et al. Impresión clínica global para pacientes con trastorno límite de la personalidad (ICG-TLP): una escala sensible al cambio. Actas Esp Psiquiat. 2007;35(4):229–35.
47. Guy W. Clinical global impressions, ECDEU assessment manual for psychopharmacology, revised. Rockville: National Institute of Mental Health; 1976. p. 218–22.
48. Poreh AM, Rawlings D, Claridge G, Freeman JL, Faulkner C, Shelton C. The BPQ: a scale for the assessment of borderline personality based on DSM-IV criteria. J Pers Disord. 2006;20:247–60.
49. Chanen AM, Jovev M, Djaja D, McDougall E, Yuen HP, Rawlings D, et al. Screening for borderline personality disorder in outpatient youth. J Pers Disord. 2008;22(4):353–64.
50. Patton J, Stanford M, Barrat E. Factor structure of the Barratt impulsiveness scale. J Clin Psychol. 1995;51:768–74.
51. Oquendo M, Baca-García E, Graver R, Morales M, Montalban V, Mann J. Adaptación española de la Escala de Impulsividad de Barratt (BIS). Eur J Psychiatry. 2001;15:147–55.
52. Ougrin D, Boege I. Brief report: the Self Harm Questionnaire: a new tool designed to improve identification of self-harm in adolescents. J Adolesc. 2013;36(1):221–5.

TFP Resources

Books

Yeomans FE, Clarkin JF, Kernberg OF. Transference-focused psychotherapy for borderline personality disorder – a clinical guide. Washington, DC: American Psychiatric Publishing; 2015.

Caligor E, Kernberg OF, Clarkin JF, Yeomans FE. Psychodynamic therapy for personality pathology – treating self an interpersonal functioning. Washington, DC: American Psychiatric Publishing; 2018.

Hersh R, Caligor E, Yeomans FE. Fundamentals of transference-focused psychotherapy – applications in psychiatric and medical settings. Cham, Switzerland: Springer; 2016.

Normandin L, Ensink K, Weiner A, Kernberg OF. Transference-focused psychotherapy for adolescents with severe personality disorders. Washington, DC: American Psychiatric Publishing; 2021.

Diamond D, Yeomans FE, Stern BL, Kernberg OF. Treating pathological narcissism with transference-focused psychotherapy. New York, NY: Guilford; 2022.

Outcome Studies

Clarkin JF, Levy KN, Lenzenweger MF, Kernberg OF. Evaluating three treatments for borderline personality disorder: a multiwave study. A J Psychiatry. 2007;164(6):922–8.

Levy KN, Meehan KB, Kelly KM, Reynoso JS, Weber M, Clarkin JF, Kernberg OF. Change in attachment patterns and reflective function in a randomized control trial of transference-focused psychotherapy for borderline personality disorder. J Consult Clin Psychol. 2006;74(6):1027–40.

Doering S, Hörz S, Rentrop M, Fischer-Kern M, Schuster P, Benecke C, Buchheim A, Martius P, Buchheim P. Transference-focused psychotherapy v. treatment by experienced community psychotherapists for borderline personality disorder: randomized controlled trial. Br J Psychiatry. 2010;196(5):389–95.

R. G. Hersh, C. De Panfilis (eds.), *Implementing Transference-Focused Psychotherapy Principles*, https://doi.org/10.1007/978-3-031-68062-5

Fischer-Kern M, Doering S, Taubner S, Hörz S, Zimmernmann J, Rentrop M, Schuster P, Buchheim P, Buchheim A. Transference-focused psychotherapy for borderline personality disorder: change in reflective function. Br J Psychiatry. 2015;207(2):173–4.

Buchheim A, Hörz-Sagstetter S, Doering S, Rentrop M, Schuster P, Buchheim P, Pokorny D, Fischer-Kern M. Change of unresolved attachment in borderline personality disorder: RCT study of transference-focused psychotherapy. Psychother Psychosom. 2017;86(5):314–6.

Sollberger D, Gremaud-Heitz D, Riemenschneider A, Agarwalla P, Benecke C, Schwald O, Küchenhoff J, Walter M, Dammann G. Change in identity diffusion and psychopathology in a specialized inpatient treatment for borderline personality disorder. Clin Psychol Psychother. 2015;22(6):559–69.

Jahn C, Wieacker E, Bender S, Krischer M. [Reduction of non-suicidal self-injury (NSSI) in adolescents with borderline personality organization treated with TFP-A]. Prax Kinderpsychol Kinderpsychiatr. 2021;70(8):728–47.

Websites

https://istfp.org/
https://borderlinedisorders.com

Videos

https://www.youtube.com/watch?v=ns6ceeBqi7o&list=PLzETDKrGS_Tjw5uGkZGZ4RHCt1RAcSiqY&index=2

https://www.youtube.com/watch?v=Y3xIolVQaSM&list=PLzETDKrGS_Tjw5uGkZGZ4RHCt1RAcSiqY&index=4

https://www.youtube.com/watch?v=-H9qZBIfjHM&list=PLzETDKrGS_Tjw5uGkZGZ4RHCt1RAcSiqY&index=14

The authors are Drs. Yeomans and Doering, who also authored the foreword.

Index

A

Accountability, 95, 96
Acute suicidal tendencies, 179
Addictive substances, 180, 181
Adherence, 51
Adolescent identity treatment (AIT), 10
Against medical advice (AMA), 208
Aggression, 31, 33, 270
Alternative model for personality disorders (AMPD), 7, 28, 35
Analysis of "transference" in the therapeutic relationship, 73
Applied transference-focused psychotherapy, 49
  approach, 14–16
  evolution of, 314, 315
Aroused-fusing transference, 292, 293
Assertive community treatment (ACT), 6
Asymmetry, 200
Attitude to Personality Disorder Questionnaire (APDQ), 126
Axis model, 273
  basic forensic module, 274, 275
  descriptive-phenomenological diagnoses, 279
  identity, superego and sexualization, 275, 276
    identity integration and impulse control, 276
    integration vs. instrumentalization of sexuality, 278
    narcissistic regulation and superego development, 277
  illness experience and treatment prerequisites, 274
  offense analysis, 275

B

Barcelona catchment area, 145
Barrat's impulsiveness scale (BIS-11), 355
Basic assumption group, 241, 260
Basic forensic module, 274, 275
Behavioral dysregulation, 350
Behavioral therapeutic, 266
Belfast self harm personality disorder service, 120
Bio, 64
Bio-psycho-social framework, 64
Bleger's theory, 341
Borderline level of personality organization (BPO), 32
Borderline ocean, 341
Borderline personality disorder (BPD), 28, 49, 241, 339
  psychoeducation for, 51
    carers of patients with, 52
    comorbidities, 66, 67
    crisis management, 74–76
    development of, 64–66
    group and treatment frame, 56, 57
    improving knowledge about disease, 52, 53
    patients with, 51
    PE program, structure of, 55, 56
    personality disorder diagnosis, 57–63
    pharmacological treatment, 67–69
    program evaluation, 76
    psychotherapy, 69, 70
    shared treatment decision making with mental health professionals, 53, 54
    TFP-informed psychoeducational program, 54
    transference-focused psychotherapy, 70–74
    warm-up exercise of meetings, 56
Borderline personality organization (BPO), 49–50, 135, 218, 337
  hallmark feature of, 34
  and reality testing, 34
  three levels of, 34

R. G. Hersh, C. De Panfilis (eds.), *Implementing Transference-Focused Psychotherapy Principles*, https://doi.org/10.1007/978-3-031-68062-5

Borderline Personality Organization Integrated Care Continuum Treatment Program (BPOTP), 218, 219
  clinical case illustration, 233–235
  contemporary standard of care, 220–222
  didactic materials, 232, 233
  establishing treatment contract, 227, 228
  goals for, 222–224
  identifying patient goals, 226, 227
  identity diffusion, 231
  involving family into treatment, 225, 226
  patient assessment in, 219, 220, 224, 225
  structure work of team, TFP principles, 229, 230
  targets for measurement, 231, 232
  teams' work coordination, 230
Borderline personality questionnaire (BPQ), 355
British Psychoanalytic Council (BPC), 115

C

Centre Psicoteràpia Barcelona – Serveis Salut Mental (CPB-SSM), 136, 218
  day hospital program
    clinicians, 138
    contemporary standard of care, 138–140
    diagnostic process, 137, 138
    indications for, 136, 137
Child and adolescent psychiatry unit (CAPU), 86
Chronic suicidality, 178
CL psychiatry, 327
Clinical Confidence with Personality Disorder Questionnaire (CCPDQ), 126
Clinical global impression (CGI)-BPD, 354
Cognitive analytic therapy (CAT), 115
Cognitive-behavioral treatment (CBT) approaches, 266
Communication
  channels of, 123
  employing three channels, 246
Community-based Departments of Mental Health (DMH), 85
Community Mental Health Team (CMHT), 111
  TFP-informed supervision to, 125
  TFP-oriented supervision for, 127
    clinical presentations, 128
    diagnosis, 127
    older patients, 128–130
Comorbid mental disorders, 171
Compassion fatigue, 198
Constraint context and projection, 295–297
Consultation-liaison (CL) service, 310
  TFP principles in, 315, 316
Containment function, 340
Countertransference reactions, 130
Crisis management, 74–76
Cross-sectional program, 138, 148

D

Day hospital (DH) program
  clinical illustration, 257–259
  clinicians working, utility for, 142, 252
  communication, monitoring various channels of, 255, 256
  contemporary standard of care, 253, 257
  CPB-SSM
    clinicians, 138
    contemporary standard of care, 138–140
    diagnostic process, 137, 138
    indications for, 136, 137
  didactic materials, 149
  goals for, 140, 141, 253
  individual TFP in, 142
  institutional/government support, source of, 148, 253, 257
  patients, 252, 253
  principles of TFP and specific modifications, 144, 145
  role play, 256
  strategies modifications, 145, 146
  tactics modifications, 146, 147
  targets for measurement, 148, 149, 257
  techniques modifications, 147, 148
  TFP-informed group therapy in, 143, 144
  treatment frame, establishing, 255
  using photograph cards, 256
  utility for, 253–255
DeanCross, 117, 118
Defenses, 31
Deficit range, 281
Delinquents, psychoanalytic tradition, treatment of, 265
Descriptive-phenomenological diagnoses, 279
Descriptive psychopathology, 267–269
Destructive impulses, 96
Developmental trauma, 65
Diagnostic and Statistical Manual of Mental Disorders, fifth edition (DSM-5), 339
  personality disorders in, 34–36

Dialectical behavior therapy (DBT), 4, 44, 69, 88, 115, 141, 223, 241, 342, 343
Differentiation, 276
Direct transference-focused psychotherapy, 118
Disorder specific treatment (DST), 13
Dominant object relations dyads, 185

E
East London NHS Foundation Trust (ELFT), 124
Ego-dystonic malignant perversion, 278
Ego-syntonic malignant perversion, 278
Emergency room (ER), 199
 using TFP principles in, 202, 203
  admission, voluntary or involuntary, 205, 206
  discharge, ER with therapeutic advice, 205
  evaluation, 203–205
Emotional expression, 346
Empathy, 31
Empty nest syndrome, 351
Evidence-based therapies, 70
Expert to expert communication, 53
Exploration, 93, 94
External reality, attention on, 96
Eye movement desensitization and reprocessing (EMDR), 223

F
Family connections intervention, 52
Family intervention
 adolescent
  parents doubt, 352, 353
  parents misinterpret, 353
  ready and affirms, 352
 clinical illustration, 355, 356
 clinicians, 338
 clinicians working, useful for
  emotional expression, regulating intensity, 346
  priority theme, choosing, 345
  strategies, 344
  technical neutrality, maintaining, 346
  therapeutic contract, 345
  treatment contract, maintaining, 345
 format for instruction, 353, 354
 gauging, measurement objectives for, 354, 355
 goals for, 343, 344
 institutional/governmental support, source of, 354
 new stage, parents begin, 353
 patients, 339–341
 standard of care, 341, 342
 techniques, 346, 347
 TFP-PF approach, phases of, 347, 348
  final treatment phase, 351, 352
  initial treatment phase, 347, 348
  intermediate treatment phase, 348–351
FO Centres for Child and Juvenile Mental Health, 338
Forensic module, 275
Forensic patient
 psychodynamic diagnostics, 300
 and psychopathology
  axis model, 273–278
  descriptive psychopathology and offense-analysis, 267–269
  prototypes and features, 271–273
  psychodynamic contexts and prototypes, 269–271
 TFFP, manual for, 300, 301
 treatment of
  forensic psychiatry, 298, 299
  institutional contexts for, 295–297
  outpatient follow-up, 299
  prisons, 297, 298
  reflective function, improvement of, 280
  structural level, reflective function and delinquency, 280, 281
  TFFP, framework and technical procedure in, 281–283
  TFFP strategies, 283–295
  transference analysis, as central mechanism of action, 279, 280
Forensic psychiatry, 298, 299
Forensic psychotherapy, 266
Fundació Orienta (FO), 338
Fusion, 276

G
General psychiatric management (GPM), 69
General therapy contract, 181, 182
Generalist approach, 4–6
Good psychiatric management (GPM), 92
GPM-oriented psychoeducation, 18
Group therapy, 187, 188, 233, 239, 240

clarification, confrontation, interpretation, 249, 250
communication, employing three channels, 246
day hospital program
clinical illustration, 250, 251, 257–259
clinicians, 252
communication, monitoring various channels of, 255, 256
contemporary standard of care, 253, 257
goals for, 253
institutional/government support, source of, 253, 257
patients, 252, 253
using photograph cards, 256
role play, 256
targets for measurement, 257
treatment frame, establishing, 255
utility for, 253–255
didactic materials, 250
format for instruction, 250
inpatient group therapy, 244, 245
institutional/government support, source of, 246
maintaining technical neutrality, 248
Munsterlingen program
clinicians, 240
contemporary standard of care, 241–243
goals for, 243, 244
patients, 240, 241
negative and positive transferences, management of, 247, 248
outpatient group therapy, 244
sessions, 187
targets for measurement, 250
utility free association in group, 246

H

Health-related concerns, 310
epidemiology, 310
healthcare utilization patterns, 311
medical comorbidity, 311
medical personnel, attitudes of, 311, 312
overarching strategies, 312, 313
Hospitalization, 209

I

Identity, 269, 275, 276
diffusion, 231
integration, 141, 276
Illness experience and treatment prerequisites, 274
Impulse control, 276
Impulsive patterns, 63
Individual TFP, 142
Informed care
accountability, 95, 96
being active/not reactive versus being neutral, 94
being thoughtful, 94
clarification, use of, 94
clinicians, contemporary standard of care for, 88, 89
corrective experiencing versus experiencing and understanding, 94
exploration versus adaptation, 93, 94
external reality, attention on, 96
first phase, 100, 101
flexible, pragmatic and eclectic, 96
goals, 89
good psychiatric management, 92
institutional or government support, 92
measurement, applications of TFP principles, 97
monitoring countertransference, 95
nature of pathology, 93
outpatient Italian Psychiatric Services, 98, 99
patients, 86, 87
phase 1, clinical case illustration of, 102, 103
phases of intervention with hierarchical goals, 99
second phase, 103–106
specific goals, 90–92
TFP principles, format for instruction, 97, 98
third phase, 107, 108
Informed consent process, 50
INHS-based standard of care, 86
Inpatient group therapy, 244, 245
Inpatient hospitalization, containment function of, 173
Inpatient TFP hospitalization, 206, 207
dealing with addictive substances, 180, 181
extended diagnostic phase, 175, 176
general therapy contract, 181, 182
indication for, 171, 172
individual inpatient TFP, 186, 187
initial phase, 175, 183, 184
inpatient crisis intervention and acute psychiatric treatment, 190, 191
inpatient treatment conditions, 208, 209
middle phase, 186
pharmacotherapy, 209, 210

religiosity and political attitude, 183
staff organization, 207
self-injuring behavior, 179, 180
sequence of, 174
sexuality and love relationships, 182, 183
suicidal behavior, 178, 179
termination phase, 188–190
TFP-based group psychotherapy, 187, 188
therapy contract phase, 176–178
treatment contact, 207
treatment focus, determining, 184–186
treatment objectives, 208
Institutional therapy (IT), 138
Institutional transference, 219
Instrumentalization, 278
Integrated care continuum
BPOTP, patient assessment in, 224, 225
clinical case illustration, 233–235
clinicians, 218, 219
contemporary standard of care, 220–222
didactic materials, 232, 233
establishing treatment contract, 227, 228
goals for, 222–224
identifying patient goals, 226, 227
identity diffusion, 231
involving family into treatment, 225, 226
patients, 219, 220
structure work of team, TFP principles, 229, 230
targets for measurement, 231, 232
teams' work coordination, 230
Integrated personality organizations, 60
Integration, 276, 278
Integrative multidisciplinary treatment (IMT), 11
Internal medicine, 327, 328
International personality disorder examination (IPDE), 152
International Society for TFP (ISTFP), 7, 115
International Society for Transference-Focused Psychotherapy (ISTFP), 116, 153
Italian National System (INHS) psychiatric care, 85

J
Justified criticism, 266, 267
Juvenile BPD, 151

K
Kernberg´s model, 151, 339
Kernberg's classification, 337

L
Level of Personality Functioning Scale (LPFS), 35
Lewisham PD Service, 118–120
Love relationships, 182, 183

M
Maternal digestive function, 295
Medical and personality disorder comorbidities
addressing medical comorbidities, 313, 314
applied TFP, evolution of, 314, 315
CL psychiatry, 327
clinical illustration, 325–327, 330–332
clinicians, 316, 317, 328
consultation-liaison service, TFP principles in, 315, 316
contemporary standard of care, 328, 329
didactic materials, 330
goals for, 324, 325, 329
health-related concerns and personality disorder pathology, 310
epidemiology, 310
healthcare utilization patterns, 311
medical comorbidity, 311
medical personnel, attitudes of, 311, 312
overarching strategies, 312, 313
institutional/government support, source of, 329
internal medicine, 327, 328
optimal medical care, promoting provision of, 321–323
patient's capacity, promoting adherence by, 323, 324
patients, 317, 318, 328
psychiatric consultation, beginning of, 318, 319
utility for, 319–321
targets for measurement, 330
utility for, 325
Medical residents, 333
Mental Community Public Health Services, 218–219
Mental health center (MHC), 5, 86
Mental health professionals, 197
clinical illustration, 212–214
contemporary standard of care for clinicians, 198, 199
didactic materials, 212
format for instruction, 212

goals, clinicians principles of TFP, 200–202
inpatient psychiatric hospitalization, using TFP principles in, 206–210
institutional/government support, source of, 211
levels of care, managing transition between, 210, 211
patients, 198
targets for measurement, 212
utility, clinicians working, 202
admission, voluntary or involuntary, 205, 206
discharge, ER with therapeutic advice, 205
ER, using TFP principles in, 202, 203
evaluation, 203–205
Mental Health Trusts (MHT), 112
Mentalization agency, 31, 279, 302
Mentalization based therapy (MBT), 44, 69, 115, 141, 223, 241
Mentalization-based therapy for antisocial personality disorder (MBT-ASPD), 267
Moral values, 31
Multi-modal therapeutic approach, 13
Munsterlingen program
clinicians, 240
contemporary standard of care, 241
mode combat escape, 242
mode dependence, 241, 242
pair formation mode, 242, 243
goals for, 243, 244
patients, 240, 241

N
Narcissism, 270
Narcissistic disorders, 311
Narcissistic personal disorder (NPD), 50, 118
Narcissistic regulation, 277
Narcissistic traits, 62
National Health Service (NHS), 14, 111
assessment, 120, 121
clinicians, 112
CMHT, TFP-oriented supervision for, 127
clinical presentations, 128
diagnosis, 127
older patients, 128–130
community mental health teams, TFP-informed supervision to, 125
diagnosis, 113, 114
different settings, application of TFP principles, 121
format for instruction of TFP principles
clarification, 122, 123
communication, monitoring three channels of, 123
contract setting, 123, 124
structuring treatment, 122
TFP-informed supervision, 122
young psychiatrists, training to, 124, 125
goals, for imparting to clinician, 115, 116
institutional/government support, source of, 117
Belfast Self Harm Personality Disorder Service, 120
DeanCross, 117, 118
Lewisham PD Service, 118–120
medication, 114
patients, 112, 113
principles of, 111, 112
psychodynamic treatment, learning, 122
staff needs, 114, 115
treatment model, 121
young psychiatrists, TFP training to, 125–127
National health systems (NHS), 5
National Institute for Health & Clinical Excellence (NICE) guidelines, 86
National Personality Disorder Development Program, 113
2015 National Personality Disorder Service Survey, 113
Negative and positive transferences, management of, 247, 248
Neurotic level of personality organization (NPO), 32
Neurotic personality organization, 33
New York State Psychiatric Institute (NYSPI), 168
Nosology, 31, 32

O
Object relations dyads, 243
Object relations theory (ORT), 28–31, 87, 135, 269, 317–320, 326
Offense analysis, 267–269, 275
Optimal medical care, promoting provision of, 321–323
Optimal parental functions, 339
Outpatient community-based multi-professional psychiatric service, 86
Outpatient follow-up, 299
Outpatient group therapy, 244
Outpatient Italian Psychiatric Services, 98, 99
Overt borderline delinquency, 271, 272

P
Paranoid transference, 290
Parasitic relationship, 341
Parasuicidality, 179
Parental functions (PF), 340
Patient's capacity, promoting adherence by, 323, 324
PE program, structure of, 55, 56
Personality disorder (PD), 31, 49, 50, 58, 85, 168, 218, 309
  in DSM-5, 34–36
  specializing generalist approach to, 4–6
Personality Disorders Institute (PDI), 27
Personality organization, levels of, 31, 32, 38
  borderline personality organization, 34
  neurotic personality organization, 33
Personality pathology, 27
  model of, 29–31
  nosology of, 30
  treatment parameters, implications for, 33
Perverted offender, 273
Pharmacotherapy, 209, 210
Photograph cards, 256
Primitive defense mechanisms, 317
Prisons, 297, 298
Program evaluation, 76
Project Air Strategy for Personality Disorders, 54
Prototypes, 271
  overt borderline delinquency, 271, 272
  perverted offender, 273
  psychopathic offenders, 271–273
Psychiatric consultation, beginning of, 318, 319
Psychiatric Hospital Munsterlingen (PHM), 240
Psycho, 64
Psychoanalytic object relations theory, 168
Psychoanalytic tradition
  in treatment of delinquents, 265, 266
  TFP, origins of, 28, 29
Psychodynamic
  contexts and prototypes, 269–271
  diagnostics, 300
  group therapy, 187
  tradition, 266, 267
  treatment, learning, 122
Psychodynamically-oriented supportive therapy, 343
Psychoeducation (PE), 18, 50
  for borderline personality disorder, 51
    Bolstering hope for change, 53
    carers of patients with, 52
    comorbidities, 66, 67
    crisis management, 74–76
    development of, 64–66
    group and treatment frame, 56, 57
    improving knowledge about disease, 52, 53
    patients with, 51
    PE program, structure of, 55, 56
    personality disorder diagnosis, 57–63
    pharmacological treatment, 67–69
    program evaluation, 76
    psychotherapy, 69, 70
    shared treatment decision making with mental health professionals, 53, 54
    TFP-informed psychoeducational program, 54
    transference-focused psychotherapy, 70–74
    warm-up exercise of meetings, 56
Psychopathic offenders, 271–273
Psychopathic perpetrators, 271
Psychopathic transference, 289
Psychopathology
  axis model, 273–278
  descriptive psychopathology and offense-analysis, 267–269
  prototypes and features, 271–273
  psychodynamic contexts and prototypes, 269–271
Psychopharmacological treatment, 153
Psycho-social mechanisms, 65
Psychotherapy, 69, 70
Public mental health system, 197

R
Reality testing, 31, 34, 269
Recapitulatory remarks, 294, 295
Reflective function, improvement of, 280
Reflective Functioning Rating Scale (RFRS), 280
Regulation, 270
Role play, 256, 257
Romantic relationships, 245

S
Sadomasochistic transference, 290, 291
Schema-focused group therapy (SFT), 69, 88, 115
Security, 201
Self-destructive chronic behavioral patterns, 63
Self harm questionnaire (SHQ), 355

Self-injuring behavior, 179, 180
Separation-individuation process, 352
Service for pathological dependences (SerPD), 86
Severe personality disorder (SPD), 86, 88, 198
Sexual relationships, 245
Sexuality, 182, 183, 270, 271, 278
Sexualization, 275, 276
Sexually sadistic transference, 292, 293
Short-term and extended inpatient psychotherapy, 167
  clinical case illustration, 193
  clinicians, 169
  clinicians working, useful for, 172, 173
    dealing with addictive substances, 180, 181
    extended diagnostic phase, 175, 176
    general therapy contract, 181, 182
    individual inpatient TFP, 186, 187
    initial phase, 175, 183, 184
    inpatient crisis intervention and acute psychiatric treatment, 190, 191
    inpatient hospitalization, containment function of, 173
    inpatient TFP hospitalization, sequence of, 174
    middle phase, 186
    religiosity and political attitude, 183
    self-injuring behavior, 179, 180
    sexuality and love relationships, 182, 183
    suicidal behavior, 178, 179
    termination phase, 188–190
    TFP-based group psychotherapy, 187, 188
    therapy contract phase, 176–178
    treatment focus, determining, 184–186
  contemporary standard of care, 170
  didactic materials, 192
  goals for, 170, 171
  inpatient TFP, indication for, 171, 172
  patients, 169
  psychoanalytic object-relations theory, 168
  targets for measurement, 192
Slightly neurotic sexuality, 278
Social reality testing, 34
Specialized Rehabilitation Service for BPO (RSBPO), 221
Split-off dyads, 61
Split personality organizations, 60
Staying connected relationship model, 18
Staying ill, 256
STIPO and its revised, shorter version (STIPO-R), 91
Structural interview (SI), 90
Structured Clinical Interview for DSM-5 Personality Disorders (SCID-5-PD), 118
Structured clinical management (SCM), 119
Structured generalist approaches, 4
Structured Interview of Personality Organization (STIPO), 90, 271, 300
Suicidality, 178, 179
Superego, 275, 276
Superego development, 277
Superego regulation, 270
Supervision, 118, 145
Systems training for emotional predictability and problem solving (STEPPS), 51, 69, 223, 241

T

Team coordination, 145
Technical neutrality, 123, 248
Tentative interpretation, 284
The "Family Guidelines" approach, 342
Thematic qualitative analysis, 126
Transference analysis, 279, 280, 283
Transference-focused forensic psychotherapy (TFFP), 267
  framework and technical procedure in, 281–283
  manual for, 300, 301
  strategies, 283
    clinical illustration, 285–287
    dominant object relationship dyad, 283–285
    idealizing transference, 291, 292
    mature affective experiences and stabilizing the mature, triangulated relationship patterns, 293, 294
    mutually defensive relational dyads, within therapeutic and offense situations, 288, 289
    paranoid transference, 290
    psychopathic transference, 289
    recapitulatory remarks, 294, 295
    reversals within therapeutic and offense situations, 285
    sadomasochistic transference, 290, 291
    sexually sadistic and aroused-fusing transference, 292, 293
Transference-focused group therapy, 188
Transference-focused offender treatment, history of
  behavioral therapeutic turn and limits, 266

justified criticism and psychodynamic, 266, 267
psychoanalytic tradition, 265, 266
Transference-focused psychotherapy (TFP), 3, 4, 12, 27, 49, 69–74, 141, 168, 218
for adolescents (TFP-A), 338
application of, 19
criticisms of, 14–16
development, 28
DSM-5, personality disorders in, 34–36
emerging areas, 8–10
evolution of, 8
individual and group psychotherapy (TFP-G) model, 223
informed group therapy, in DH, 143, 144
informed psychoeducational program, 54
informed supervision, 122
model of change, 72
object relations theory, 29–31, 135, 136
oriented psychiatric consultation, 324
oriented supervisions, 98
original modification of, 19
origins of, 7
for parental functions (TFP-PF), 337
personality organization, levels of, 31, 32
borderline personality organization, 34
neurotic personality organization, 33
psychoanalytic tradition, origins of, 28, 29
rationale of, 6, 7
specializing generalist approach, 4–6
specific mental health settings, principles in, 18
specific patient populations and treatment contexts, principles to, 11, 13, 14
teaching and supervision of, 44
theoretical integration, 9
therapeutic family intervention, 20
to community mental health teams, 12, 125
trainees and practicing clinicians, principles to, 10–12
treatment approaches, 45
treatment model and clinical approach, 36
case formulation, 37, 39
interpretive process, 40–44
model of change, 36, 37
patient assessment, 37
therapeutic neutrality, 40
treatment structure, 39, 40
utilization of core aspects of, 45
volume, 17
Transference-focused psychotherapy for parental functions (TFP-PF), 343
initiative, 338
phases of, 347, 348
final treatment phase, 351, 352
initial treatment phase, 347, 348
intermediate treatment phase, 348–351
program, 338
Transgressive perversion, 278

U
University Hospital of Cologne Day Hospital Program
clinical illustration, 160, 161
contract setting, 156
diagnostic process, 151, 152
clinicians, 152–154
didactic materials, 160
goals for imparting, 154
institutional/government support, source of, 159
strategies modifications, 154–156
targets for measurement, 160
techniques modifications, 158, 159
TFP principles, format for instruction, 160
treatment staff and adolescent patients, contract between, 156, 157
treatment staff and parents, contract between, 157, 158
utility for, 154

V
Vulnerability, 200

GPSR Compliance

The European Union's (EU) General Product Safety Regulation (GPSR) is a set of rules that requires consumer products to be safe and our obligations to ensure this.

If you have any concerns about our products, you can contact us on ProductSafety@springernature.com

In case Publisher is established outside the EU, the EU authorized representative is:

Springer Nature Customer Service Center GmbH
Europaplatz 3
69115 Heidelberg, Germany

Batch number: 10732076

Printed by Printforce, the Netherlands